THE COMPLETE
SWIMMING POOL REFERENCE

About the Author

Tom Griffiths, EdD, is the Director of Aquatics and Safety Officer for Intercollegiate Athletics at The Pennsylvania State University. He oversees five large swimming pools and a state-of-the-art fitness center and is responsible for safety for athletic and recreational sports on the University Park campus.

Dr Griffiths teaches swimming pool management and operation courses for the National Recreation and Parks Association (NRPA) and the National Swimming Pool Foundation (NSPF). He is a prolific writer, speaker, and safety consultant.

THE COMPLETE SWIMMING POOL REFERENCE

Tom Griffiths, EdD
Director of Aquatics
Safety Officer for Intercollegiate Athletics
The Pennsylvania State University
University Park, Pennsylvania

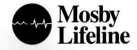

A *Harcourt Health Sciences Company*
St. Louis Philadelphia London Sydney Toronto

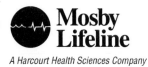

A Harcourt Health Sciences Company

Mosby, Inc.
11830 Westline Industrial Drive
St. Louis, Missouri 63146

0-8016-7182-5

01 02 03 04 / 9 8 7 6 5 4

To William R. "Wild Bill" Campbell,
my mentor, who has already forgotten more about
swimming pools than I'll ever know.

To Steve Shinholser, of American Pool Service,
my stellar student/athlete who taught me much
about diving, pools, and life.

To my girls, Roni, Kendra, and Rachel,
who appreciate my profession
as much as I do.

PREFACE

This book combines technical aspects of pool operations manuals with practical information of water safety texts. The book is written for all those who own, operate, or otherwise work at swimming pools, including lifeguards, pool operators, pool managers, swimming coaches, diving coaches, swimming instructors, and even residential pool owners.

The *Complete Swimming Pool Reference* is written clearly and concisely; even complicated topics are easy to understand. With 24 comprehensive chapters included, there is something for every aquatic professional. Chapter 14, *Water Parks*; Chapter 17, *Preventive Lifeguarding*; Chapter 18, *Legal Liability and Risk Management*; and Section IV, *Pesticides Safety and Education* introduce new information of vital importance to pool professionals. This work also includes a variety of references and resources to assist readers who wish to study a topic in more depth.

ACKNOWLEDGEMENTS

The editors wish to acknowledge the reviewers of this book for their invaluable help in developing and fine-tuning the manuscript.

Walter Dennis Berry, BS-HPER, MA
Director of Student Life
Office of Student Affairs
Washington College
Chestertown, Maryland

Paul Crutchfield
Administrative Assistant
City of Spokane, Washington

Carvin DiGiovanni
Technical Director
National Spa and Pool Institute
Alexandria, Virginia

Mark A. Hokkanen, MST
Director of Aquatic and Wellness Center
Oklahoma City Community College
Oklahoma City, Oklahoma

Wallace A. James
Mechanical Engineer
Certified Risk Evaluator
President, Con-Serv Associates, Inc.
Humboldt, Iowa

Fontaine C. Piper, PhD, EdS, MS, BSE
Associate Professor of Exercise Science
Northeast Missouri State University
Adjunct Associate Professor of Anatomy
College of Osteopathic Medicine
Kirksville, Missouri

Special appreciation is extended to the McCoy Natatorium staff at Penn State University, particularly Frank Bennett, Joan Emel, Bob Gates, Fred Horner, Janice Kocher, Sam Schillero, and Chuck Spicer for their help, support, and efficient operation of the Penn State pools through the years. Finally, sincere thanks is extended to Herb Schmidt, Associate Athletic Director at Penn State University, for his encouragement and support of my professional growth and development.

CONTENTS

Section VI: Pesticide Safety and Education

INTRODUCTION

Swimming attracts more than 125 million participants annually; this figure represents nearly half of the US population. For years, swimming has been the most popular participant sport in the United States. Only walking has surpassed its popularity in recent years.

According to National Spa and Pool Institute estimates, there are nearly 10 million pools in this country. Six million are privately owned, residential pools. Homeowners maintain an additional three million hot tubs and spas. The number of public and semi-public pools in this country is approaching one million.

People frequent pools for a variety of reasons: fitness, relaxation, instruction, competition, and therapy. Today's swimming facilities do not just accommodate lessons and lap swimmers but are multidimensional fitness centers encompassing all age groups.

Despite the increasing number of pools and spas, and our growing population, drownings have remained constant at 7000 to 8000 individuals a year, indicating improved water safety. Fortunately, only 10% of these drownings occur in swimming pools, but tragically almost half of these drownings involve small children.

Ironically, we build pools in this country to promote health, fitness, and safety, but several risks and hazards are produced with the construction of swimming facilities. This book can help maximize the health and safety benefits of aquatics while reducing hazards and risks. Safe, enjoyable, and clean swimming pools can result if the guidelines in this book are followed.

There are many good texts available that can assist the swimming pool owner, operator, or other employees. Some texts are technical and written primarily for swimming pool technicians who need precise information on pool chemistry and filtration. Concerning safety, The American Red Cross is the leader on lifeguarding and water safety and produces excellent works on these subjects. Residential pool owners are often refered to pamphlets published by swimming pool chemical companies that are easy to follow and understand.

The Complete Swimming Pool Reference attempts to accomplish the almost impossible task of combining the most valuable elements of technical, practical, and water safety publications to produce a book that can be used by anyone in aquatics.

It is hoped that anyone associated with a pool, whether it be public or private, will find this book informative and helpful. The needs of homeowners, hotel/motel managers, park directors, pool operators, lifeguards, coaches, and parents are addressed. *The Complete Swimming Pool Reference* includes many other references and resources that will allow the reader to gain additional information concerning pools and spas. All readers will benefit from this book, from professional pool technicians who service swimming facilities to homeowners who relax in their hot tubs.

How to Use this Book

The information presented in this book progresses from very simple ideas to more complex swimming pool issues. The novice pool owner or operator may wish to concentrate on the earlier sections before moving on to the filtration and chemistry chapters. Conversely, the experienced pool person may wish to skim the initial chapters and spend more time on the later sections in the book. Additionally, some readers will prefer to concentrate on the maintenance and operations sections of the book, while others may want to focus on the safety and human relations portions.

Before addressing each chapter, the reader should carefully read the key terms defined at the outset of each section and then turn to the review questions at the end. Reviewing the key terms and questions will aid the reader in attending to the most critical aspects of each chapter. The answers to the review questions start on p. 00. Appendix B contains a "Personal Pool Profile" that can be completed so the information read can be applied directly to the reader's particular pool.

In addition to this book, there are several other valuable sources of swimming pool and water safety information. The American Red Cross, The US Consumer Product Safety Commission, The National Pool and Spa Institute, National Swimming Pool Foundation, YMCA, and the National Recreation and Parks Association are just a few organizations that can provide the reader with additional information on swimming pools and spas. Addresses and phone numbers can be found in Appendix A2.

Every pool owner and operator must understand fully the local health codes and ordinances that regulate swimming facilities in their region. This book is not intended to replace or supersede local swimming pool regulations; *The Complete Swimming Pool Reference* only serves as a general guide and helpful reference for those who own or operate swimming pools and spas. The reader must also understand that many state health codes regulating swimming pools are out of date. Much of what is found in these pages is more up-to-date.

SECTION I
POOLS

This initial section covers the basic physical components of swimming pools. Chapter 1 contains a brief, general description of swimming pools, including a classification of different types of pools. Topics introduced are circulation, pool configurations, construction materials, finishes, decking, and equipment. Safety, signage, and supervision are also introduced in this section, and chemical balancing is mentioned briefly. These topics are discussed in detail later in the book.

Chapter 2 specifically addresses the residential pool. This chapter is a comprehensive treatment of private pools, and the emphasis in this chapter is on safety. Layers of protection and pool barriers are important aspects of this chapter. Topics like filtration, circulation, and water chemistry will be presented in Sections II and III.

Chapter 3 discusses public pools in detail. Different types of pools are discussed, as well as construction materials and pool equipment. Ladders, lights, finishes, markers, barriers, programming, and security are covered in this section. Special considerations for outdoor pools are also discussed. Pool areas such as the entrance, locker rooms, first aid room, staff room, and concession areas are also included in this chapter. Chapters 1, 2, and 3 cover swimming pools in general terms, and Sections II through V contain specific, in-depth information regarding pools.

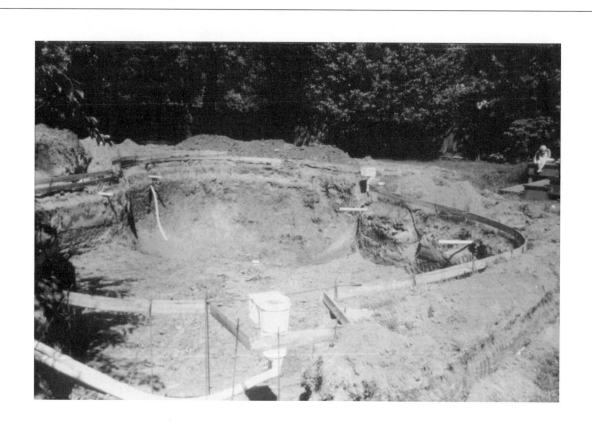

1

A POOL PRIMER: BASIC CHARACTERISTICS OF SWIMMING POOLS

Key Concepts

- *Classifications*
- *Basic Water*
- *Aggressive Water*
- *Signage*
- *Diving Hopper*
- *Safe Diving Envelope*
- *Circulation Components*
- *Pool Finishes*
- *Pool Decks*
- *Pool Equipment*
- *Chemical Balance*

This book contains detailed information on all aspects of swimming pool safety and operations. The basics of swimming pools will be presented simply and clearly first, before they are discussed in depth. Regardless of what recommendations are made in this text, it is important to remember that they are general guidelines. Local swimming pool ordinances and health codes establish the standard of care in specific regions of this country but are often out of date and provide minimum standards only. Local ordinances and health codes should not be violated or ignored, but in some instances this text will recommend higher standards. Good common sense should not be overlooked and is also required for running a clean, safe pool.

On first glance a swimming pool appears to be a quiet, calm, and still body of water. A pool expert often refers to the perfectly calm pool as a "quiescent pool." But in reality, whether busy or slow, a swimming pool is a dynamic system of moving water that continually flows from the pool for treatment and returns cleaned, heated, and sanitized. In fact, a pool

is a recycling system whereby the entire volume of water passes through a filtration plant several times each day. As the water travels through the filter it is cleaned of dirt and other organic debris. Before it returns to the pool, however, it is often heated and must be sanitized using a powerful chemical. A clean, clear, germ-free pool requires tremendous attention. Large or small, every pool is required to filter and chemically treat its water through this process. When a pool is not filtering or there is an absence of chemical disinfectant in the water, the pool must be closed immediately. Without filtration and disinfection, the water will turn cloudy and bacteria will grow, thus becoming unsafe for all who enter the pool.

Classifications of Swimming Pools

Public, semi-public, and private are three different ways of categorizing pools. For the purposes of this text, these classifications are defined as follows.

Public pools

A public pool is usually a larger pool (more than 1800 square feet) that is owned or operated by some legal entity and is made available to anyone who pays a small entry fee. However some public pools do not charge admission (Fig. 1-1).

Semi-public pool

This pool is similar to the public pool but has specific entry restrictions like that of a fitness center, country club, or hotel/motel pool. Members must qualify and often pay to join before entry into the swimming complex.

Residential pools

For the purposes of this text, residential pools are private pools that are not regulated by the health

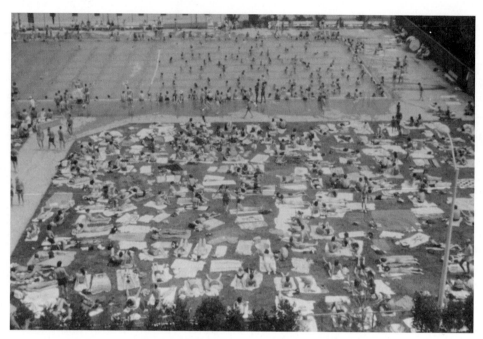

Fig. 1-1.   A well-used outdoor pool.

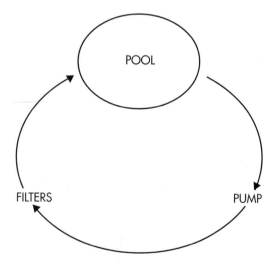

Fig. 1-2.   Swimming pool circulation simplified: a closed loop.

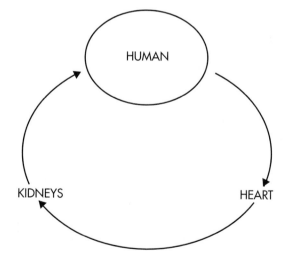

Fig. 1-3.   Swimming pool circulation is similar to the human body's circulation.

department or some other regulatory agency. Residential pools are not intended for commercial use and are not owned by more than three families. Specific dimensions are covered in Chapter 2. Public and semi-public pools are usually inspected by a health official, whereas residential pools are not.

There are further subclassifications of swimming pools, each of which fall under the public, semi-public, or residential categories. These include community and neighborhood pools, agency pools (YM/YWCAs, JCCs, Boy Scouts, Girl Scouts, etc.), school pools, hotel/motel/apartment/condo pools, water parks, and spas/hot tubs. Because of their popularity, residential, community, and hotel/motel/resort pools will be discussed in detail later in this text .

Circulation

Although all swimmers see the pool, few have the opportunity to become familiar with the pool's plumbing. Although this aspect of swimming may not be exciting to all pool owners and operators, an adequate understanding of **filtration** and **chemical disinfection** is a must if good, clean water is to be maintained. For the sake of discussion, a swimming pool plant functions like a closed loop system. Although swimming pools are not technically "closed loops" (most of the water stays in the system much of the time), they will be considered closed loops in this text for ease of understanding (Fig. 1-2)

To help understand how a swimming pool functions, one should consider how the human body works. The heart circulates blood in the body much the same way a **centrifugal pump** recirculates swimming pool water. The kidneys remove toxic wastes from the blood just as filters remove debris from the pool water. Just as the veins and arteries carry blood to and from the heart, so does a series of influent and effluent pool pipes (Fig. 1-3). When we discuss water chemistry later in this book, you will learn that pool water can be either basic and scale forming or aggressive and corrosive. Using the human body as an analogy once again, scale forming water serves to block the pool's plumbing like bad cholesterol blocks arteries. On the other hand, corrosive water eats away at the swimming pool plant in the same fashion that cancer deteriorates the human body.

More specifically, the basic components of a swimming pool and its circulation system include the following:

1. Vessel or swimming pool basin
2. Surge or balancing tank (in larger pools)
3. Pump
4. Hair and lint strainer (except on vacuum filters)
5. Filter or filters
6. Heater (if necessary)
7. Chemical disinfectant system

The water circulates by leaving the pool from outlets around the perimeter found in either surface gutters or skimmers. To a lesser extent, some water also leaves through the main drain or bottom outlet. The pool pump then either pushes or pulls the water through the filters. If necessary, the water is heated and then must be chemically treated before returning to the pool by way of inlets located on the pool bottom or pool walls. Typically, hundreds of gallons a minute flow through the filtration plant to be filtered, heated, and chemically treated during this process. Refer to Fig. 1-4 for a flow chart illustration of water circulation.

In addition to the pool and the filtration system, knowledgeable pool owners and operators should be familiar with different types of swimming pool construction, pool finishes, decking, accessories, and pool equipment.

Pool Configurations

A variety of shapes and sizes of pools is available. After years of large pools being built to accommodate many different types of activities, pools are now being downsized for lap swimming, safety, and construction costs. Most pools have a shallow and a deep end. Typically, the shallow end of a swimming pool is approximately 3.5 feet deep. Competition pools with starting blocks located in shallow water should be moved to the deep end. Headfirst entries must be prohibited from the pool deck in less than 5 feet of water, because 95% of all serious diving injuries occur in this depth. Many aquatic professionals are now recommending 9 feet of water for headfirst entries from the pool deck.[1] The deep end of the swimming pool ranges from 8 to 13 feet, although "diving" from a board should not be permitted into less than 11 feet. In public pools the preferred depth is 12.5 feet or adults may be seriously injured by striking the bottom. Diving does not refer to untrained, unsupervised recreational divers entering the water headfirst. Headfirst entries should be used instead of the term *diving* so as not to confuse this with the sport of competitive springboard diving.

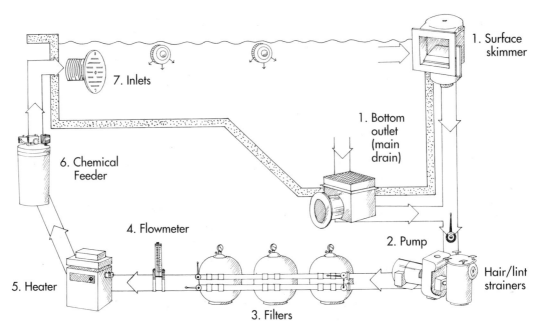

Fig. 1-4. Circulation components. (Illustrator, Nancy Bauer.)

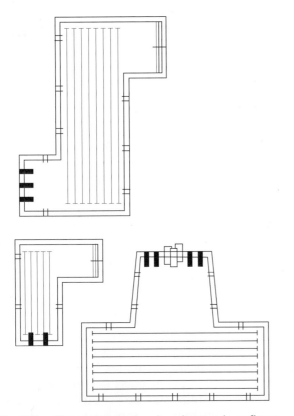

Fig. 1-5. Some standard swimming pool configurations. (From Gabrielson M: *Swimming pools: a guide to their planning, design, and operation*, ed 4, Champaign, III 1987, Human Kinetics.)

Regardless of the type of pool, diving from a board should be permitted into a safe diving envelope only. According to the American Red Cross, a safe diving envelope is an underwater area that has adequate depth and distance to allow any diver to maneuver safely underwater without striking the bottom or slope of the pool. This important concept is discussed in greater detail in Chapter 16.

A straight, rectangular pool is the most common pool, and when other shapes like T, Z, or L are observed, it is usually an attempt to entertain other activities in the pool without interfering with lap swimming or swim team practice. Creative pool designs are usually built with increased programming in mind (Fig 1-5).

Diving hopper or spoon-shaped pools

Diving hoppers or spoon-shaped pools refer to the deepest section of the pool, which was constructed to accommodate diving. To do this a steep slope must be created between the shallow and deep areas of the pool[1] (Fig. 1-6). Although the American Red Cross addresses the dangers of diving in diving hoppers or spoon-shaped pools, the National Spa and Pool Institute (NSPI) makes no mention of these hazards. While this is one way of accommodating more than one activity in a rectangular-shaped pool, it does create some problems. The slope itself is problematic. Nonswimmers can slide down the slope into deeper water, and springboard divers can hit the slope with their heads following a dive. Black or red lines should be painted across the bottom of the pool to alert swimmers and divers of this slope. A surface line or **life-line** should cross the pool on the surface to prevent novice swimmers from entering the diving area. While this is a common design for YMCA, high school, and even college pools, a separate diving well often provides more safety and greater programming options.

Pool Construction

There are two basic types of pool construction, above-ground and in-ground swimming pools.

Above-ground pools are usually constructed with aluminum or galvanized panels, although a recent trend is toward inflatable rubber pools. In-ground pools are constructed of a variety of materials including different types of concrete, fiberglass, metal, vinyl, and even wood.

Pool Finishes

Regardless of what type of pool finish is selected, the color of the pool basin or finish should be white in almost all cases. A white underwater finish provides excellent visibility for safety and aesthetics. White pool basins full of water appear blue, although many naturalistic pools today are using dark bot-

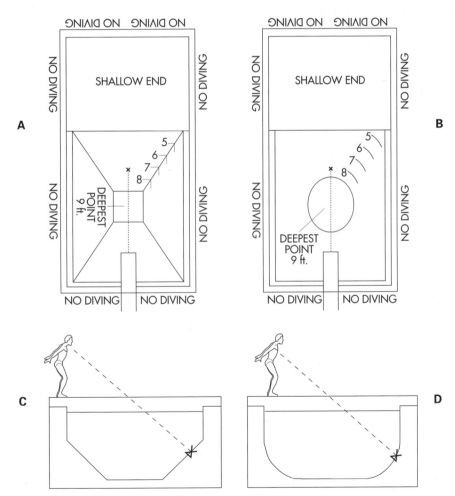

Fig. 1-6. **A,** Top view of hopper-bottom pool. **B,** Cross-section of hopper-bottom pool. **C,** Top view of spoon-shaped pool. **D,** Cross-section of spoon-shaped pool. (From American Red Cross: *Swimming and diving,* St. Louis, 1992, Mosby.

toms. Outdoor pools using concrete will often have a plaster finish. Many indoor pools are finished with tile. Ceramic tile is the most versatile finish, but not surprisingly it is also the most expensive. Residential pools are now using vinyl liners, which are both popular and reasonably priced. Stainless steel and fiberglass pools are also available. Of course, there are advantages and disadvantages of each pool finish selected.

Decking

Many different materials can be used for deck areas surrounding the pool. Whatever surface is used, however, it must be nonslip. Also, the deck must be a flat surface free of depressions or dimples that can collect water and must be sloped away from the pool for proper drainage. Decks cluttered with furniture and other pool equipment can often obstruct views of the pool and create hazards. Some decking materials that have worked well include brick, tile, wood, flagstone, terrazzo, concrete, indoor/outdoor carpeting, cocoa mat, flow-through tiles, and exposed aggregate concrete.

Please note that matting or carpeting often remains wet, thus promoting algae and fungi growth. Rubber, interlocking, self-draining deck tiles are becoming very popular, but they must also be cleaned regularly.

Whatever the deck surface, it must be hosed down regularly to be debris-free, and care must also be taken to prevent algae from growing. Calcium hypochlorite (granular chlorine) works well in this application, as well as sodium hypochlorite (liquid chlorine).

Pool Equipment
Ladders, Steps, and Handrails

Ladders should be either recessed into the pool wall or should be the removable type. Ladders, handrails, and steps should not protrude into lap lanes to prevent accidents. Loose-fitting ladders should be corrected immediately. Ladders and handrails should be made of stainless steel or some other corrosion-resistant material. To prevent trips, slips, and falls, ladders and steps must have nonslip surfaces and the edges should be clearly marked with a contrasting color or colored tile.

Diving Boards and Slides

Before either apparatus is installed, adequate depth must be determined for each piece of equipment. Smaller slides at public and residential pools should probably be reserved for children under 12 years of age because older, larger individuals might discharge from the slide with too much force. Larger, water-park slides are designed for all ages. Regardless of the age of the slider or size of the slide, feetfirst sliding is the only way to go. Headfirst slides must be prohibited for all. Sliders must be certain that no other swimmers or sliders are in the discharge area. Diving boards should be reserved for flat-bottom, deeper pools. Whenever possible, pools should be constructed to allow diving or sliding into a portion of the pool outside the general swim area or lap lanes. Rules and regulations concerning their use must be prominently posed.

Signage, Safety, and Supervision

Vigilant supervision is the key to swimming pool safety, regardless of the size of the pool or audience it attracts. Clear, concise signage prominently displayed is also a must. Water depths must be clearly marked both on the decks and on the pool walls. No diving and shallow water warnings must also be clearly displayed. Contrasting, colored letters and numbers must be at lease 4 inches high. Rules and regulations must also be displayed (see Appendix D2). Some signage experts strongly suggest using highway type signs around the pool with contrasting colors like red and white, or yellow and black, which connote danger. Likewise, diamond- or octagonal-shaped signs may also convey danger. Pool signs similar to shapes and colors observed on our highways might be more recognized by swimmers and divers. Graphics should be used whenever possible, particularly in multicultural areas.

Whenever a hazard is created at the pool it should be repaired or removed immediately. Accidents at the pool are usually the result of a combination of irresponsible actions on the part of the pool patron, inadequate supervision, and a failure to warn. "Walk-abouts" during the early morning hours and the last thing in the evening can greatly reduce hazards and safety violations. Safety checks should be performed hourly in busy pools.

Chemical Balance

The purpose of the disinfectant (usually chlorine) placed into the water is to keep the water germ free and also clear for aesthetics and safety. Chlorine accomplishes this through sanitation (germ killing) and oxidation (burning up organic material). The immediate concern of any pool owner or operator is to keep appropriate chlorine or bromine and pH levels in the pool. Chlorine is the most popular disinfectant, although there are many different types and forms of oxidizers other than chlorine. pH levels buffer the disinfectant and usually relate to bather comfort. In addition, the water must be balanced, which requires readings in temperature, total alkalinity, and calcium hardness (see Chapter 9). Balanced water not only keeps swimmers comfortable but also protects the pool shell and all related equipment.

pH and chlorine levels are the primary concern of the pool operator, who keeps the water comfortable for pool patrons, that is, user-friendly. Temperature, total alkalinity, and calcium hardness levels are also important but change more gradually.

Balanced water is friendly to the pool's plumbing, and to a lesser extent the swimmers in the pool. As one's understanding of basic water chemistry increases, water quality problems tend to decrease.

Summary

This chapter briefly describes and summarizes basic characteristics of swimming pools. Other more detailed information regarding pool basics may be found in the references listed. Pool shapes, sizes, construction materials, equipment, circulation, chemistry, and safety are introduced. Regardless of what type of pool is owned or operated (public, semi-public, or residential), local ordinances and regulations regarding swimming pools must be understood, followed, and wherever possible, surpassed. In addition, The National Spa and Pool Institute is a good resource for swimming pool publications and dealers; call (800)-359-SWIM.

References
1. American Red Cross: *Swimming and diving*, St Louis, 1992, Mosby.

Bibliography
Gabrielson AM: *Swimming pools: a guide to their planning, design, and operation*, ed 4, Champaign, Ill, 1987, Human Kinetics Publishers.
Kowalsky L(editor): *Pool/spa operators handbook*, San Antonio, 1991, Swimming Pool Foundation.
Mitchell P: *The proper management of pool and spa water*, Decatur, Ga, 1988, BioLab.
Recreonics: *Buyers' guide and operations handbook*, 1991, Indianapolis, Ind, Catalog number 41.
Williams KG: *The aquatic facility operator's manual.*,Hoffman Estates, Ill, 1991, National Recreation and Park Association, National Aquatic Section.

Review Questions

1. What is the difference between a semi-public pool and a public pool?

2. List two different types of semi-public pools.

3. Private pools are primarily what type of pool?

4. What agency regulates residential pools?

5. List five components of a circulation system.

6. In what depth of water do most headfirst injuries occur?

7. List three characteristics of a good pool deck.

8. Concerning swimming pool chemistry, what is the difference between sanitation and oxidation?

9. What is the disadvantage of a spoon-shaped pool?

10. Are chlorine readings required to determine water balance?

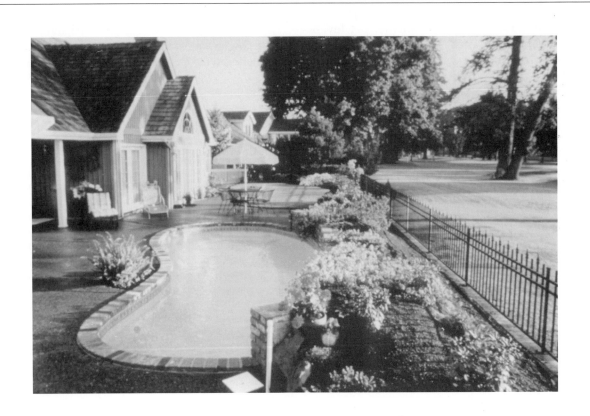

2

RESIDENTIAL POOLS

Many homeowners agree that nothing is more satisfying than having a pretty, blue pool in the backyard. Whether filled with active people or just sitting there quiet and calm, a pool significantly adds to the quality of life. A swimming pool greatly enhances both exercise and entertaining. In her book,*Pools*, Klein describes swimming pools as "... a place for rest, relaxation, rejuvenation, and exercise."[1]Although local health codes and ordinances regulate public pools, they often do not apply to residential pools.

Swimming attracts more than 125 million participants annually. According to the National Swimming Pool Institute, there are nearly seven million residential pools in the United States. While this number includes in-ground and above-ground pools, it does not include the three million hot tubs and spas home-

owners enjoy. Of all the newly constructed swimming pools in the United States each year, approximately 60% are privately owned, residential pools.

Oxtoby-Smith, a New York based market research company, reports the following five major reasons why homeowners consider purchasing a pool.[3]
1. Clean swimming water—55%
2. Great fun—47%
3. Add value to home—29%
4. Help beat the heat—29%
5. Help keep physically fit—19%

Many pool owners appreciate the recreation and relaxation a swimming pool provides. Some acquire a swimming facility for fitness or therapy. Others maintain a pool to teach their children to be water safe. The fitness movement of the 1970s and development of inexpensive "prefab" pool packages both have contributed greatly to the growth of home pools in this country. The introduction of the vinyl liner pool has also kept the price down on home pools. The pools of today are no longer playthings for the rich. In-ground pool costs are similar to new car costs, and prices vary the same way new car models do. For both pools and automobiles, there are some very expensive luxurious models, and there are also some very inexpensive and more practical models. Above-ground pools are much less expensive than in-ground pools. During recessionary periods, while in-ground pool construction tends to decline, above-ground pool purchases remain stable.

Most residential pools run safely and do not experience any problems. However, several risks accompany pool ownership. "Swimming pool time" should be "leisure time" instead of "worry time."[2] Fortunately, the two most feared risks, drowning and spinal cord injury, can be easily avoided. While home pool drownings usually involve small children, spinal cord injuries most often affect adults. According to a

How the Pool Industry Sees Its Market*

DEMOGRAPHICS

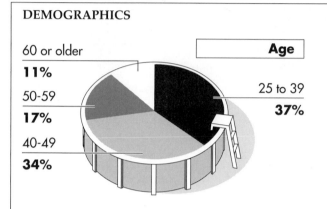

Age

60 or older
11%

50-59
17%

40-49
34%

25 to 39
37%

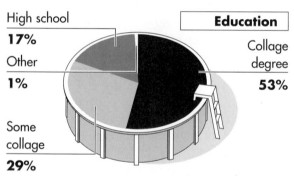

Education

High school
17%

Other
1%

Some collage
29%

Collage degree
53%

Marital status

Single
14%

Married
86%

MARKET PENETRATION

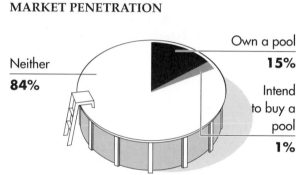

Neither
84%

Own a pool
15%

Intend to buy a pool
1%

ATTITUDES ABOUT POOLS

Reason to buy	Percent of non-owners who strongly agree
Clean swimming water	55%
Great fun	47%
Add value to home	29%
Help beat the heat	27%
Help keep physically fit	19%
Reason not to buy	
Safety hazard for children	51%
Expensive to care for	41%
Expensive to buy	24%
Require too much space	24%
Dealers are disreputable	7%

*Figures from a telephone survey of 997 homeowners with family income over $40,000, the core market for swimming pools and spas. The survey was conducted in May by Oxtoby-Smith, a market research firm, for the National Spa and Pool Institute, a trade group.

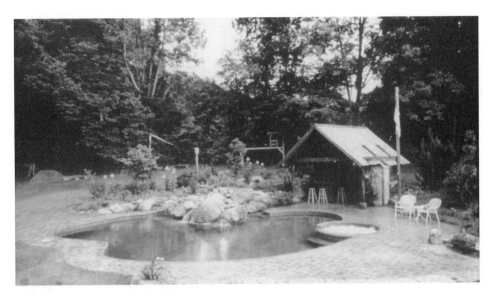

Fig. 2-1. A well-designed and maintained residential pool. (Courtesy Bomanite, Madera, Calif.)

survey by Oxtoby-Smith, the leading cause for not purchasing a residential pool is that many homeowners perceive pools as a safety hazard for their children. In fact, more than half of the respondents in this survey cited the safety issue for not purchasing a pool.[3] This chapter is dedicated to teaching homeowners how to make residential pools safe for their families (Fig. 2-1).

According to the National Spa and Pool Institute[3]:

A residential pool shall be defined as any constructed pool, permanent or nonportable, that is intended for noncommercial use as a swimming pool by not more than three (3) owner families and their guests and that is over twenty-four inches (24") in depth, has a surface area exceeding 250 square feet and/or a volume over 3,250 gallons"

Safety

More than half of all swimming pool drownings occur in privately owned residential pools. Tragically, toddlers between the ages of 1 and 3 years are usually the victims of home-pool drownings. A 2-year-old boy is the most likely candidate, and between 300 and 400 small children drown annually in backyard pools. Thousands are sent to the hospital each year as a result of near-drowning incidents, and many of these accidents lead to permanent brain damage. Child drownings occur quickly and quietly, without warning. Children in trouble cannot cry out for help, because all their energy is spent attempting to breathe.

When it comes to safeguarding children around a swimming pool, it is important to note that no one safety practice or piece of equipment is fool proof. For this reason pool owners are advised to have a system of safety precautions, so that if one fails, another will come into effect. This "layering" of safety techniques and mechanisms is perhaps the best method of protecting children around a pool.

Supervision

The most effective way for parents to protect their children from drowning in their own backyard is to practice vigilant supervision. Parents of most young drowning victims claim they left their child unsupervised for less than 5 minutes. *A child can drown in less than 1 minute.* Some children have drown while the parent in charge left the pool to answer the phone. Children must never be left alone around a pool for any length of time. More important, parents must not be distracted from watching their children. Just because adults are stationed around the pool does not mean children are safe in the water. Too

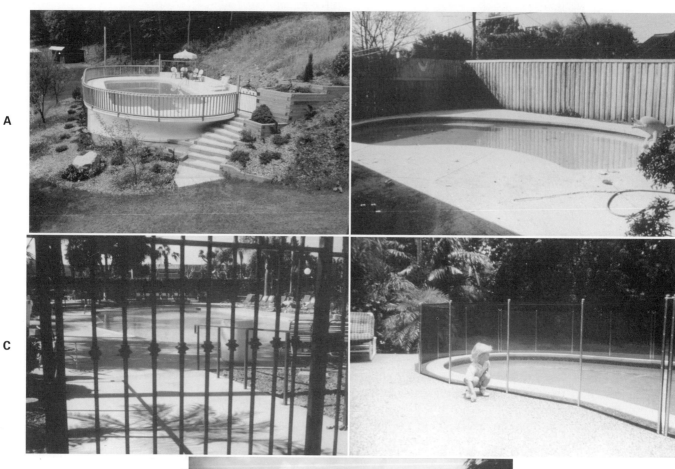

Fig. 2-2. **A, B,** and **C,** Effective fencing and gates. **D** and **E,** See-through mesh fencing specifically designed for small children can be installed and removed in minutes. (**A,** Courtesy Lynn Smith, Clearwater Swiming Pools, Centre Hall, Penn; **D** and **E,** courtesy Protect A Child, Pool Fence Systems.)

often, adults talk, read, or even sleep while kids are in the pool. Some parents use flotational devices on their children instead of supervising them. Inflatable swimming aids can deflate. Other swimming aids have been known to slip off of the child.

Parents should also refrain from placing too many furnishings and toys around the pool. A pool deck cluttered with swimming accouterments can obstruct the parents' view of the water, thus impairing supervision and delaying rescue efforts. When the pool is not in use, all toys and floats should be removed from the pool so that they do not lure a child into the water.

Pool Rules

Swimming pool rules and regulations must be clearly marked and observed at poolside. Clearly stated rules will help to eliminate water rescues. "No Running," "No Horseplay," "No Diving," and "No Glass" are just a few that should be mandated. "Never Swim Alone" is one rule that must be enforced by the family. If children have had swimming lessons, this does not necessarily mean that they are water safe and do not require supervision. In fact, for some individuals, swimming lessons make them overconfident and careless around the pool.

Barriers

According to the U.S. Consumer Product Safety Commission (CPSC), nearly half of all children who drown in residential pools were *last seen inside the house*. Although close supervision is the key to drowning prevention, barriers also help to keep small children out of the water. There are several types of swimming pool barriers homeowners can use, but proper fencing is perhaps the best protection. (Fig. 2-2)

Proper fencing for swimming pools is one of the most controversial topics in the swimming pool industry. While the CPSC advocates very stringent fencing requirements, many pool builders and owners often find these recommendations too difficult and expensive to achieve.

The CPSC and some states recommend installing a fence on all four sides of the pool, and the house is not allowed to serve as one side of the fence. Pool fences should be a minimum of four feet high, but

many experts recommend a height of 6 feet. The fence should be composed of vertical slats, free of footholds or handholds that can aid children in climbing it. Slats must be placed no greater than 4 inches apart to prevent toddlers from squeezing through. Chairs, benches, and tables should be kept well away from the fence.The proper installation of fence gates is of paramount importance. Gates should be self-closing and self-latching so that after anyone enters or exits the pool, the gate automatically closes and latches. The latch should be between 48-and 54-inches high and should be located on the pool side of the fence. This forces a child to reach up and over the top of the fence to manipulate the latch. Gates must never be propped open. (Fig. 2-3) If this latching arrangement poses a problem for those in wheelchairs, an alternative safe latching mechanism may need to be used.

Whenever possible, the house should not serve as one side of the barrier protecting children from the pool. If the house is a part of the barrier, additional precautions are required. All exit doors and windows leading to the pool should be kept locked whenever small children are in the house. Additionally, windows and doors should be equipped with an audible warning device that is set to sound off whenever an exit from the house to the pool is opened. To use these exits without tripping the alarm, adults can temporarily cancel the alarm for a single opening of a door or window by using a touchpad or key located well out of the reach of children. Pool alarms that emit a loud signal when the pool water is disturbed are becoming popular. Alarms are available in wave motion, electronic detector, and photoelectric sensor varieties. For more information concerning these alarms, a local pool supply company should be contacted.

Pool Covers

There are two basic types of pool covers: safety covers and thermal blankets. Safety pool covers come highly recommended for every homeowner with a swimming pool. These covers are usually a nylon mesh material that allows rainwater to pass through but keeps most debris out. Safety covers are often "locked" in place and should support a minimum of 225 lbs per square foot. Some automatic pool covers have a key-operated electric motor switch with a power disconnect.

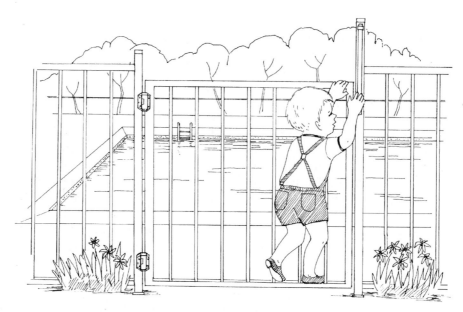

Fig. 2-3.   Child-proof latching device. (Illustrator, Nancy Bauer.)

Insulating covers or blankets are usually made of a solid material. Because more than 50% of a pool's heat is lost through evaporation, a pool cover significantly slows this process and saves both utility and chemical costs. Providing a barrier between the water and the air minimizes the loss of water, heat, and chemicals through evaporation.

All pool covers and blankets must be completely removed before entry into the pool. Partial removal of pool covers can lead to entrapment and drowning (Fig. 2-4). Pool safety covers are extremely valuable when the pool is not in use or the homeowners are away. Sturdy pool covers not only prevent children from entering the water, but they also protect against vandalism.

CPR

While close supervision and effective pool barriers will prevent most child drownings, pool owners must be prepared for emergencies. Anyone owning a pool should have certification in cardiopulmonary resuscitation (CPR). Recovery rates are much higher for drowning victims when CPR is applied immediately, as compared with resuscitation efforts that are deferred to the rescue squad. The following lists additional rescue techniques and equipment that will be helpful in making effective rescues at home.

Telephone

A specially installed or portable phone should be at poolside. 911 (or the local rescue squad number if different) must be clearly marked on the phone, and a highly visible "phone" sign should be posted so that neighbors and friends can find it easily in an emergency. Emergency procedures should also be prominently displayed by the phone (Fig. 2-5).

Rescue equipment

When a rescue must be made, even one involving a small child, entering the water is not recommended because a double-drowning may result. There are many different types of rescue equipment including a long pole (10 to 12 feet long), a large ring buoy with throwing line attached, and any number of extremely buoyant, flotational devices. Many rescue devices can be made inexpensively by reusing household items. For instance, an empty plastic milk jug with clothesline rope attached to the handle makes for an excellent "throw-rope." And of course, every pool should have a first-aid kit. A written, emergency action plan that can be practiced is the best guarantee that appropriate efforts will be carried out promptly.

Diving and other headfirst entries

Currently, the preferred minimum depth for competitive diving is 11 feet, while the preferred depth is 12.5 feet of water directly below the tip of the board

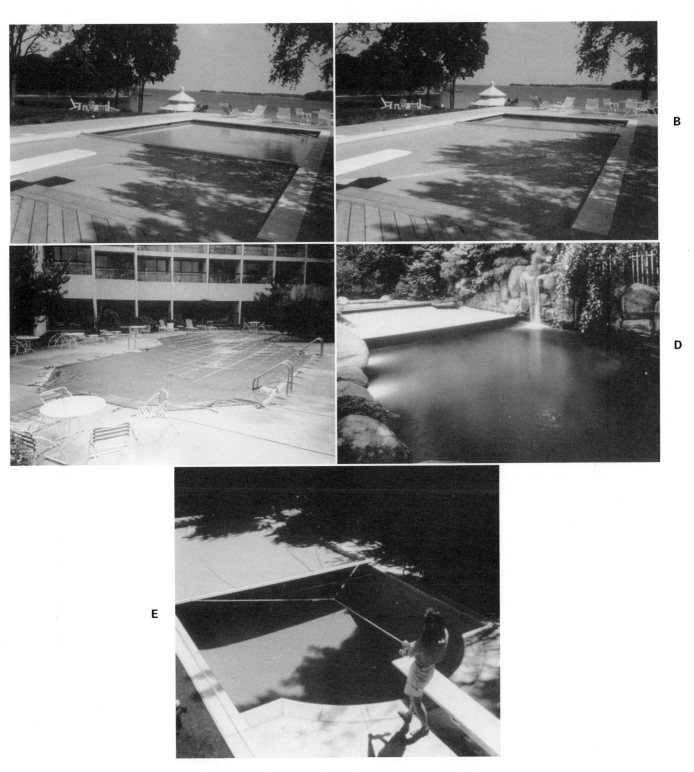

Fig. 2-4. Automatic pool cover and manually attached security covers. (**D** and **E**, Courtesy Vover Pools, Salt Lake City, Utah.)

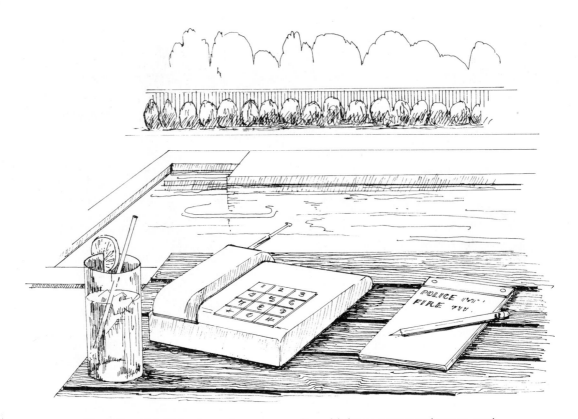

Fig. 2-5. Poolside phone for emergencies with important numbers posted.

(plummet) and extended out in front of the board for 16.5 feet. Diving from a springboard requires a safe diving envelope that allows a diver to safely maneuver underwater. Diving from a springboard requires a safe diving envelope that allows a diver to safely maneuver underwater. Diving from springboards also requires supervision regardless of the pool. For the sake of this discussion, diving takes place from a springboard, whereas headfirst entries occur from platforms other than springboards. Chapter 16 discusses diving in depth. The "diving" that occurs in residential pools is the headfirst entry variety rather than true springboard diving, even though a springboard may be used.

The greatest risk of neck injuries to adults (95%) in residential pools is caused by entering the shallow end of the pool head-first and hitting the pool bottom forcefully. Of all the sport-related spinal cord injuries that occur each year, most of these are a result of untrained individuals entering headfirst into natural shallow water, and most of these injuries happen in the open water environment, not in swimming pools.

Ironically, victims of spinal injury are most often healthy, athletic males between the ages of 13 and 35. This group is at risk more than any other because they have the ability to strike the pool bottom with tremendous force. In addition, more than half of these victims have high blood alcohol contents. Risk analysis also indicates that drowning and near drowning accounts for 75% of the total risk for aquatic facilities, whereas "diving" accounts for only 8%.[4]

Although many water safety experts teach people how and where to dive safely, entering home pools head-first from the side, a diving board, or a slide can be dangerous. Adults should always enter the water feet-first on their first entry into the pool, whether it's from the side of the deck or the diving board. When entering the water headfirst, adults should use a long, shallow dive and steer up to prevent hitting the bottom..

Both 1993 NCAA and U.S. Diving competitive diving rule books require a minimum of 11 feet under the 1 board for competitions but prefer 12 feet. NCAA and U.S. Diving have never experienced a cat-

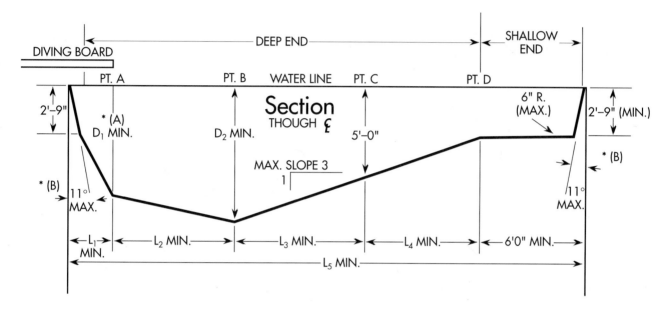

*IMPORTANT—A. MINIMUM DEPTH UNDER DIVING BOARD OR JUMP BOARD
B. TYPE I POOLS SHALL HAVE PLUMB WALLS AS SHOWN IN ARTICLE 3.6.5

POOL TYPE	MINIMUM DIMENSIONS							MINIMUM WIDTH OF POOL		
	D_1	D_2	L_1*	L_2	L_3	L_4	L_5	PT. A	PT. B	PT. C
0	See 3.5.5, 3.5.6	DIVING EQUIPMENT IS PROHIBITED								
I	6'-0"	7'-6"	1'-6"	7'-0"	7'-6"	6'-9"	28'-9"	10'-0"	12'-0"	10'-0"
II	6'-0"	7'-6"	1'-6"	7'-0"	7'-6"	6'-9"	28'-9"	12'-0"	15'-0"	12'-0"
III	6'-10"	8'-0"	2'-0"	7'-6"	9'-0"	6'-9"	31'-3"	12'-0"	15'-0"	12'-0"
IV	7'-8"	8'-6"	2'-6"	8'-0"	10'-6"	6'-9"	33'-9"	15'-0"	18'-0"	15'-0"
V	8'-6"	9'-0"	3'-0"	9'-0"	12'-0"	6'-9"	36'-9"	15'-0"	18'-0"	15'-0"

*See 3.5.2

Fig. 2-6. NSPI minimum diving depths for residential pools. (From ANSI/NSPI: *Standards for residential swimming pools*, Alexandria, Va, 1987, The Institute.)

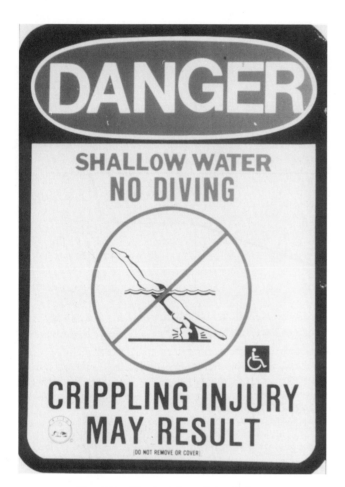

Fig. 2-7. Typical "no diving" sign.

astrophic diving injury in a supervised facility. Since 1972 the National Federation of State High School Associations (NFSHSA) has allowed high school competitive springboard diving in a minimum of 10 feet of water without ever having a catastrophic neck injury. NFSHSA recommends a 12-foot depth for newer pools but continues to sanction events in older, 10-foot pools.[5]

Although depth is an important factor, supervision is the key in preventing diving accidents. NSPI states that diving should be allowed in only those residential pools that are in total compliance with their minimum standards for residential pools (Fig. 2-6). Basically, all "dumb dives" must be prohibited in residential pools. These "dives" include diving through inner tubes, catching balls while entering head-first,

doing acrobatics, and distance dives. When these types of entries are allowed, diving into unsafe depths may result. For instance, a "diver" out of control could hit the sides or the upslope of the pool where the water is shallow.

It must be emphasized, however, that more injuries are caused by swimmers entering very shallow water headfirst rather than divers injuring themselves on diving boards. And having a diving board in a residential pool at least indicates to guests where the deep end is located. Like many hotel/motel pools, some homeowners attempt to place "big pool" equipment in a small pool. Often, there is simply not enough space and water depth to safely accommodate diving boards or slides in a private pool. If homeowners are planning to have a diving board, they must be certain that the minimum standards for safe diving are met and supervision is constant and vigilant. While these accessories are fun for children to use, they can be quite dangerous for adults, particularly at a party. Some pools may have sufficient water depth directly under the tip of the diving board, but unfortunately, showoffs can enter the water near the sides or the upslope where the water is shallow.

Diving boards and slides may not a good idea for some residential pools. If they do exist in a residential pool and sufficient depth and distance are not available, these accessories should be removed. If, however, the owner decides to keep this equipment in the case of marginal depths and distances, children under 12 years of age ONLY should be allowed to use diving boards or slides, and supervision is a must. Most victims of headfirst entries are males 13 years of age and older without formal training. If individuals older than 12 years cannot be kept from using the equipment in this case, it should be removed. Younger children are usually not large or strong enough to hit the bottom in 9 to 10 feet of water. Headfirst entries and sliding must always be supervised.

If headfirst entries are banned at a pool, effective signs prohibiting diving should be posted conspicuously around the swimming facility (Fig. 2-7). Headfirst entries should *NEVER* be attempted in an *ABOVE-GROUND POOL*.

Pools and parties are almost synonymous. Of those few serious neck injuries that do occur in pools, many occur during these events. Typically, someone has too much to drink, behavior becomes boisterous, the "diver" miscalculates a "dive" while showing off, and a broken neck results. Dangerous headfirst entries come from almost any platform: the pool deck, the diving board, the pool fence, and even the roof of the house. As the height of the dive increases or as the water depth decreases, the chance of serious injury becomes greater.

When planning a pool party, home owners should separate the alcohol from pool activities. One possible alternative might be to have swimming first, then serve drinks only after the pool has been cleared and closed. Hiring a trained lifeguard, whether or not alcohol is served, is always a good practice. Rules should be spelled out in writing beforehand, and the lifeguard should be responsible for enforcing them. Sending a copy of these rules with the invitation is also a good idea. If a residential pool is used at night, adequate lighting is a must. Good illumination is needed so that swimmers can easily read safety signs, see pool walls and bottom clearly, and walk on the pool deck safely. Lighting experts should be consulted before installing backyard lights for the pool. The Illuminating Engineering Society requires 10 footcandles for outdoor recreational pools, although 30 footcandles is preferred by many pool experts.[6]

Above-Ground, On-Ground, and In-Ground Pools

When it comes to selecting a pool, the homeowner has three basic choices: should the pool be constructed above, on, or in the ground? According to NSPI, an above-ground pool is a removable pool of any shape that has a minimum water depth of 36 inches and a maximum water depth of 48 inches at the wall. The wall is located on the surrounding earth and may be readily disassembled or stored and reassembled to its original integrity.[7] The above-ground pool tends to be smaller and much less expensive than the in-ground pool. The above-ground pool also has one constant depth; this pool does not provide for both shallow and and deep water. Because these pools are small and shallow, activities in the pool must be carefully monitored to prevent accidents. Headfirst entries must never be allowed in an above-ground pool. This pool also appears more temporary than permanent. Construction materials include aluminum, galvanized steel, and even wood.

But perhaps the fastest growing above-ground pool construction material is plastic. Pool plastics are much the same as automobile plastics; raw plastics combined with polymer resins to produce advance composites like PVC or polypropylenes. These composites enhance strength, flexibility, anticorrosion, UV resistance, and in addition are appealing to the eye. Some above-ground pools are characterized by large, freestanding, and interlocking panels, while others are one continuous roll that is supported by uprights and channels. A vinyl liner is then added to these structures to hold the water. A more recent type of above-ground pool is the large inflatable rubber variety. The lifespan for above-ground pools may be less than 10 years (Fig. 2-8).

The above-ground pool is the least expensive and

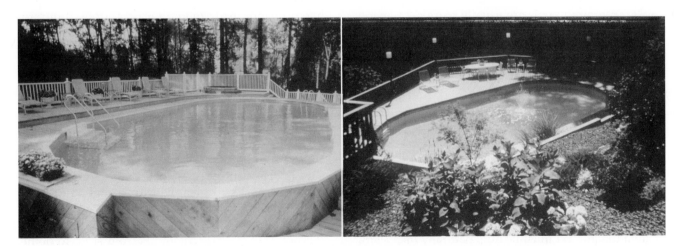

Fig. 2-8. Well-planned above-ground pools. (Courtesy NSPI, Alexandria, Va.)

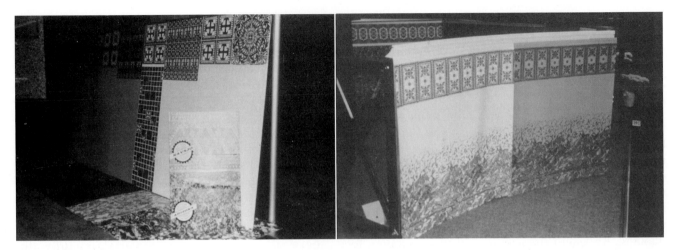

Fig. 2-9.   Vinyl liner samples.

most affordable pool in th United States. The average household income for above-ground pool purchasers as compiled by NSPI in 1991 is $39,000 as compared with $81,000 for in-ground pool purchasers. Although these figures will change over time, in-ground pools will probably remain roughly twice as expensive as above-ground pools.[4]

An on-ground residential swimming pool is a removable pool package whose walls rest fully on the surrounding earth and has an excavated area below the ground level where diving and the use of a water slide are prohibited. The slope adjacent to the shallow area shall have a maximin slope to 3:1 and the slope adjacent to the side walls shall have a maximum slope of 1:1.8

While above ground pools tend to be temporary pools, on-ground pools are usually more permanent. On-ground pools are constructed with rigid walls that come in sections. With this rigid wall design comes increased durability and flexibility in size and shape. Sturdy decking is often attached to the wall panels, providing increased strength and permanence. In addition, on-ground pools can be easily identified by fixed piping and electrical equipment for filtration and disinfection, whereas above-ground pools often lack these features.[4]

In-ground pools are more permanent and aesthetically pleasing structures. NSPI simply defines an inground swimming pool as any pool whose sides rest in partial or full contact with the earth.[9] A large hole in the ground must be dug, naturally increasing construction costs over the above-ground pool. While concrete residential pools offer the homeowner strength and durability, they are quite expensive to build.

More recently, vinyl liner in-ground pools have become popular. A vinyl liner in-ground pool looks just like a concrete pool but has a sand bottom and paneled sides that swimmers do not see. The bottom underneath the liner is usually shaped using sand, cement, or vermiculite to form a solid base. As a result this type of pool is very attractive and lasts longer than an above-ground pool but costs significantly less than a concrete in-ground pool. Although the vinyl liner usually lasts a minimum of 10 years, it does eventually wear out and needs to be replaced periodically. Vinyl liners are not that difficult or expensive to replace. The vinyl liner in-ground pool has probably made owning a pool a possibility for many homeowners who never thought they could afford one. In general, in-ground pools can last 30 to 40 years (Fig. 2-9).

Swimming Pool Chemicals

Pool chemicals must be kept out of the reach of children. In addition, storing pool chemicals in the garage or an all-purpose shed with gardening supplies is not a good idea. Fertilizers and automotive supplies can cause fire or explosions when mixed with certain pool chemicals.

When transporting chemicals from store to home, pool owners should use a separate cardboard or plastic box to protect the car and passengers from chemical spills. The driver should exercise special care to avoid excessive speeds, turns, and stops. Chemicals should never be left in the car unattended for any period of time. They should be quickly moved to the proper storage area.

Chemical containers must be stored separately and must not be stacked on top of one another. Lids must be sealed tightly. Pool chemicals should also be kept up off the floor. If at all possible, pool chemicals should be stored in a separate, clean, cool, dry, and well-ventilated building. A small utility shed can be built or purchased for this purpose, but it should be used exclusively for pool supplies.

Before using chemicals, be sure to read and follow the directions. Never mix chemicals, and avoid using the same scoop for different chemicals. Never add chemicals to the pool when swimmers are present and always use eye and face protection when working with chemicals.

Electrical Safety

All electrical outlets near the pool should be protected by ground fault interrupters (GFI), which are designed to prevent electrical shock. However, electrical appliances should be kept away from the pool. Only battery-operated radios should be allowed near the pool. If outdoor stereo speakers are used, all other stereo components, including amplifiers, should be kept indoors or well away from the pool.

All lighting fixtures and other electrical appliances must be checked regularly for routine maintenance. Before making any electrical repairs, the power must be turned off. Better yet, a licensed electrician should be called whenever there is a question about electricity, particularly in a wet environment. Above all, repairing underwater pool lights requires an expert, and all other electrical components must be kept away from the pool.

All electrical appliances should be installed according to the National Electrical Code (NEC) and any federal, state, or local codes that also apply.

Pool Maintenance Simplified

Several new developments in the swimming pool industry have helped homeowners maintain clear and clean pools with less stress and strain. Automatic cleaning systems and pool covers are just two new items that have simplified pool maintenance. In addition to security and energy savings, a pool cover, regardless of type, prevents airborne debris like dust, dirt, and leaves from entering the pool. So a pool cover not only keeps heat in the pool and prevents chemicals from being evaporated, but it also keeps organic debris from entering the water. A solar blanket type of pool cover will certainly pay for itself in a short period of time.

Several different types of automated pool cleaners are also available to homeowners. These devices were developed to save the pool owner time in vacuuming the pool bottom. Most of these devices are designed to operate at night or whenever the pool is free of swimmers.Before purchasing an automatic pool cleaner, the homeowner must be certain that the pool will not have trespassers in the evening. Theft of the machine can occur easily at night. Also, if the machine is tampered with while still in the water, electrocution could result, but this is extremely rare.

Hose bibs should be installed near the deck so that deck cleaning can be performed conveniently. The hose bib must not, however, create a trip hazard.

Indoor Pools

Some residential pools are constructed inside the home. In this case excellent ventilation in and around the pool enclosure is important to remove excess heat and humidity; otherwise damage to the home may result.

Insurance

Experienced and potential pool owners alike should check with their local insurance carrier to be certain they have adequate liability coverage in case an accident does occur in the pool. Most standard homeowner insurance policies automatically extend liability coverage to include swimming pools. This is good news, because for the most part pools are covered by the existing policy, and no additional insurance costs are charged to the homeowner. However, a homeowners policy should have liability coverage for a minimum of $300,000. Older policies may have a liability limit of $100,000. If a catastrophic injury does occur, $100,000 may not cover all expenses, and therefore increased liability coverage is warranted.

Homeowners may also wish to examine a liability umbrella policy, which covers homeowners for up to a million dollars and extends liability coverage to include automobiles.

Summary

For a safe, healthy, and enjoyable home-pool atmosphere, always remember the 10 commandments of swimming pool safety:

- Vigilant supervision
- Pool telephone
- Clearly stated pool rules
- Written emergency procedures
- Proper chemical storage
- Effective pool barrier
- CPR certification
- Lifesaving equipment
- Never swim alone
- Electrical safety

The American Red Cross videos, *Home Pool Safety*: *It Only Takes a Minute* and *Water, The Deceptive Power* are available at local American Red Cross chapters to assist home pool owners in safeguarding their pools. The American Red Cross also offers a variety of swimming and safety courses that aid in promoting water safety. Just because children have had swimming lessons does not mean they can be left unattended at a pool.

For those interested in purchasing a pool, NSPI offers pertinent publications and a list of dealers who are members of their organization; call (800)395-SWIM.

References

1. Klein K: *Pools.*
2. Guardex: Hydrotech Chemical Corp, Marietta, Ga.
3. Burrow C: All about swimming pools, *The New York Times*, September 13, 1992.
4. ANSI/NSPI: *Standards for public swimming pool* Alexandria, Va, 1991, The Institute.
5. Gabriel J (editor): *Diving safety: a position paper*, Indianapolis, Ind, 1992, US Diving.
6. True S: Personal communications, Kansas City, Mo, January 23, 1993.
7. R-P6: *Current recommended practice for sports lighting*, New York, 1989, Illuminating Engineering Society.
8. NSPI: Pool and spa marketing study for 1991, Alexandria, Va, 1992, The Institute.
9. Gabrielson AM: *Swimming pools: a guide to their planning, design, and operation*, Champaign, Ill, 1987, Human Kinetics Publishers.

Bibliography

American Red Cross: *Swimming and diving*, St Louis, 1992, Mosby.

Kowalsky L (editor): *Pool/spa operators handbook*, San Antonio, 1991, National Swimming Pool Foundation.

Mitchell KP: *The proper management of pool and spa water*, Decatur, Ga, 1988, BioLab.

NSPI: *The sensible way to enjoy your pool*, Alexandria, Va, 1983, The Institute.

Recreonics: Buyers' guide and operations hand book, 1991, Indianapolis, Ind. Catalog number 41.

Williams KG: *The aquatic facility operator's manual*, Hoffman Estates, Ill, 1991, National Recreation and Park Association, National Aquatic Section.

Review Questions

1. Of all newly constructed pools, what percentage are residential pools?

2. Explain the difference between an above-ground and an in-ground swimming pool?

3. Regarding water safety, what age group is a major concern at residential pools?

4. List three different "layers" of protection for residential pools.

5. What characteristics should a good fence have that is installed around a pool?

6. What precaution must be taken before swimming in a pool that uses a pool cover?

7. Is a separate telephone at poolside important?

8. Is "diving" headfirst into an above-ground pool permissible as long as the "diver" protects the head?

9. Are above-ground swimming pools usually removable?

10. What type of in-ground pool construction has significantly reduced the cost of owning a pool?

11. What should protect all electrical outlets near a pool?

12. List five important rules for safe chemical handling and storage.

13. Will purchasing a pool significantly increase the cost of homeowners insurance?

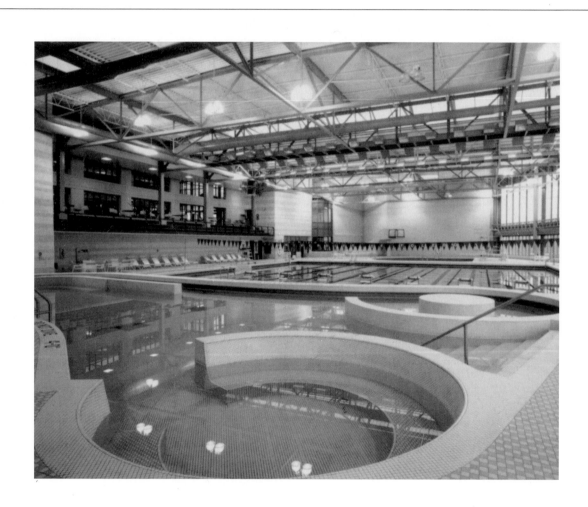

3

PUBLIC POOLS

The primary purpose of the public pool is to provide a variety of aquatic opportunities to the public at a minimal cost. By definition, a public pool is any pool other than a residential pool, which is intended to be used for swimming or bathing and is operated by an owner, lessee, operator, licensee or concessionaire, regardless of whether a fee is charged for use.[1]

For the sake of this discussion public pools may also double as school, YMCA, park and recreation pools, or similar types of agency pools. While the residential pool chapter was written mostly for the residential pool owner, this chapter will primarily address the public pool employees, whether they are the pool manager, coach, instructor, or lifeguard. Standards for public pools are provided by local municipalities or health departments. In addition, the National Spa and Pool Institute in Alexandria, Virginia, publishes recommended standards for public pools and is a good source of information.

Residential pools normally do not provide lifeguards, whereas at public pools, lifeguards are often an integral part of the system. Another important distinction between private and public pools is that public pools are regulated by local ordinances and health codes, making the management of these facilities more involved.

Because public pools are designed to offer a variety of aquatic opportunities to many different individuals, pool sizes and configurations vary. The most popular community pools usually have creative pool designs that allow for different activities occurring simultaneously. The trend today, however, is to build shallow (5 feet or less) rather than deeper (10 feet or more) pools. Zero depth pools, which create a walk-in or beachlike entry, are also becoming popular.

Pool designs must be dictated by programs and priority user groups. A pool cannot be successfully designed or programmed without the target audience in mind. For example, a swimming pool located in a senior citizen community better have lots of warm, shallow water; deep water is of little value to this group.

ADA

Public Law 101-336 or the Americans With Disabilities Act (ADA), which went into effect on January 26, 1992, extends the Civil Rights Act of 1964 to include disabled citizens. The ADA prohibits discrimination against those individuals with disabilities in public places, including pools. This law entitles all Americans equal opportunity and full enjoyment of public services, facilities, employment, goods, and

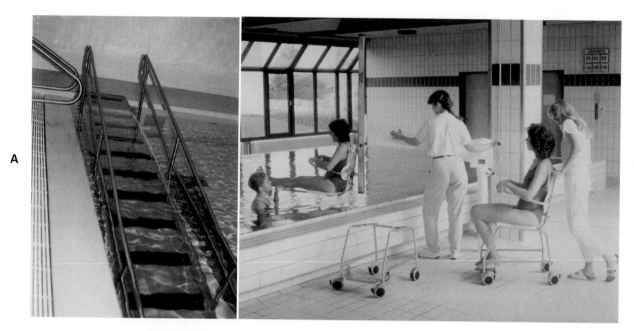

Fig. 3-1. **A,** Removable stainless steel access ramp may be needed to comply with the ADA. **B,** Chair lifts may be used when pool space is at a premium. (**A,** Courtesy AFW Company of North America, Olean, NY; **B,** courtesy Arjo, Morton Grove, Ill.)

opportunities. Only private clubs and religious organizations are exempt from this law. Public pools and spas are significantly affected by this law. The law may require changes in pool policies and procedures, elimination of architectural barriers, and the addition of services and equipment to aid the disabled. Some pool modifications might include handrails, ramps, chair lifts, wider doorways, nonslip surfaces, improved lighting, and assistants who can aid the disabled (Fig. 3-1). Those overseeing public pools must be familiar with the ADA. Every public pool operator should be familiar with the ADA requirements. A copy of the ADA can be obtained by writing:

U.S. Senate Subcommittee on Disability Policy, 113 Senate Hart Office Building, Washington, D. C. 20510.

Swimmer Loads

Every public pool should have an enforceable maximum user load that must not be exceeded. State or local pool codes normally establish swimmer loads for public pools and may use any one of a variety of formulas. The criteria used to determine swimmer loads may vary between indoor and outdoor pools,

shallow and deep portions of pools, deck surface area, and water surface areas. For example, one swimmer load requirement might read "no more than one swimmer per 20 sq. ft. of surface area" In this case the entire surface area of the pool would be calculated and then divided by 20 sq. ft. to determine how many people are allowed to be in the pool at one time. It is the responsibility of the pool manager or operator to calculate the maximum swimmer load according to the local code and together with the lifeguards, enforce it.

Public pools must also determine how much of their programming time is going to be devoted to instruction, recreation, and competition.

These priorities must be spelled out as specifically as possible (Fig. 3-2).

Special Use Pools

Whenever possible, separate pools should be constructed for separate programs so that conflicting programs do not run into each other. Additionally, different pools can maintain different water temperatures, which is beneficial to different user groups. Special use pools that have been used successfully include the following.

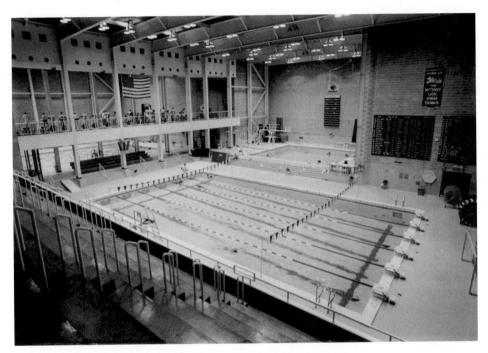

Fig. 3-2. A racing, diving, and instructional pool all under one roof.

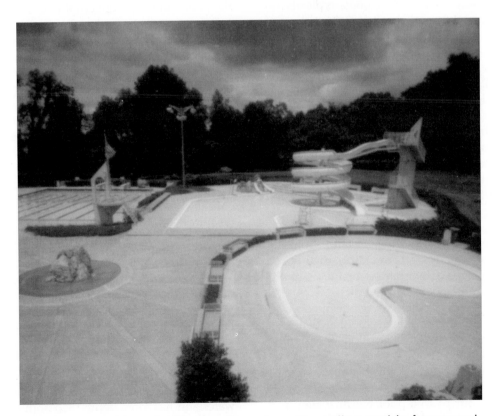

Fig. 3-3. A multiuse family aquatic center with wading pool in foreground. (Courtesy Paddock Swimming Pool, Rockville, Md. Photographer, Dan Cunningham.)

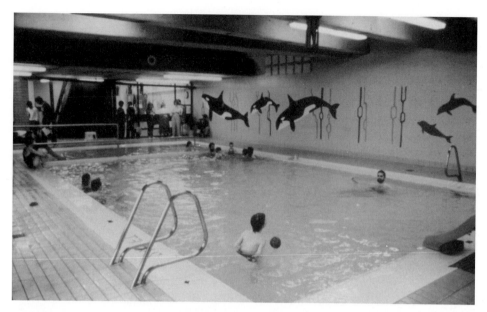

Fig. 3-4. Instructional pool used for teaching activities. (Courtesy Mark Hokkanen.)

The wading pool

A wading pool is simply a pool that has shallow depth used for wading. Wading pools typically do not exceed depths of more than 2 feet (24 inches) of water depth. It is intended for use by toddlers and young children under the age of 5 years. Many refer to this pool as the "kiddy pool" or "familiarization pool" (Fig. 3-3).

The water depth at the perimeter of this pool should not exceed 18 inches. Walls should not extend more than 6 inches above the water surface. Wading pools with a walk-in entry (zero depth) are becoming increasingly popular because families with children find them easier to use. This pool should be completely separated and apart from the main pool. The greater the distance of the wading pool from the main pool, the less likely a small child will wander off into the deeper pool; however, distance from the main pool also creates supervision problems. Whenever possible, a 4 foot barrier or fence should separate the wading pool from other pools.

At some public pools parents have been asked to supervise their children in this pool rather than lifeguards. This is a questionable practice. If assigning lifeguards to wading pools is not possible, then guards should regularly check on this pool as a part of their normal guarding rotation. Older children should be kept out of this pool because they can injure smaller children. If smaller children are not being properly supervised by their parents or other responsible adults, the child should be removed from the pool and the parents should be consulted.

Protective covers and antivortex plates on pool outlets and drains are extremely important in the kiddy pool, otherwise small children may become entrapped on them. The wading pool should have a separate filtration and disinfection system but does not necessarily hold true for older public pools. Concerning wading pool circulation, the recommended turnover rate for wading pools is 2 hours.

The instructional pool

This pool is typically a shallow, warm water pool that is used primarily for water play and swimming instruction The advantage of the instructional pool is so learn to swim programs, aquacize, and similar activities can take place while the main pool is being used by the swim team or other large groups. Sizes and shapes of instructional pools vary, but the maximum water depth should be between 3.5 and 5 feet. Because of the shallow depth of water in this pool, head first entries must be prohibited (Fig. 3-4).

The competition or main pool

This pool has traditionally been the focal point of aquatic programming (Fig. 3-5). It contains the most water and has more depth than both the instructional and wading pools. While most older competition

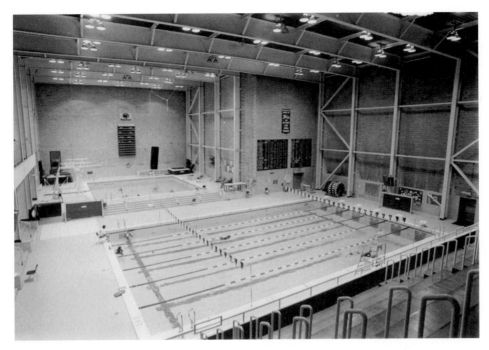

Fig. 3-5. Separate racing pool and springboard diving pool.

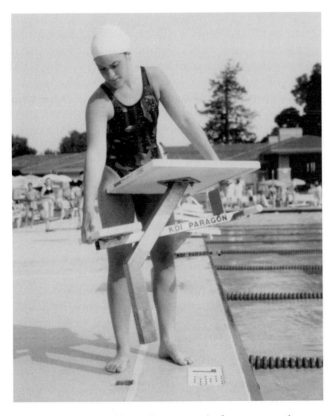

Fig. 3-6. Removable racing start platform can reduce headfirst injuries. (Courtesy KDI Paragon, Pleasantville, NY.)

pools have a minimum depth of 3.5 feet, the recommended minimum depth for competitive pools is now between 4 feet and preferably 5 feet to prevent neck injuries caused by improper racing starts. This is where the bulk of aquatic activity occurs and usually contains the racing course for swim team practice and meets. Many lap swimmers gravitate towards this pool. The NCAA and U.S. Swimming organizations should be contacted for dimensions and other recommendations if competitive swimming is to take place in this pool. If starting platforms (blocks) are used in this pool, they should be located at the deep end of a pool. Although the NCAA (1993) requires a minimum of 4 feet, deeper water (minimum 5 feet) provides a greater margin of safety. When not being used by team members, starting blocks should be either covered or removed from the pool deck to prevent injuries. If they cannot be removed, patrons must be prevented from using them (Fig. 3-6).

The diving pool

The benefit of a separate diving pool is that deep water activities are removed from the main pool, thus eliminating conflicts between swimmers and divers and other deep water activities. By having a separate diving well, a flat bottom profile can be constructed and sufficient water depth provided to prevent neck

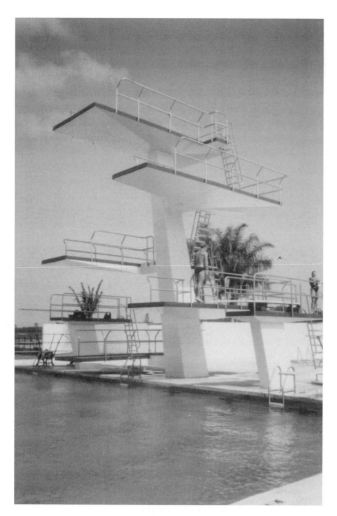

Fig. 3-7. Separate diving well with competitive spring boards and towers. (Courtesy KDI Paragon, Pleasantville, NY.)

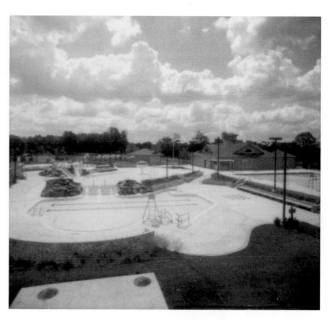

Fig. 3-8. Multiuse family aquatic center or leisure pool. (Courtesy Paddock Swimming Pool, Rockville, Md. Photographer, Dan Cunningham.)

and back injuries. If competitive diving is permitted in this pool, the preferred depth is 12.5 feet for 1 m diving boards. Before constructing a diving well, the NCAA, U.S. diving, or FINA regulations should be followed.

The diving well is often used by springboard divers, but when the diving boards are not in use, other activities like SCUBA diving, synchronized swimming, lifeguarding, and water safety courses may be conducted there.

Another advantage of the diving pool is that the depth is constant without any slopes. The constant depth should be a minimum of 12.5 feet and can be as much as 17 feet if towers are a part of the facility. Although the diving pool enhances diving safety and

improves programming throughout the entire aquatic facility, it is often the most underused pool in the complex, because only accomplished swimmers use it and participants are unable to stand up in it (Fig. 3-7).

Specific information about diving boards, stands, rules, and regulations will be discussed in the diving chapter.

Although separate pools are ideal for both programming and safety, they are more expensive to construct and maintain than one large pool. Separate pools require separate filtration systems, heaters, surge tanks, and disinfection systems. If only one pool can be built, several areas in the pool should be able to be separated from the main pool to allow for activities in addition to lap swimming.

Multiuse family pools

As the traditional pools just mentioned age in this country, they are increasingly being converted into multiuse family centers that include whirlpools, waterfalls, fountains, slides, and other activities for families with small children (Fig. 3-8). Pools designed for competitive and instructional programs only are rapidly becoming things of the past. Multiuse family pools are becoming so popular that their attendance rates far surpass traditional pools. For more information concerning this new concept in swimming pools contact the National Recreation and Parks Association and the World Waterpark Association.

Areas outside the pool but within the aquatic facility are important for the functioning of any aquatic facility. They include the entrance, deck area, bathhouses, and snack bar.

Pool Entrance

The entryway to a swimming pool serves many functions of which only one pertains to admission. This is often "control central" for aquatic facilities and should include ample office and storage space.

The entry area is where the admission policy to the pool is enforced and also the ideal place to disseminate information to the pool patrons. Rules and regulations should be posted in this area along with pool staff pictures and certifications.

This is also a good location for the first aid kit, telephone, and public address system. This is an ideal place to keep files on accident reports, health department forms, and all other records and documentation. This area should also provide ample shade and protection from inclement weather. A public telephone is desirable in this area. If patrons are not pro-

vided with a public phone, the pool phone will be overused and hinder the functioning of the pool office. The pool entrance should not be a place where lifeguards are permitted to congregate. Not only does this practice create a poor public image, but a traffic control problem often results when guards are allowed to "hangout" at the pool entrance when not on duty.

Pool Decking

The deck area must be constructed with a nonslip surface and should surround the entire perimeter of the swimming pool. Pool decks must be designed to remove pool splash-out water, deck cleaning water, and rainwater without leaving any standing water. Adequate sloping of the decks to drains or perimeter areas is important to protect against puddling and algae growth. Outdoor pools normally have larger decks than indoor pools. The wet areas of a pool deck are located within 10 feet of the water's edge. Walking and lounging should be provided for ondeck areas located away from the wet areas. "NO DIVING" signs should be placed on all pool decks adjacent to water depths of less than 9 feet. These

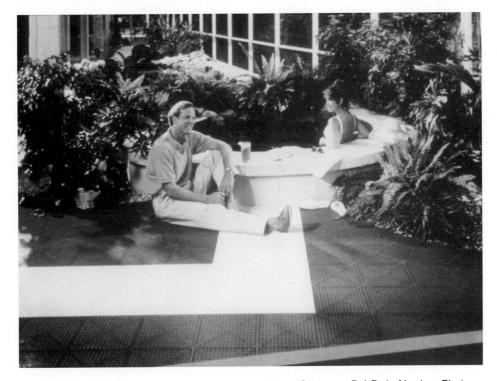

Fig. 3-9. Nonslip interlocking vinyl deck tiles. (Courtesy Dri-Dek, Naples, Fla.)

signs must be within 18 inches of the pool edge, and the letters must be at least 4 inches tall. Contrasting colors are also recommended for these signs. Hose bibs should be installed around the perimeter of the pool deck to ease cleaning of the entire pool deck area.

As mentioned previously in Chapter 2, there are a variety of construction materials. If concrete decks are to be installed, they should conform to the standards recommended by the American Concrete Institute. Attractive, nonslip, flow-through decking

materials are rapidly becoming a big business within the pool industry. Vinyl and rubber decking tiles as well as runners are available to place over existing decks to increase attractiveness and safety (Fig. 3-9).

Many facility operators believe that they have inadequate deck space. A spacious deck not only allows for better administration of swimming meets and other events but also provides an unobstructed view of the water, thus promoting water safety. Painted decks or carpeted decks often lead to problems (Fig. 3-10).

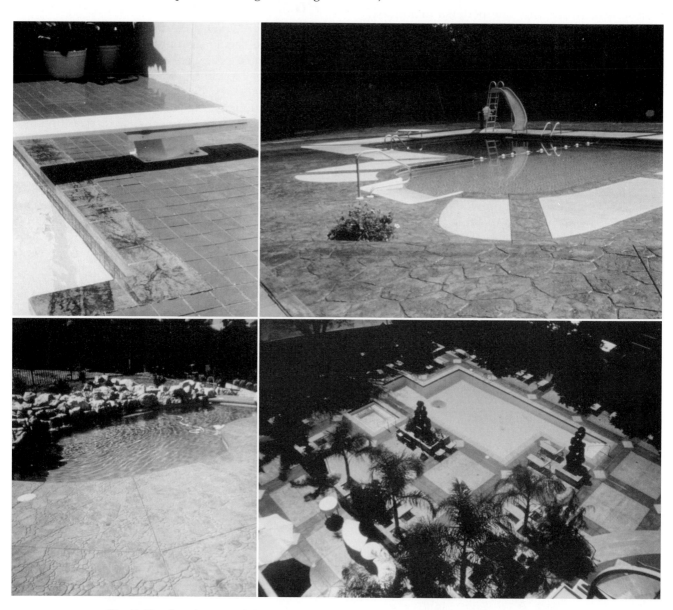

Fig. 3-10. Spacious pool decking combining a variety of materials including concrete, stamped concrete, and brick. (Courtesy Bomanite, Madera, Calif.)

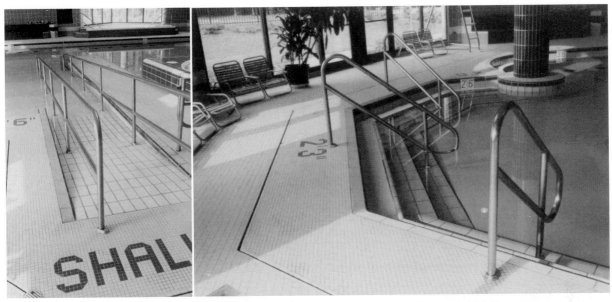

Fig. 3-11. Ramps and steps with stainless steel handrails. (Courtesy KDI Paragon, Pleasantville, NY.)

Ladders and Steps

All pools should have at least two means of entering and exiting with both the shallow and deep ends of the pool being served. A good rule of thumb to follow is to have an entry/exit device every 75 linear feet of pool wall. Ladders must be constructed of corrosion-resistant material like stainless steel. All ladders should be recessed to eliminate hazards to patrons swimming past them. Each ladder should have two handrails or hand holds. The steps on the ladder must be nonslip. Recessed steps built into the wall must also have two hand rails or holds and nonslip steps and the recessed treads should drain into the pool to prevent an accumulation of dirt. For specific dimensions of ladders and steps, local and state codes should be consulted. Whenever actual stairways are used in a pool, they should be either recessed from the swimming area or removable. Once again, the steps must be non-slip (Fig. 3-11).

Coping

Pool copings refer to the construction joint or cap that connects the vertical pool wall to the horizontal pool deck. It is imperative that pool copings are watertight so that water does not pass to the ground

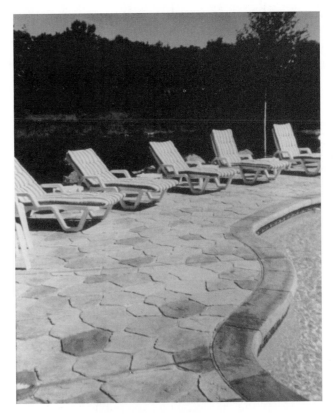

Fig. 3-12. Coping divides the deck from the pool. (Courtesy Bomanite, Madera, Calif.)

Class	Application
I*	International, professional and tournamenty
II	Collage and Diving
III	High school without diving
IV	Recreational
*Televised	

Recommended Illuminance Criteria for Above-Pool Lighting					
Class	**Surface in Horizontal Footcandles**			**Vertical Footcandles**	**Uniformity (Maximum to Minimum)**
	Indoor	Outdoor	Deck	Platform	
I*	70		50	70*	2.0
II	50	30	20	30	2.5
III	30	20	10		3.0
IV	30	10	10		4.0
*The plateform in the principal viewing direction should have 70 to 100 footcandles without direct glare to the divers.					

Fig. 3-13. Above-pool lighting recommendations. (Courtesy IES of North America, New York.)

beneath or behind pool walls. Copings must also be constructed with a permanent, nonslip surface. Pool copings are often constructed of concrete, stone, or tile. Copings also serve as hand holds for swimmers entering and exiting the pool (Fig. 3-12).

Lighting

Lumens and footcandles are two terms used to measure illumination.

In general, lumens describes the magnitude of brightness coming off the light fixture or bulb, whereas footcandles refers to the light that reaches the surface below. Footcandles are measured by a light meter.

Generally, the Illuminating Engineering Society (IES) recommends 50-footcandles for indoor competition pools and 30-footcandles for public recreational pools. Indirect lighting is usually used for smaller indoor pools with low ceilings, whereas direct light-

ing must be used in large indoor complexes with high ceilings. Whichever lighting is used, glare must not be produced on the surface of the water. Outdoor pools typically require less light than do indoor pools. See Fig. 3-13 for specific recommendations.[2]

Underwater Lights

All underwater lights must be installed according to the National Electrical Code. Ground Fault Interrupters (GFIs) are also an important requirement. A licensed electrician should be consulted whenever installing, repairing, or replacing lights. Whenever underwater lights are being handled, circuit breakers must be turned off. Mishandling of underwater lights may lead to electrocution.

Underwater lights come in two basic types, dry niche and wet niche.

The dry niche light is a light unit placed behind a watertight window in the pool or spa wall. This light

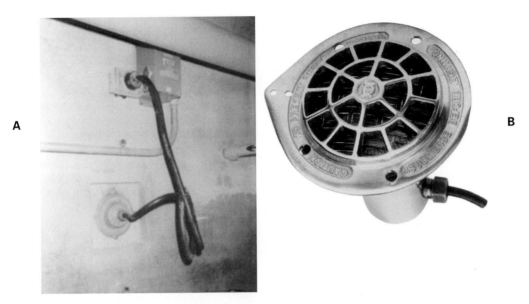

Fig. 3-14. **A,** Dry niche underwater lighting fixture. **B,** Wet niche underwater lighting fixture. (Courtesy KDI Paragon, Pleasantville, NY.)

can be removed, replaced, or repaired without entering the water. The dry niche light is often handled in the filter room or around the pool shell. A tunnel is created in the pool wall, under the pool deck, and houses the light and fixture. A glass lens separates the dry niche light from the pool water. A bulb with too much wattage can damage the lens. In addition, the lens may break if the light is turned on when the water level in the pool falls below the lens.

A wet niche light is a watertight fixture and water-cooled fixture placed in a submerged wet niche in the pool or spa wall and is accessible only from the pool or spa (Fig. 3-14). This light must be removed from the pool and placed on the pool deck for repairs. With the wet niche light, both the light and the person repairing it get wet. As a result many individuals prefer working with dry niche lights. Wet niche lights are cooled by the surrounding pool water and may explode if lighted out of the water.

Lighting fixtures should be between 2 and 3 feet below the surface of the water with an additional level of lights at 8- and 10-foot depths for deeper pools.[2]

Pool Finishes

Although there are many different types of pool finishes, some are not appropriate for public pools.

Most public pool finishes should be light or white in color for good visibility. Of all the pool finishes, perhaps plaster is the most popular, particularly with concrete pools. Plastered pools are often referred to as marbledust, "Marcite," and "Marblelite." This pool finish may have to be replastered about every 8-10 years. Tile as a pool finish is very durable but also extremely expensive. Once a pool basin is tiled, it rarely, if ever, needs to be repaired or replaced. Often, because of the great expense of tile, pools will combine plaster and tile applications. The tile in this case would be reserved for the water line on the pool wall or racing lines on the pool bottom. Rubber-based paints can also serve as a pool finish. Paints used in this fashion should be chlorinated rubber-based paints that are resistant to pool chemicals and unbalanced water. These paints are popular when used for renovation projects. Epoxy paints are quite expensive, but they form a hard, impervious surface that many public pools require. Painted pool finishes will have to be repainted frequently, about every 5 years. Regardless of the type pool finish employed, it must provide good visibility, ease of cleaning and a nonslip surface. Although vinyl-lined pools are popular in private residences, they are usually not compatible with public pool use, because the finish is somewhat slippery and vinyl may not be able to withstand heavy swimmer loads.

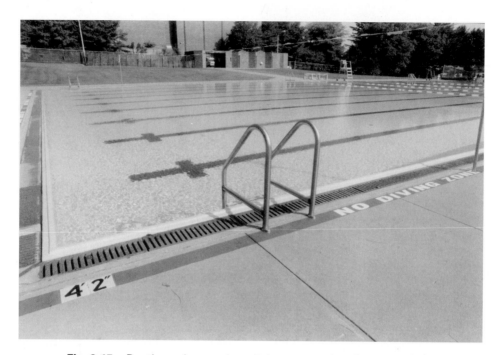

Fig. 3-15.   Depth markers and no diving zone painted on pool deck.

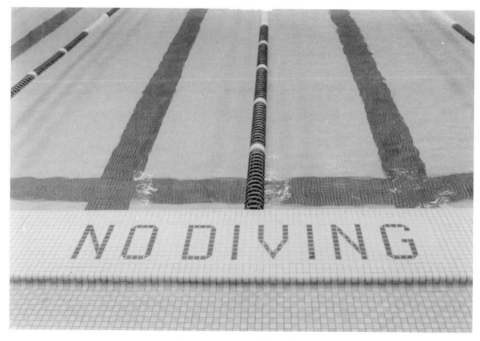

Fig. 3-16.   No diving markers.

Depth Markers

Depth markers are an integral part of every pool but particularly for public pools. These markings may be painted or tiled but they must plainly and conspicuously identify the water depth (Fig. 3-15). These signs must appear both on the vertical pool wall just above the water line and horizontally on the pool deck or coping close to the water's edge (no more than 18 inches away from the water). Depth markings must be clearly visible both to the swimmer in the water and the patron on the pool deck. Depth markings on the pool deck must be slip-resistant and appear at the minimum and maximum water depths and wherever the slope of the bottom changes. Depth markers should appear periodically on the pool deck but should not be placed more than 25 feet apart. In addition, a depth marker should be placed whenever a 2-foot change in water depth takes place, but local codes and pool ordinances must be checked before installation of these markers.

Depth markers must be a minimum of 4 inches high (6- to 8-inch numbers are preferred) with the numbers being a contrasting color from the background. The depth markings should be permanently installed, and whenever possible, meters as well as feet should be indicated.

Safety Markings

Depth markings are an important public pool requirement in many states, but additional signs and markings should be used at public pools. Headfirst entries from the side of the pool must be prohibited in less than 9 feet of water. If any headfirst entries are permitted in water depths between 6 and 9 feet, it should be for supervised, shallow-water, racing starts only. Diving warnings must be given to all pool patrons often and at regular intervals wherever the water is shallow. **"NO DIVING"** signs should be placed on the deck near depth markings. It may be wise to make these warnings larger than the depth markers. Some pools incorporate a no-diving zone by painting a red or orange line around the edge of the deck (Fig. 3-16).

Because headfirst accidents can have such catastrophic results, additional precautions against headfirst entries into shallow water should also be taken. These suggestions will be further discussed in the diving chapter of this book.

Warning lines should be painted or tiled on steps or the pool bottom whenever a significant change in

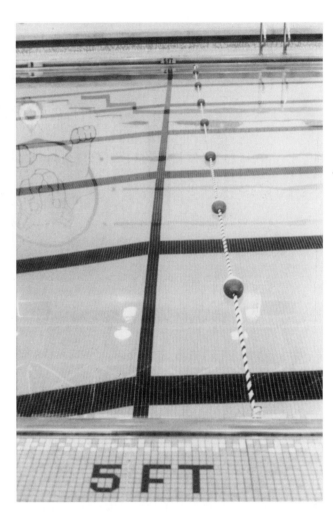

Fig. 3-17. Warning lines on pool bottom. (Courtesy Tim Gervinski.)

depth occurs. These warning lines should be approximately 4 inches in width and colored black, dark blue, or red (Fig. 3-17). A boundary line should be placed on pool bottoms to divide deep from shallow water. A buoyed line (lifeline) should also be installed across the surface of the pool above the break point and about 2 feet closer to the shallow end of the pool. Warning lines on pool steps, edges, ledges, and other possible obstructions are very helpful in cautioning swimmers of abrupt changes in depth or surface structures.

Pool rules and regulations should be posted at the entrance of the pool, in the locker rooms, and at various locations where these rules are particularly pertinent (Fig. 3-18). Typical pool rules prohibit running, glass, unsupervised swimming, general horseplay, and boisterous behavior. Other signs are also needed

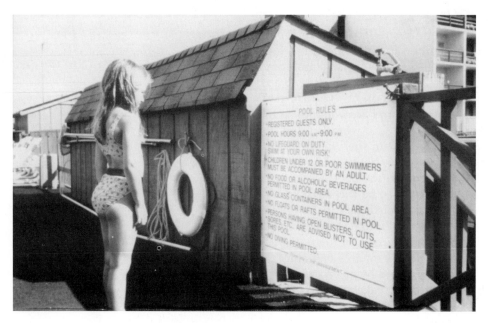

Fig. 3-18. Posted pool rules.

to explain policies like dress codes, the use of flotational devices, smoking, and the like. Whenever possible, a written copy of pool rules and regulations should be given to each member of the pool.

General signage at any pool is extremely important. Rules and regulations not only help to prevent lawsuits, but more important, they also help to prevent accidents from occurring. Particularly in geographic locations with a multicultural character, graphic signs using illustrations as well as written messages can be more effective.

As mentioned in the previous chapter, using contrasting colors similar to highway warning signs should also be helpful in conveying the appropriate message.

Lifeguarding Equipment

Many states require that elevated lifeguard chairs be maintained at public pools. Though elevated chairs do give lifeguards an improved vantage point from which to supervise swimmers, lifeguards have been known to injure themselves climbing in and out of the chairs. Lifeguard chairs may either be permanently installed in the pool deck or be of a portable variety. Although the portable lifeguard chair provides many advantages, it does take up more deck space.

Lifeguard chairs must be strategically placed to avoid blind spots and glare from the sun. Chairs should also be positioned closer to sections of the pool that have greater risks. Whenever possible, shade and water should be provided at each chair. First aid kits, gloves, and face shields to protect lifeguards from bloodborne pathogens should be located at every chair. If a water rescue must be initiated from the elevated chair, guards must be trained and reminded not to dive into the water from the chair. Many good lifeguards have been seriously injured by diving from lifeguard chairs. A good rule of thumb used to determine the number of lifeguard chairs is one elevated chair per 2000 square feet of pool surface area. Local swimming pool codes should be checked, however, before elevated lifeguard stands are purchased or installed (Fig. 3-19).

In addition to elevated chairs, lifeguards and pool patrons must have rescue equipment conveniently and conspicuously available to them. Lifesaving equipment should include the following:

- A strong, light pole at least 12 feet long with a large, blunt hook located at one end, often called a shepherd's crook.
- A ring buoy or other throwing device with a line attached. The rope should be at least 50 feet long.
- An emergency telephone with important numbers listed. This phone should be restricted to emergency use only.
- A backboard for use of trained individuals in case of a neck or back injury (Fig. 3-20).

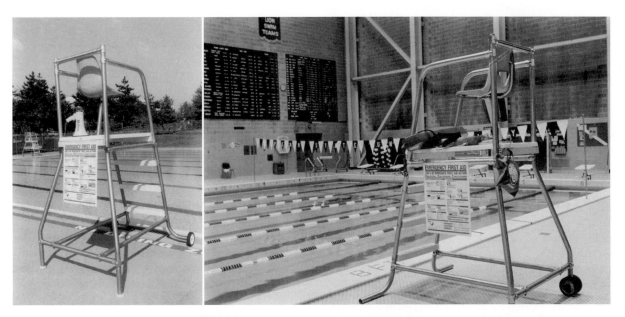

Fig. 3-19. Portable, elevated lifeguard chair.

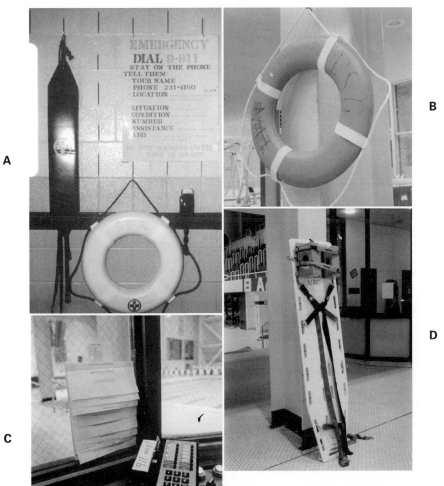

Fig. 3-20. **A,** Rescue tube, ring bouy, and emergency procedure posted. **B,** A large ring bouy. **C,** Emergency telephone with important numbers and procedures listed. **D,** Backboard for care of spinal injuries. (A, Courtesy Tim Gervinski.)

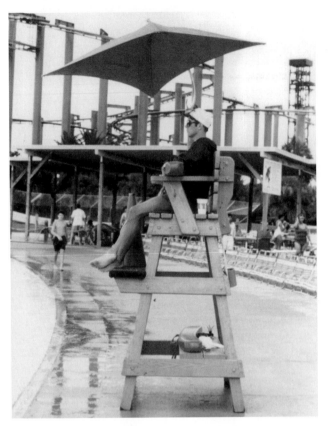

Fig. 3-21. Elevated lifeguard protected by umbrella from both sun and rain. (Courtesy Water Safety Products, Melbourne Beach, Fla.)

Outdoor Pools: Special Considerations

Outdoor pools are faced with additional problems that are often not concerns for indoor pools. These concerns are many and varied.

Indoor pools are protected from the ultraviolet rays of the sun. Unfortunately, outdoor pools are bombarded with these damaging rays, which dissipate chlorine levels and also promote algae growth. When pools are located in sunny, hot regions, it is extremely difficult to keep sufficient levels of chlorine in the pool. For this reason many outdoor pool operators are moving toward the use of stabilized chlorines which are not affected by the ultraviolet rays of the sun. Stabilized chlorines are therefore able to withstand the sunlight and remain in the water longer, thus saving money and avoiding low chlorine levels. The use of stabilized chlorines save significant sums of money. Stabilized chlorines also have some disadvantages associated with them and will be discussed in detail in Chapter 7. It must be pointed out that some states ban the use of stabilized chlorines in public pools.

Outdoor pools often have increased trouble with algae growth. This is not only due to the sun but also caused by wind, rain, and other organic materials being blown into outdoor pools. Sunlight does have a significant effect on algae growth.

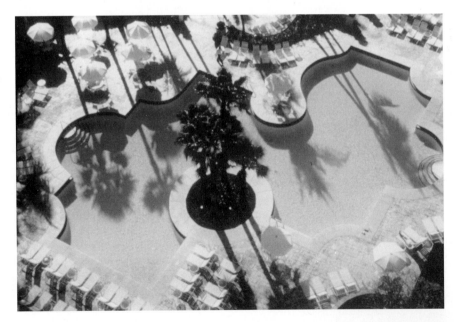

Fig. 3-22. Swimming pool furniture on spacious pool decks. (A, Courtesy Bomanite, Madera, Calif.)

Outdoor pools need to provide shaded areas for lifeguards and patrons alike. With all the information available on skin cancer today, it would be irresponsible not to provide protection from the harmful rays of the sun. Although large beach umbrellas are often the simplest remedy in this regard, they can often become airborne during windy conditions and have, in fact, caused serious accidents. When umbrellas are used for shade, extra care must be taken to fasten them down securely and they must also be taken down when a storm is approaching (Fig. 3-21).

Lounge chairs are often provided at outdoor pools. Pool furniture is moved and abused greatly during the course of a season. Sturdiness and stacking ability are two basic requirements for selecting pool furniture. Cleaning pool decks and lounging areas becomes extremely difficult if chairs cannot be stacked. Also, lounging areas should be kept away from the wet deck areas and as far away from the pool deck as possible so as not to cause sight obstructions of the pool or impede rescue efforts. Whenever possible, lounging areas should be kept separate from pool and deck areas (Fig. 3-22).

Pool cleanliness

Outdoor pools are typically more difficult to keep clean because so many more undesirable materials may enter the pool. Leaves, grass clippings, and other foreign objects are of particular concern. Leaves not only clutter the pool bottom but can easily clog skimmers and gutters, thus reducing proper filtration. Pollen, dirt, dust, rodents, and other small animals often find their ways into outdoor pools. Once again, these are not only unsightly but also reduce the flow of water back to the filters.

Experienced pool operators increase the surface skimming of their pools as more objects find their way into the pool. With increased skimming action less debris will sink to the bottom. If a large amount of debris does make it to the bottom of the pool, pool operators will then take more water from the bottom outlet (main drain) to pull the undesirable material out of the pool.

A good pool cover, as well as wind screens, can also help reduce the amount of undesirable matter going into the pool. Whenever possible, trees and shrubs and even lawns should be kept well away from the pool edges to prevent leaves and clippings from entering the pool.

Barriers

The entire aquatic facility must be bordered on the perimeter by a strong, durable fence or wall, preferably 8 feet in height. Fencing requirements vary in different states and for different types of pools. It is imperative that at least the minimum fencing requirements are met. All barriers must be designed to deter unauthorized entry and should not have any external

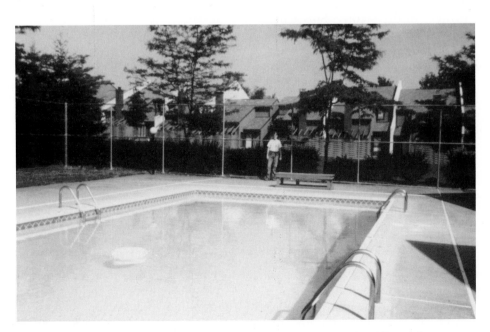

Fig. 3-23. An 8-foot chain-link fence securing a semi-public pool.

handholds or footholds. Fences must be checked on a regular basis for holes and other openings. Signage located periodically on the fence should warn trespassers about unlawful entry. A large double-doored gate must be available for the entry of emergency vehicles and chemical deliveries (Fig. 3-23).

Lighting

Outdoor pools should have adequate lighting for security reasons, even if night-time swimming is not planned. A night watchman is also a good idea if trespassers and vandalism are a possibility. It is not uncommon for this night watchman to provide other pool services such as vacuuming and bath-house clean-up. When lighting is planned for evening swimming and programs, care must be taken so that excessive glare is not produced on the surface of the water. Glare at night will inhibit the lifeguards' ability to watch and protect patrons.

Food Concessions

Anytime food is served at a swimming facility, whether it is sold on the premises or brought in by patrons, it must be consumed in special areas reserved for eating and drinking only. Smoking should also be banned at most swimming facilities. It is interesting to note that U.S. Swimming bans smoking anywhere in an aquatic facility during a swimming competition. Keeping an aquatic facility clean can be a nightmare if eating and drinking are allowed to take place anywhere in the facility. Snack bars should provide for eating with tables and refuse cans clearly marked and kept away from the pool decks. Fencing and signage also helps in keeping food and drink away from the pool and deck areas. Above all, glass must be kept out of the facility. Particularly with outdoor pools, as food and drink consumption increases, so will bees and flies.

There are two basic ways of dispensing food at pools: self-service vending machines or full-surface snack bars. While many public pools (full-service) enjoy the profits of a full-surface snack bar, there are also several disadvantages, including personnel and hygiene concerns. Food and drink at an outdoor pool will also attract bees and flies.

Public pools must have a minimum of one drinking fountain, but preferably one per 2000 square feet of pool surface area, whether or not food and beverages are served. Because this type of pool may produce burns, bee stings and cuts, additional training and first aid equipment may be required of the staff.

Programming

An important aspect of the public pool that is not normally a part of a private pool is programming. Once again, to program correctly, pool management needs a clear set of priorities. Some things that must be programmed are:

Vacuuming (very early in the morning to allow dirt to settle)

Lessons (mid mornings and late afternoons)

Team practice (early morning after vacuuming and early evenings)

Recreational swims (all other times)

Lap swimming (before and after people go to work and whenever possible during the day)

Special groups and shows

Each of these activities should be prioritized with those individuals in charge.

Security

Securing the pool from trespassers and vandals after the pool closes is a difficult but important task. Not only someone can get seriously hurt after hours, but a great potential for vandalism also exists. There are several things that can be done to safeguard the outdoor pool at night:

A security light

Every outdoor pool should have a bright light illuminating the surface of the pool and surrounding areas. With such a light, police officers and security guards can simply drive by and look at the surface of the water. Surface water that shows any sign of activity may indicate that someone has been in the pool.

Electronic devices

Several electronic devices help defend against unauthorized entry into the pool. Water sensors can detect almost any water disturbance and can activate an alarm at the local police station. Closed-circuit television cameras, electronic eyes, and many other electronic burglar alarm type devices can protect the pool but can be expensive.

A night watchman

Hiring someone in the evening to watch the pool at first glance appears to be a boring and expensive proposition. If, however, the person assigned to security in the evening can also perform duties like pool vacuuming and bathhouse cleaning, this situation may even save the pool money. A night watchman is a good idea for many outdoor pools. It should be remembered that this employee need not make arrests or physically deal with intruders but rather simply call police upon unlawful entry. Lifeguard and desk attendants have often filled-in this capacity.

Locker Rooms

Locker rooms, showers, and toilet facilities are an integral part of every aquatic facility. A wonderful experience at a swimming facility can be easily ruined by a bad impression of the locker room facility.

Dressing and sanitary facilities should be provided with separations for each gender and without interconnections. These rooms must be well lighted, drained, and ventilated. Mold, fungus, and algae are prone to grow if special precautions are not taken. Locker rooms and sanitary facilities must also be planned to allow for daily housekeeping and regular maintenance.

Partitions separating dressing rooms, showers, and toilets in aquatic facilities are often troublesome areas. Partitions must be constructed of durable materials, yet because of the high humidity content and general wetness in this area, they must not be prone to water damage and mold. In addition, partitions should be installed so that cleaning walls and floors with hoses, mops, and brooms is not only possible but convenient .

All locker room and shower floors must have a nonslip surface yet smooth enough to ensure ease of cleaning. Carpet, runners, and the like, while making for a nonslip surface, often create slip hazards and are difficult to clean. Ample floor drains must be installed to provide for proper drainage. Floors must be sloped toward drains not less than one-fourth inch per foot, with an adequate number of floor drains for proper and complete drainage.

Tiled floors are excellent for locker rooms, but of course they are very expensive. The grout between individual tiles helps tremendously in making tile floors nonslip. Although larger tiles are more aesthetically appealing to many, they are often more slippery than floors composed of smaller tiles. If individual tiles are larger than the foot size of swimmers, the floor becomes more slippery. This is because larger tiles allow swimmers' feet to hydroplane on water before hitting the grout between tiles. Smaller tiles

provide recessed grout that allows water to drain from individual tiles and also provides a roughened surface for swimmers.

Concerning lavatories and urinals for male swimmers, one lavatory (sink) and one toilet for the first 100 users and one additional for every 200 users is a good rule of thumb to follow. These fixtures should be roughly doubled for female swimmers. Local and state codes should be consulted to be certain a facility is in compliance.

A minimum of two shower heads should be made available for each gender, and for every additional 50 swimmers, a shower head should be added. The water temperature at discharge should not exceed 90° F, and the flow rate of each shower head should not exceed 2 gallons per minute. Thermostats and water heaters for showers should not be accessible to users.

Soap dispensers should be available at each lavatory but must be made of an unbreakable material. Likewise, only unbreakable mirrors should be located above each lavatory. Sanitary napkin dispensers should be available in all female facilities. All plumbing fixtures must be in accordance with local plumbing codes. Fixtures should be easy to clean and resistant to corrosion.[3]

Electrical outlets in locker room areas deserve special attention. All outlets must be installed with GFIs and located away from wet areas and lavatories. Wall-mounted hair and hand dryers are preferred over the personal handheld variety.

Spectator Areas

Whenever possible, spectator and visitor areas should be isolated from decks and swimming pool areas. Shoes and street clothes are not compatible with wet deck areas and can cause problems in both traffic control and deck sanitation. If spectators must be allowed within the pool perimeter and deck area, they should be kept separated from areas used by bathers. If possible, spectators should have separate toilet facilities. At least one drinking fountain should be available for spectators and guests.

Operation and Management

As mentioned earlier in this chapter, all facets of aquatic administration are affected by the American Disabilities Act (ADA).

Hiring and supervising personnel, programming, facility management and many other areas of pool management, must follow ADA guidelines. All pool owners, operators, and staff must become familiar with this law to mainstream disabled individuals into aquatic facilities and programs.

Every public pool should be maintained under the direct supervision of a properly trained swimming pool operator. The pool operator must be trained in sanitation, safety, pool maintenance, record keeping, and legal liability. Many states require the pool operator to be certified, and some municipalities train and certify pool operators working in their region. The National Swimming Pool Foundation and the National Parks and Recreation Association offer excellent training and certification in Pool Operations.

Lifeguards should be required at every public swimming facility. They should be properly attired and easily recognized. Lifeguards should be certified in lifeguarding techniques, first aid, and CPR, but more important, the pool manager or operator should specifically train lifeguards for the facility that they will be working. This key link between pool operator and lifeguard must not be overlooked. Both preseason and in-service training is required. Lifeguards require adequate rescue equipment and frequent breaks. More information will be presented on lifeguards in the Lifeguarding Chapter.

Job descriptions must be given to all employees, including lifeguards. Written and oral instruction are needed for all procedures, including water rescues and other emergencies. These instructions are also needed for the maintenance of pool water, including chemical disinfection and adjustments, filtration, backwashing, vacuuming as well as water testing, just to name a few.

Pool rules, regulations, policies, and priorities must be written and posted in a conspicuous place. Pool patrons should also receive a written copy. Lifeguards and pool personnel must also understand and enforce all rules as well as OSHA and right-to-know laws.

Swimmer loads are determined by criteria established by the local health department or other regulatory agency. The maximum allowable number of swimmers in a pool at one time can be determined by pool surface, depth, water volume in gallons, and other factors. Indoor and outdoor swimming facilities usually have different swimmer loads. Pool management must know and observe swimmer limits pre-scribed for their pools. Swimmer limits are sometimes written on the pool permit. A good general rule of thumb is one lifeguard for every 25 swimmers. Depending on the type and skill level of the pool patrons this lifeguard-to-swimmer ratio may be increased or decreased.

All required pool applications and permits must be submitted with the state or local authority. Pool permits must be renewed annually.

Public pools must be maintained in accordance with local and state codes. And must pass all inspections by the regulatory agency to remain open. Permits are often revoked or suspended when the pool constitutes a health or safety hazard to the user. The pool operator should close the pool immediately upon discovering any unsafe condition. While the pool is closed, the hazard must be removed, repaired, or replaced before the pool is reopened to the public. For example, if a rung on a ladder is loose, it must be tightened immediately, or someone might slip and fall while exiting the pool. If an antivortex plate is missing, the spa or pool must be closed until replaced, ect.

Pool management would also be wise to meet regularly with fire, police, ambulance, and EMT officials to be consistent with emergency care procedures. Lifeguards and the emergency response team should be trained to work well together. All pool records should be kept for a minimum of 5 years. More on swimming pool management and operations will discussed in Chapter 19.

First Aid Room

Every public pool should have a first aid room that is reserved for emergencies only and is fully stocked with emergency equipment and supplies. The larger the facility, the larger the first aid room should be. The first aid room should have a cot, several blankets, a sink, and if at all possible, a shower and toilet. Lifeguards and other employees should not use this as a staff room.

Some large water parks even station a registered nurse in the first aid room during operating hours. Spine boards and other emergency equipment required by local codes should also be kept here. The first aid room may be an ideal place to post all staff first aid and CPR certifications. When questions concerning the requirements of the first aid room arise, the local health department or another regulatory agency should be contacted. Bloodborne pathogen information and protective equipment should be located in this first aid room.

The location of this room is important. Not only should it be visible to all patrons, but it must also be readily accessible to emergency vehicles. It should have immediate access to outside streets. A phone dedicated for emergency use only should be located in the first aid room. Emergency numbers and procedures should be posted clearly and conspicuously near the phone.

Staff Room

Whenever possible a separate staff room should be available for lifeguards and other employees to rest and relax, away from the swimming pool patrons (Fig. 3-24). At an outdoor facility, this becomes very important in getting the lifeguards out of the sun. If a separate building or room is not possible, perhaps a

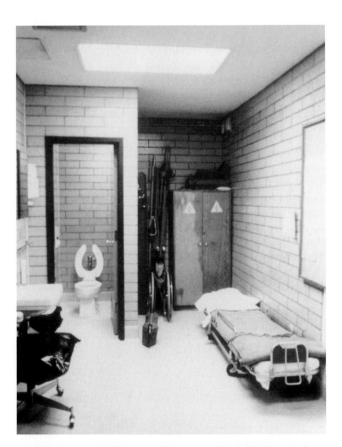

Fig. 3-24. Staff room. (Courtesy Mark Hokkanen.)

tent would be helpful. A refrigerator, couch, and reading materials particularly those that related to water safety and emergency care would be beneficial. Employees, only should be allowed in this facility.

Hotel, Motel, and Resort Pools

Although hotel, motel, and resort pools are public pools, technically, it would be more accurate to describe these facilities as semipublic. While admitting the public, the usual entrance restriction is that the swimmer be a guest of the hotel, motel, or resort. According to a survey of frequent travelers conducted by *U.S. News and World Report*, 92% of the respondents expected to have a swimming pool at their hotel, motel, or resort. More important, the swimming pool was more heavily used than other amenity. In another study conducted by Holiday Inns, the swimming pool was found to be the most important factor in the selection of a vacation hotel.[4]

The hotel, motel, and resort pools are mentioned separately in this chapter not only because of their popularity but because they have special problems associated with them. Apartment and condominium pools have similar concerns as the hotel or motel pools except for the transient clientele.

A common problem that exists with many of these facilities is a design problem. Many hotel, motel, and resort pools are smaller pools with many "big pool" amenities placed in them. Many of these types of pools have diving boards and slides even when they do not have sufficient surface area or depth to allow for these activities. Another safety concern with these pools is the clientele that use the pool. The following generalities often exist at many hotel, motel, and resort pools.

- Transient clientele
- May not understand rules
- Alcohol consumption
- Very old
- Partying
- Very young
- Unfamiliar with pool
- No lifeguard on duty

It is wise to discuss these variables further to better understand some of the risks associated with hotel, motel, and resort pools. Many individuals who use these pools are either on vacation or attending professional meetings. Because they are away from home, they are unfamiliar with the pool dimensions

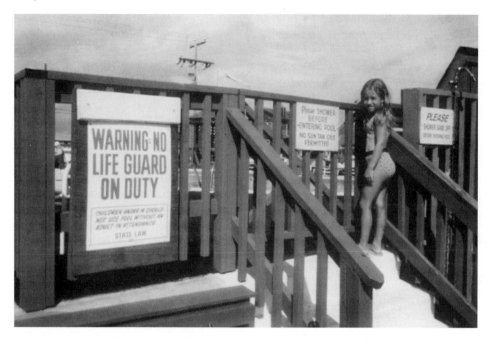

Fig. 3-25.   Hotel/motel pool. No lifeguard on duty sign.

and safety practices in the locality of the hotel. Alcohol is often consumed. In addition to traveling professionals, these pools attract retired individuals as well as young families with small children who are vacationing. As a result, a very heterogeneous or mixed ability group is found in a relatively small body of water. To make matters worse, lifeguards are not on duty more often than not (Fig. 3-25). Because the pool is designed to be aesthetically pleasing to guests, child barriers are often missing, thereby making it easy for children to wander into the pool. Hotels, motels, and resorts may not have any knowledgeable staff to run the pool.

For the reasons mentioned above, this special category of pool probably needs extra attention and may require the services of a professional pool company that can manage the pool properly. Another alternative would be to get staff members trained and certified as pool operators through the National Swimming Pool Foundation, the National Recreation and Parks Association, the YMCA, or some similar organization.

Summary

Public pools require diligent planning, management, and supervision. All those working in and around the water should be trained in several areas, including first aid, CPR, lifeguarding, water safety instruction and certified pool operations. For specific certification requirements, local authorities responsible for swimming pools should be contacted.

References

   1. ANSI/NSPI: *Standard for public swimming pools*, Alexandria, Va, 1992, The Institute.
   2. RP-6: *Current recommended practice for sports lighting*, New York, 1989, Illuminating Engineering Society. Alexandria, Va., 1992, The Institute.
   3. *Pool and Spa News*: May 7, 1990.

Bibliography

American Red Cross, *Swimming and diving*, St. Louis, 1992, Mosby.
Clayton R D, Thomas D G: *Professional aquatic management*, ed 2, Champaign, Ill, 1989, Human Kinetics.

Gabriel J: *Diving safety: a position paper*, Indianapolis, Ind, 1992, US Diving.

Gabrielson AM: *Swimming pools: a guide to their planning, design, and operation*, ed 4, Champaign, Ill, 1987, Human Kinetics.

Johnson R: *Swimming pool operations*, Harrisburg, Penn, 1989, Pennsylvania Department of Community Affairs.

Kowalsky L (editor): *Pool/spa operators handbook*, San Antonio, Tex, 1991, National Swimming Pool Foundation.

NSPI: *Pool and spa market study for 1991*, Alexandria, Va, 1992, The Institute.

NSPI: *The sensible way to enjoy your pool*, Alexandria, Va, 1983, The Institute.

Pope J R Jr: *Public swimming pool management.* I and II. Alexandria, Va, 1991, National Recreation and Park Association.

Williams K G: *The aquatic facility operator's manual*, Hoffman Estates, Ill, 1991, National Recreation and Park Association, National Aquatic Section.

REVIEW QUESTIONS

1. Starting blocks for competitive swimming should always be located at which end of the swimming pool?

2. Headfirst entries from the pool deck should never be allowed in a depth of water less than how may feet deep?

3. What is the difference between a dry niche and a wet niche underwater pool light?

4. List three types of pool finishes.

5. List some good characteristics of effective pool safety markings and signs.

6. List five special problems for outdoor pools that indoor pools do not usually experience.

7. List three different security problems for outdoor pools.

8. What is the ADA and who is it designed to assist?

9. List five concerns for hotel/motel/resort pool operators.

SECTION II
MECHANICAL

Section II addresses the mechanical aspects of swimming pools, specifically circulation and filtration. Chapter 4 discusses the principals of swimming pool circulation. Particular attention should be paid to the concepts of swimming pool "turnovers." Components of the circulation system are also be discussed and include pool outlets, surge tank, hair and lint strainer, pump, filters, heater, chemical feeders, and other pool gauges, valves, and meters. Although good descriptions are given in this chapter for each of the circulation components, trained electricians, plumbers, and pool engineers can offer invaluable experience to novice pool owners and operators.

Chapter 5 deals specifically with swimming pool filtration. The three basic types discussed are sand, diatomaceous earth, and cartridge filters, although a variety within each category are evaluated. The reader should visit a swimming pool dealer to closely examine the various types of filters firsthand. The filter photographs and illustrations provided in Chapter 5 can certainly aid the reader in better understanding filtration, but seeing filters in person is a valuable experience. Filtering rates and backwashing techniques are an important part of the chapter.

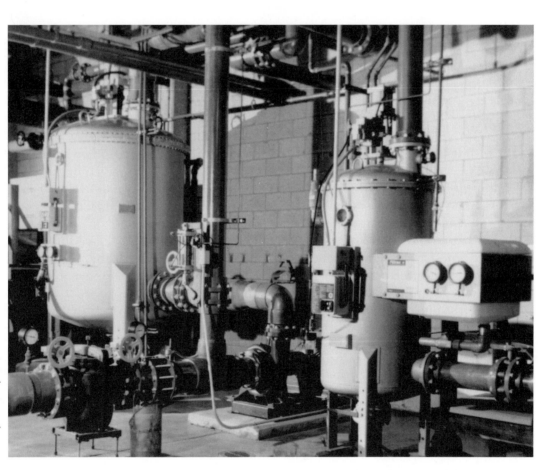

4

CIRCULATION

Key Concepts

- *Turnovers*
- *Pool Outlets*
- *Surge Tanks*
- *Hair and Lint Strainers*
- *Pumps*
- *Pool Inlets*
- *Guages and Valves*
- *Gutters and Skimmers*
- *Weirs*
- *Heater*
- *Chemical Feeders*
- *Filters*

Swimming pool water must be circulated continuously through filters whenever the pool is open for swimming, and for most pools circulation should be maintained 24 hours a day. The circulation system must be capable of drawing water from the pool and then distributing cleaned, heated, and treated water evenly throughout the pool. The circulation process, which was briefly discussed in Chapter 1, is expanded here. Several different pieces of equipment and apparatus are responsible for pool circulation. They include the following:

1. Pool outlets
2. Surge or balancing tank
3. Hair and lint strainer
4. Pump
5. Filters
6. Heater
7. Chemical feeders
8. Pool inlets
9. Gauges, valves, and meters

Turnovers

Collectively, the equipment above is responsible for swimming pool circulation. More important, however, pool circulation equipment must maintain certain "turnover" requirements. Many states require that public pools "turnover" every 8 hours, but the trend appears to be moving towards a 6-hour turnover. This means that in a pool that contains 120,000 gallons, an equivalent amount of water must pass through the filtration plant and return to the pool every 6 hours, or four times a day. This does not mean, however, that every drop of water in the pool must be filtered every 6 hours but rather that 120,000 gallons must be recirculated. In fact, during one turnover less than half of the water in the pool actually goes through the filter, according to Gage and Bidwell's Law of Dilution. As depicted in the following illustration, turnover rate is crucial to water clarity in a swimming pool (Fig. 4-1).

To determine a given pool's turnover rate, only the pool volume and the flow rate, as indicated by the flow meter in gallons per minute (GPM), are needed. In most pools the turnover rate is expressed in hours, whereas in hot tubs and spas the turnover is expressed in minutes.

To determine the turnover rate (TR) for swimming pools the following formula is used:

$$\text{TR in hours} = \frac{\text{gallons of pool water}}{60 \times \text{flow rate in GPM}}$$

To determine the turnover rate for hot tubs and spas, the following equations should be used:

$$\text{TR in hours} = \frac{\text{gallons of spa water}}{\text{flow rate in GPM}}$$

Water clarity depends on good turnover rates. Proper turnover rates are particularly important to public pools with high swimmer loads. Without adequate turnovers swimming pool water will not stay clear. Some suggested turnover rates are found in Table 4-1.

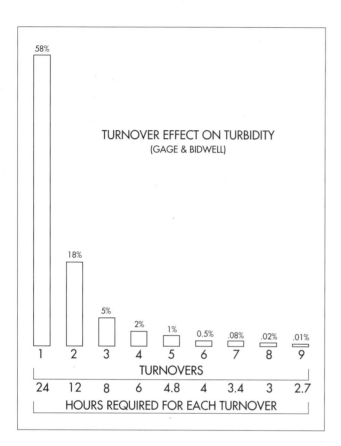

TURNOVER EFFECT ON TURBIDITY
(GAGE & BIDWELL)

Fig. 4-1. 95% of the pool water is filtered in three turnovers according to Gage and Bidwell's Law of Dilution.

Table 4-1.	Ideal Turnover Rate	
	Light-Moderate Swimmer Loads	**Heavy Swimmer Loads**
Public Pools	6-8 hrs	4-6 hrs
Public Spas	< 30 mins	10-20 mins
Residential Pools	8 hrs	6 hrs
Residential Spas	< 30 mins	< 30 mins

Hydrotech publishes useful turnover/flow rate graphs for pools and spas (Fig. 4-2). By studying these graphs, flow rates needed to achieve desired turnover rates for pools and spas can be easily determined without performing the math provided on p. 53. By simply matching the water volume of a given pool in the column on the left with the desired turnover rate on the right, required flow rates can be found below this intersection on the bottom of the graph. For example, a 80,000 gallon pool that needs a 6-hour turnover would require a flow rate of 222 GPM.

The sequence of how the water flows during circulation will now be discussed.

Pool Outlets

Pool outlets are the exit points through which water leaves the swimming pool. The water is filtered and heated when necessary, and is then treated before returning to the pool. This is where the circulation process begins. Most of the water leaving the pool goes through a perimeter gutter or skimmer sys-

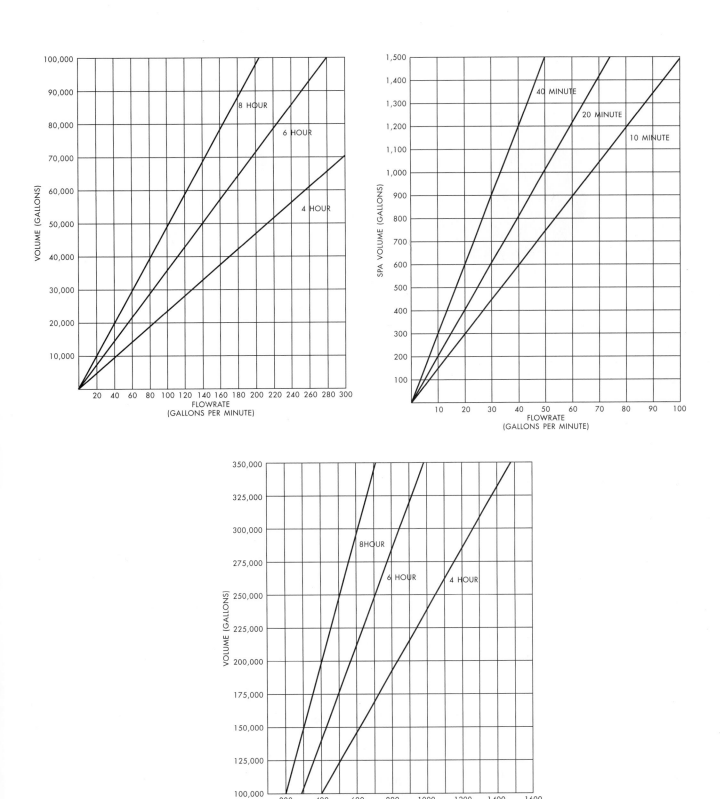

Fig. 4-2. The proper management of pool and spa water. (Courtesy BioLab, Decatur, Ga.)

A

B

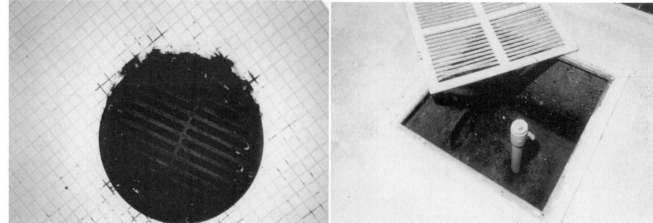

Fig. 4-3. **A,** Main drain on an indoor pool. **B,** Main drain with detached grate on an outdoor pool. (Note hydrostatic pressure relief valve in center.)

tem. The swimming pool vessel is designed to collect slightly more water than it can actually hold. Therefore water is continually flowing out of the vessel, predominantly from the surface instead of the bottom. Some states require that 10% of all water leaving the pool exits through the main drain or bottom outlet.

The system of surface overflow should be designed to handle the bulk of water returning to the filtration system, because the surface is where the majority of contaminates are located. Surface overflow of water is often referred to as the perimeter overflow system or surface collection.

Many states recommend that 75% of the water leaving the pool vessel should come from the surface, while only 25% should come from the bottom outlet (main drain). Some jurisdictions state that *no less* than 50% of the water leaving the pool must come from the surface, while *no more* than 50% should come from the bottom outlet. Please note, the term *main drain* is somewhat of a misnomer, because draining the pool occurs rarely and is not the only function of this outlet. As mentioned above, the main drain also serves as an important outlet for pool water circulation.

The main drain serves as the bottom outlet for swimming pool circulation but is less significant when compared with the surface skimming action. It is not recommended to place the bottom outlet directly under a diving board because divers will be tempted to play with the drain grate, and divers have been known to get their fingers caught in these drains. The surface area of the grates covering the drain should be much greater (about 10 times) than the orifice of

returning water to the filters. This will dissipate suction and prevent bathers from getting stuck to the outlet.

The bottom outlet must be located in the deepest part of the pool. Two bottom outlets are preferable to one. The bottom grate must always be secured in place (Fig. 4-3).

Gutters vs skimmers

Although they both remove water from the surface of the pool, gutters and skimmers are significantly different in design. *Gutters* are troughs that are installed continuously around the perimeter of the pool. In general, larger public pools tend to have gutters, whereas smaller pools (residential, hotel, motel, etc.) tend to use skimmers. Usually, the larger the gutter, the better the skimming action. There are many different types of gutter designs. Two basic design differences in gutters are below deck and deck level gutters.

Deck level gutter systems are becoming popular because they produce great skimming action and a flat pool surface that is ideal for competitive swimming. There is little chance for waves to splash back into the pool once the water reaches the deck level gutter. A popular deck level design is the rimflow gutter, which is characterized by a large surge trench that surrounds the pool and collects surface water through slotted coping stones or grates on the deck level (Fig. 4-4). The water level and deck level are the same in this design. Because the skimming action is superior in these designs, rimflow gutters are quite loud as a result of all the water pouring into the perimeter trench located just below the deck.

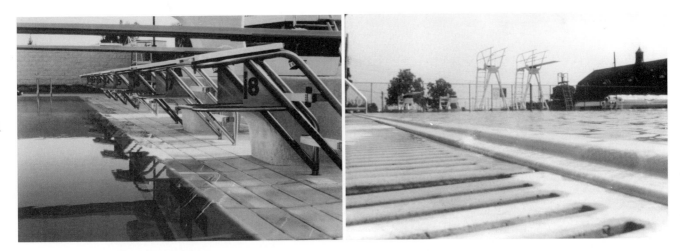

Fig. 4-4. **A,** Wide, competitive perimeter overflow gutters under racing platforms. **B,** Perimeter overflow gutter at large, outdoor pool. (**A,** Courtesy KDI Paragon, Pleasantville, NY.)

Another deck level overflow system, the roll out gutter, is similar to the rimflow gutter but does not have a large surge trench. Because swimmers do actually step into the roll out gutter to enter the swimming pool, the surface should be nonslip. Additionally, because a large surge trench is not available, a more turbulent, choppy pool may result.

Recessed gutters are found below the deck level (Fig. 4-5). They are found more often in indoor pools and work in the same manner as a deck level return, but they are located inside the pool walls just below deck level. Typically, in a pool with a recessed gutter the water surface lies 12 to 18 inches below the deck. Older pools have small gutter troughs, whereas newer pools, particularly those built for competitive swimming, have wide, deep troughs.

Skimmers are individual exit ports or boxes located intermittently around the pool. While the lids covering skimmer baskets are located on deck level, the skimmer baskets are located below deck level and just below the water surface of the pool. The lids or cover plates of skimmers can often be displaced, creating a safety hazard. Bathers walking on the pool deck will step on these lids, so they must be secure and have nonslip surfaces. The removable baskets found in each skimmer box collect leaves, grass, and other large debris that can hamper circulation and filtration. Skimmer baskets that are neglected (not cleaned regularly) often hinder good skimming action. Skimmers are usually placed every 500 to 800 square feet of water surface area or about 20 feet apart. Local codes must be checked before installing skimmers to at least meet but hopefully exceed their

minimum requirements. Skimmers are inexpensive to install but cannot skim surface water as well as the gutter system. Although a skimmer system is fine for smaller pools, a gutter system is recommended for large public pools. Some states do not allow skimmers in swimming pools with surface areas greater than 1600 square feet.

Weirs are doors or flaps that maintain a one-way skimming action by regulating the flow of water into the skimmer basket and are an integral part of the skimmer system (Fig. 4-6). Once debris enters a skimmer basket, the weir prevents it from returning to the pool if the skimmer is flooded. When the weir is in place, the flow of water is controlled fairly well. Too often, however, weirs are pulled out by children or simply float out from the throat of the simmer. Without the weir in place, skimmers do not work as effectively as they should.

Weirs must also be equipped with a Styrofoam flotational device and will not function properly without it. Children should be warned about playing with weirs because being one-way gates, weirs can trap arms and hands in the skimmer.

Whether a gutter or skimmer system is utilized, the water level in the pool is of paramount importance if these surface overflow systems are to work effectively. The water level must be maintained at the top of the gutter line. In the case of skimmers, the water level should be maintained at least 3 inches up the weir but no more than half-way above the opening. Water allowed to rise above these recommended levels will flood either the gutter or skimmer.

Conversely, when the water level is too low, water

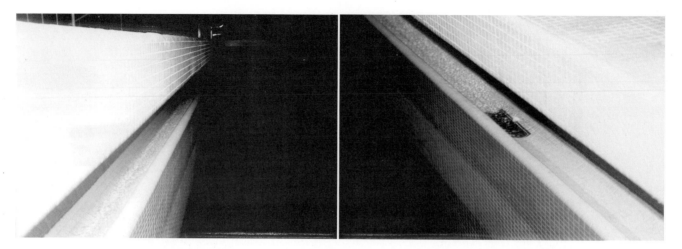

Fig. 4-5. Recessed gutter with good skimming action on indoor pool. (Courtesy Steve Manual.)

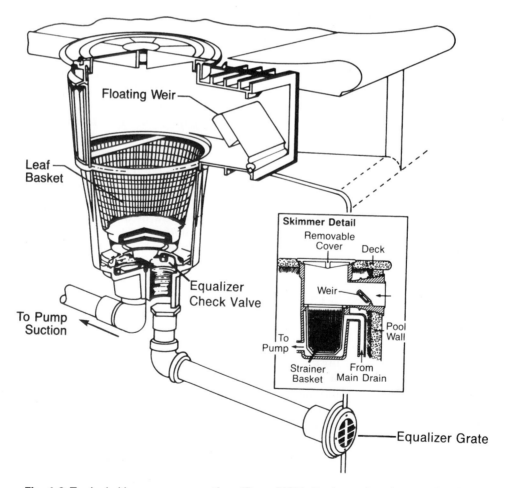

Fig. 4-6. Typical skimmer cross-section. (From NSPI: *Basic pool and spa technology*, ed 2, Alexandria, Va, 1992, The Institute.)

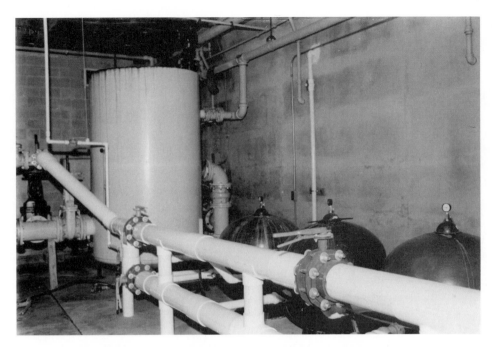

Fig. 4-7. Large surge/balancing tank for public pool.

will not be skimming at all into the gutter or skimmer. Dry skimmers and gutters result in all the water returning to the filters through the bottom outlet, which is not desirable and is even illegal in some states.

An ideal water level is one that allows for optimum skimming action by maintaining a "thirsty" gutter. A "thirsty" gutter aggressively pulls water out of the pool, over the lip, and into the gutter drains. It should look and sound like a miniature waterfall. In fact, a thirsty gutter with good skimming action is often a noisy gutter; water cascading out of the pool through the surface collection system can be heard clearly from the pool deck. To produce this effect, the water level in the gutter must be below the level in the pool.

Conversely, "thirsty" skimmers will probably suck air, which may in turn damage the pump. There should always be an ample amount of water in skimmer baskets. Many skimmers also contain throttle plugs to regulate the flow of water. To ensure consistent skimming action, some skimmers must be throttled. Skimmers closest to the pump tend to have the strongest suction. These skimmers need to be throttled back. Skimmers located farthest from the pump have much less draw, so they need to be opened fully.

When gutters or skimmers are flooded by a water level in the swimming pool that is too high, water must be removed from the pool by opening the appropriate valves and sending water to waste or sewage treatment plant. If the water level in the pool is too low, water must be added to the pool from the local water source. This addition of new water is called "make-up" water.

There are many other types of surface overflow systems, including recessed gutters and prefabricated gutters, but the functions are the same. Some work better than others, usually because of the size of the gutter trench.

The Surge (Balancing) Tank

Pools with gutters should have surge or balancing tanks, which are designed to hold a large volume of displaced swimming pool water in reserve (Fig. 4-7). Surge tanks must be large enough to to hold a large capacity of water so that when the pool load is suddenly increased, water will not be lost. Without a sufficiently sized surge tank, water in the pool displaced by swimmers would overflow the surge tank and enter the waste stream. Balancing tanks with float valves prevent overflows from occurring. Pools with skimmers do not have these tanks.

The purpose of surge tanks is twofold: to hold a

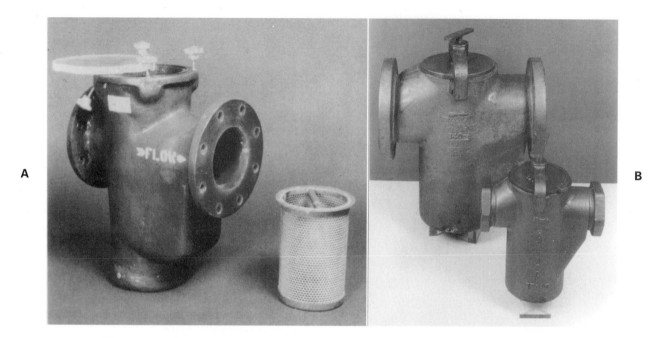

Fig. 4-8.   **A,** Fiberglass cover on hair and lint strainer allows pool operator to check basket without stopping filtration. **B,** Cast iron strainers with flange. (Courtesy Brock Enterprises, Hamden, Conn.)

reserve capacity of water when a large number of bathers enter the water and to protect the pump by maintaining a water level in the tank that is above the suction port of the pool pump. This second benefit protects the pump from surges of water flowing into the pump and also prevents the pump from sucking air. Skimmer pools do not normally have surge tanks, and consequently an auxiliary pipe can be added to the bottom of the skimmer and connected to the pool wall to prevent the skimmer from sucking air. If the water level in the skimmer gets too low, water is then pulled through this pipe to prevent the pump from sucking air.

The surge tank is an important component of the circulation system, because pool pumps require a constant source of water with little resistance to suction and free of air. The water in the surge tank is lower than the water level in the pool when the pump is running. The float valve in the surge tank helps to balance the water coming into the tank, regulating flows between the gutters and the bottom outlet. An open concrete pit in the filter room may also serve as the surge tank.

The surge tank works in the following fashion. Outgoing pool water flows by gravity from the pool vessel through the surface collection system and the bottom outlets and into the surge tank. When the gutters are flooded, more water is taken from the skim-

mers. When the pool is quiet and the skimmers are almost dry, more water is taken from the bottom outlet. Although there are wide variations in the amount of water in the surge tank, the main function of this component is to keep the suction into the pump constant.

Hair and Lint Strainer

Perhaps one of the most important yet most neglected components of the circulation system is the hair and lint strainer (Fig. 4-8). This device is simply a mesh basket located in the circulation system just in front of the pool pump to protect the pump from large visible debris. The only circulation systems that do not require hair and lint strainers are vacuum filters, because the pump follows the filter. Therefore, in a vacuum system, the pool pump is protected by the filter bed. Pressure and vacuum filter systems will be discussed in detail later in this section.

The hair and lint strainer is often neglected because cleaning it can be messy. Although it is easy to clean the hair and lint strainer, the pool operator often gets wet, and what is found in the basket is often unpleasant (hair, lint, band-aids, goggles, bathing caps, dentures, etc.). Most health codes require extra hair and lint baskets on hand so that a clean basket can replace the dirty one immediately without stopping filtration. When checking the hair and lint strainer, the pump must be turned off and valves on either side of the basket need to be closed on flooded suction systems. These baskets should be checked whenever the filters are backwashed and whenever the pumps are turned off. A dirty hair and lint strainer can just about stop a filter flow rate, thus leaving the pool with no filtration at all. Also, if the lid on the hair and lint strainer is not replaced securely, air might be sucked into the system. Finally, since many hair and lint strainers are located next to the pump, they can be filled with water to prime the pump when restarting the system.

The Pool Pump

Before discussing the pool pump itself, it is important to discuss the *placement* of the pool pump. Quite simply, if the pump is located just before the filters, the filtration system is a pressure system. On the other hand, if the pump is located after the filters, the filtration system is a vacuum system. In the pressure system the pump pulls the water from the pool or surge tank and pushes water into the filters. In the vacuum system water is drawn from the filters, and the pump then pushes the water back to the pool. Vacuum and gravity filter systems do not require a hair and lint strainer because the filters screen any foreign objects that could harm the pump.

Pump placement is also important for maintenance and repairs. If indoors, the pump should be positioned as close to the pool as possible. It should be placed in a cool, dry place and secured on a rigid platform. Care must be taken to keep water, dust, and chemicals well away from the pump. If the pump is kept outdoors, it is important to shield the pump from the elements, particularly the sun and rain, and maintain good ventilation as well.

The pump is the heart of the pool's circulation system, but many pool owners and operators do not understand how a swimming pool pump works. To maintain clean, clear swimming pool water, a pump must move the water through the pipes and filters. As the water travels through pipes, valves, and fittings, however, friction or resistance to flow is created. Additionally, some portions of a circulation system are higher than others, thus requiring additional force to move the water. Pool pumps must overcome gravity and the resistance to flow in order to circulate water effectively.

Swimming pools use one of the many types of centrifugal pumps exclusively. The centrifugal pump is quite simple with only one moving part, the impeller. Centrifugal pumps take water from the suction side into the center or eye, where the impeller spins and imparts velocity to the water inside the pump (Fig. 4-9). The impeller then throws water off its edges at a high velocity. The pump casing converts this water velocity energy to water pressure, which is required to move the pool water through the filters and back to the pool.

Because the pump impeller fits snugly in its casings, the hair and lint strainers become very important in protecting the pump from damage caused by foreign objects in the water (Fig. 4-10).

An important benefit of using a centrifugal pump is that if a valve is closed on the pressure side of the pump, no damaging pressures develop. As pressure increases in a centrifugal pump, the power required by the pump decreases significantly. As a result the water spins and churns within the pump and is not supposed to cause damage to the piping, but much depends on the location of valves. The pump may eventually overheat if the discharge valve remains closed, but pipes and filters should not be damaged by excessively high water pressures. It must be mentioned, however, that circulation pipes have cracked, filter lids have been popped, and when pump temperatures get too hot, PVC piping has actually melted.

Pump sizing and pipe sizing

The discussion of pool pumps and pipe sizing go hand in hand, because both are dependent upon each other for performance. Selecting the best pump and piping for any pool is best left to the manufacturer's recommendations and certified engineers. Feet of head (a measurement of resistance to flow) and the recommended flow rate in gallons per minute are the two criteria needed to select the correct pump for any pool. Pipe diameters, lengths, elbows, and fittings are all considered when determining feet of head. A typical swimming pool may have anywhere from 40 to 60 feet of head.

A common problem with pool pumps is the piping in relation to the horsepower of the pump. In general, the suction pipe should be at least as large, if not larger, than the pump pipe connection. The smaller the pipe, the greater the resistance. Suction side piping must be kept as straight as possible with as few elbows and obstructions as possible. The pump's efficiency is compromised and resistance is increased

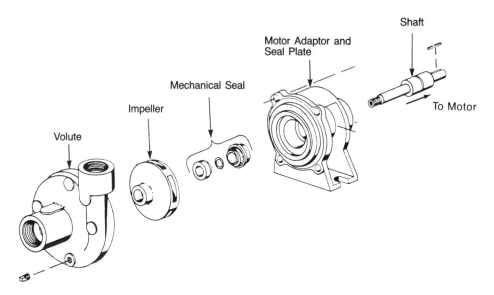

Fig. 4-9. Centrifugal pump, exploded view. (From NSPI: *Basic pool and spa tecnology*, ed 2, Alexandria, Va, 1992, The Institute.)

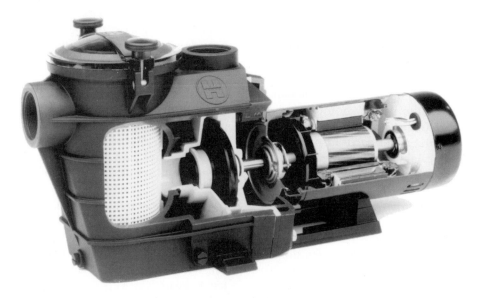

Fig. 4-10. High performance residential pool pump. (Courtesy Hayward Pool Products, Elizabeth, NJ.)

with too many additions to the suction side piping. Contact the pool pump's manufacturer or dealer for complete pipe sizing information.

Whereas undersized pool pumps "burn up" early, oversizing pool pumps causes channeling of filter beds and the breakage of filter laterals.

The two important factors needed to size pool pumps properly are GPM and total dynamic head. Feet of head must be measured on both sides of the pump, the vacuum side and the pressure side.

To evaluate an existing pump's size, the following exercise is helpful. The pressure side of the system is downstream from the pump. By using a pressure gauge to measure the pressure in pounds per square inch (PSI), and multiplying this number by a constant of 2.31, the feet of head for the pressure side can be found.

The suction side of the system is located upstream of the pump. By using a vacuum gauge or manometer on the suction side, the vacuum can be measured in inches of mercury. The vacuum gauge reading is multiplied by a constant of 1.13 to find suction feet of head.

The total feet of head for this system is determined by adding the pressure feet of head to the vacuum feet of head. Using the required flow rate in GPM and the total feet of head requirements, a pump curve is referred to. The point at which both GPM and total feet of head intersect on a pump curve determines the pump size needed.

For pools that require the pump to be located below the pool level, a *flooded suction pump* is used because it has more "pushing" power and achieves 1750 RPM. Pumps located above the pool must have more "pulling" power, so *self-priming pumps* that achieve 3400 RPM are used in this instance.

Although the process of pump and pipe sizing is quite simple, a registered engineer, licensed electrician, or local swimming pool supplier can be quite helpful. Before constructing or renovating a pool, these individuals should be consulted to determine the appropriate pump size for the pool in question.

The Filter

If the pool pump is the heart of swimming pool circulation, then the filters are the kidneys. The filters remove suspended particles from the water, which is essential in reducing turbidity and increasing water clarity. Suspended particles that the filters remove

include but are not limited to dirt, dust, hair, and oil. It is important to note that filters DO NOT remove dissolved particles or bacteria. Basically, the pool filters simply strain unwanted solids from the water before it is returned to the pool. The basics of filtration will be discussed here, and the specifics of each filter will be discussed in detail in Chapter 5.

As mentioned previously, placement of the pool pump determines whether the filter system is a pressure system or a vacuum system. In a pressure system the pump is located before or upstream of the filters, whereas in a vacuum system, the pump follows the filter. When looking at a pressure filter system, not only does one see the pump upstream of the filter, but the filter media is enclosed in a tank, under pressure. The vacuum system can be detected easily because the pump is downstream of the filter, and often the vats or tanks are open, allowing the media to be viewed. The vacuum system in not under pressure.

Regardless of the type of filter system or media used, the process of filtration remains the same. The filter surface area or bed creates small pores where dirt lodges and is unable to pass through. It is important to note that dirt can also trap additional dirt: therefore a dirty filter is often an effective filter. When the water can no longer flow efficiently through the system because of the accumulated dirt, the filter media must be cleaned or replaced.

Filters will produce clear, clean water when properly sized, installed, and operated. The effectiveness of any type of filtration system, as evidenced by water clarity, depends on several interrelated factors: the filter media, the amount of filter area, the flow rate, and the turnover rate.

Filter medias can be divided further into two types: permanent and temporary media. Permanent media is a filter media that can be reused and does not have to be replaced on a regular basis. Sand is the most common permanent filter media. Temporary media is a filter media that must be replaced after each filter cleaning or backwashing. The most popular temporary media is Diatomaceous Earth or simply DE For the purposes of this text, the discussion of filter medias will be presented in the following order: Sand, DE, and Cartridge

Sand filters

Many types of sand filters are available for swimming pool use. Sand is a low-maintenance media that lasts for years. It is easy to clean and relatively inexpensive to purchase. Sand filters use a specially grad-ed sand, shaped like triangles, that when poured into a filter creates tiny caves, crevices, or pores which trap dirt as pool water flows through the sand bed. Advantages of sand filters include the permanent media, low cost, and ease of operation. There are three basic types of sand filters: sand and gravel, high rate pressure sand, and vacuum sand. Sand filters will be discussed in detail in Chapter 5.

Diatomaceous earth filters

Diatomaceous earth (DE) filters use the fossilized remains of aquatic marine life called *diatoms*. These skeletal remains look like microscopic snowflakes and perform a superior job of filtering because they have the ability to trap more dirt and screen finer particles than sand. The advantage of DE is the high water clarity it produces because of its ability to screen out even the smallest of particles. The disad-vantage of this system is that the media is temporary, needing to be replaced after each filter cleaning. The cleaning of DE filters also tends to be more labor intensive. Some suggest that DE may become more difficult to dispose of in the future.

Detailed information regarding DE filters is dis-cussed in Chapter 5.

Cartridge filters

Cartridge filters represent the latest technology in swimming pool filtration. Whereas Sand and DE fil-ters use natural media, the cartridge media is artifi-cial. The filter media in a cartridge system is a syn-thetic fabric. The cartridge filter system is small and does a fine job of removing particulate matter. Perhaps the greatest advantage of this system is that water is not wasted during backwashing; cartridge filters are simply hand-cleaned. The disadvantage of this system is that the filters are difficult to keep clean.

The Heater

Particularly in a multiuse pool, water temperature is perhaps the most critical variable of all swimming pool factors because different populations require different water temperatures for comfort. A change by only a few degrees in water temperature is signifi-cant for patrons, whereas this is not the case for air temperature. When a swimmer is immersed in water, body heat is lost approximately 200 times faster than when simply surrounded by air of the same tempera-

ture. This helps to explain why swimmers get chilled so quickly in water. A pool that is too cold will not attract patrons. A pool that is too warm will not only drive the more competitive swimmers away but will also cost additional money to heat.

It is important to note the following temperature ranges for a variety of aquatic activities:

Competitive swimming—79° to 81° F
Youth instruction—82° to 86° F
Senior citizens and
    special populations—84° to 86° F
Therapeutic swims—86° to 90° F

As you would expect, these temperature ranges make it difficult to please all patrons, particularly when only one body of water is available. When these activities are conducted indoors, the air temper-ature should be maintained about 4° to 6° warmer than the water temperature.

Pool heaters are sized to raise water temperature for a given volume between 20° and 40° F. The rise in temperature should be gradual, approximately 1° per hour. When undersized, a pool heater will heat the water too slowly; when oversized, the cost of installa-tion and operation will increase. Also, an oversized heater requires a lot of space.

The fuel source will vary in geographic regions. Smaller pools often use propane heaters, which are designed to heat the water quickly. In some areas solar heaters make a good heat source.

The following information contains basic informa-tion that pool operators may need when dealing with the pool heater.

Thermostat

The thermostat regulates the heater, which in turn heats the pool, and is a temperature control device that shuts off the heater when the water temperature reaches the desired temperature. Turning the dial to the highest setting will not speed up the heating process. It is best to set the thermostat for where the water temperature should be and be patient while waiting for results. Only the person in charge of the pool should be allowed to touch the thermostat.

By-pass valve

Swimming pool heaters are not designed to heat all the water being circulated. The by-pass valve main-tains a constant flow of water through the heat exchanger, thus preventing damage to the heater components. If the by-pass valve is fully open, no pool water is being heated; when the by-pass valve is completely closed, all the swimming pool water is targeted for the heater, overloading and perhaps damaging it.

British Thermal Unit

The British thermal unit (BTU) is a measurement used to define the capabilities of heaters. One BTU is capable of raising the temperature of 1 pound of water by 1° F.

Heat exchanger

The heat exchanger is a device with coils, tubes, or plates that absorbs heat from any fluid, liquid, or air and transfers that heat to another fluid (pool water) without intermixing.

Proper water balance (see Chapter 6) is of paramount importance to the operation and longevity of pool heaters. Corrosive water will destroy heater components, whereas scaling water will clog heating elements.

When a pool heater malfunctions, sometimes the solutions are simple. They include the following:

1. No water flow to the heater. The filter, hair and lint strainer, skimmer, or main drain may be blocked.
2. No fuel. The heater's fuel line may be clogged or the fuel tank may be empty. In the case of an electric heater, check the circuit breaker.
3. Thermostat. This control device may either be turned down or broken.
4. The timer switch. Many pool heaters are on a timer. Be certain the toggle switch is turned "on."

Whether sizing a new heater or repairing an existing heater, it is important to contact a swimming pool supply company or a heating specialist. If electrical work is required, a licensed electrician should be contracted.

Chemical Feeders

Swimming pools are equipped with a variety of chemical feeders that add chemicals to the pool's circulation system to maintain proper chemical levels (Fig. 4-11). Faulty feeders can lead to unacceptable chemical levels leading to pool closure. Erosion feeders, diaphragm pumps, and peristaltic pumps are three of the most common pool feeders.

Erosion feeders are relatively new to the swimming pool industry and operate simply. Solid, slow dissolving chemicals like bromine sticks, and calcium hypochlorite or Trichlor tablets are placed into a special canister in the circulation line through which pool water circulates through the container and slowly dissolves the solid chemical. Chemicals like Dichlor are not placed in an erosion feeder because they dissolve quickly. NOTE: Never add chemicals other than those specified by the manufacturer. The improper use of chemicals in an erosion feeder may lead to a fire or dangerous explosion.

Although erosion feeders are simple devices, finding the proper placement and plumbing for the feeder is not so easy. The high chemical concentration coming from the erosion feeder can damage circulation equipment located downstream. However, placing the erosion feeder away from the pump may cause poor flow through the feeder. Before installing an erosion feeder, more than one pool specialist should be consulted concerning the installation.

Diaphragm and *peristaltic pumps* have been used to feed chemicals to pools for many years (Fig. 4-12). The chemicals that these pumps are adding to the circulation system should be covered or their gases might corrode the pump. The pump should also be kept away from the chemical vat. Peristaltic pumps seem to be easier to operate because they have no ball and check valves that are notorious for clogging and needing service.

Without discussing the specific mechanics of each pump, the following description may be useful. The chemical feeder head is located between two lines of plastic tubing. One line is suction tubing, and the other line is pressure or discharge tubing. The chemical feeder head is designed to first create a vacuum in suction tubing, which pulls liquid chemical from a vat into the head and then pushes the chemical through pressure tubing that is connected to the circulation system. Many problems associated with chemical feeders can actually be attributed to the plastic feeder lines. Each line has a one-way check valve that becomes dirty and must be cleaned or replaced regularly. The end of the suction line that is immersed in liquid is called the foot strainer. The foot strainer is easily clogged, needs to be cleaned often, and may need to be replaced periodically. At the end of the discharge tube is the injector, which also must be cleaned or replaced often.

Both diaphragm and peristaltic pumps need to be cleaned regularly because being positive feed pumps, the feed lines can become pressurized and cause chemical spills if the valves and injectors become clogged.

Additionally, the plastic lines themselves often become clogged. The best preventive maintenance for

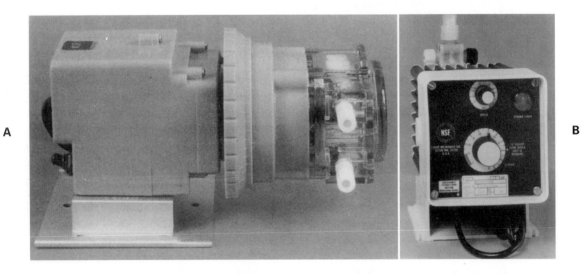

A   **B**

Fig. 4-11. **A,** Peristalic chemical feed pump is virtually non-clogging because chemicals do not contact pump parts. **B,** Positive displacement diaphragm chemical feed pump used for liquid chlorine, corrosive acids, and thick polymers. (Courtesy Brock Enterprises, Hamden, Conn.)

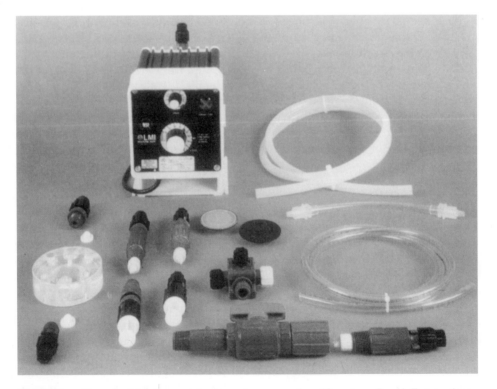

Fig. 4-12. Chemical feed pump parts and accessories. (Courtesy Brock Enterprises, Hamden, Conn.)

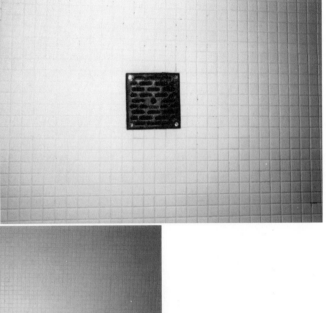

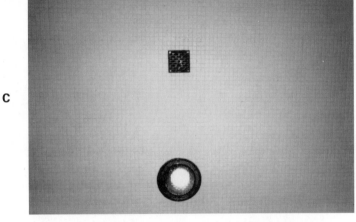

Fig. 4-13. **A,** Bottom inlet for outdoor pool. **B** and **C,** Side wall inlet for indoor pool. (Courtesy Steve Manual.)

the tubing, valves, and injectors is running a muriatic acid solution (10%) through the chemical feeder and its lines. This must be done with extreme care, however, because muriatic acid and chlorine must not be mixed together. If periodic acid cleaning does not help, the lines and valves should be replaced. Chemical feeders that pump soda ash slurry, DE slurry, and liquid chlorine are particularly susceptible to clogging. Newer pumps have built-in, fresh water flushing devices that prevent clogging. Gas chlorinators are detailed in Chapter 7.

Inlets

Swimming pool inlets are the last items in the circulation loop through which heated and chemically treated water is finally reintroduced to the pool (Fig. 4-13). The best distribution is accomplished through pool bottom or floor inlets. Wall inlets are also used, particularly in smaller pools. Inlets must have covers in place that are designed to better distribute the water and can be adjusted to direct flow. Inlets can be tested by adding dye in the skimmers or gutters; inlets that are clogged will not show dye coming through them. Blocked inlets can mean pool closures in some states. Inlets are usually made of chrome-plated bronze or plastic, or other corrosion-resistant material.

Valves, Meters, and Gauges

Numerous valves, meters, and gauges are found in a pool's circulation system. All are important in maintaining and adjusting the water circulation of the swimming pool. Valves control the flow of the circulating water and may be ball, gate, butterfly, and

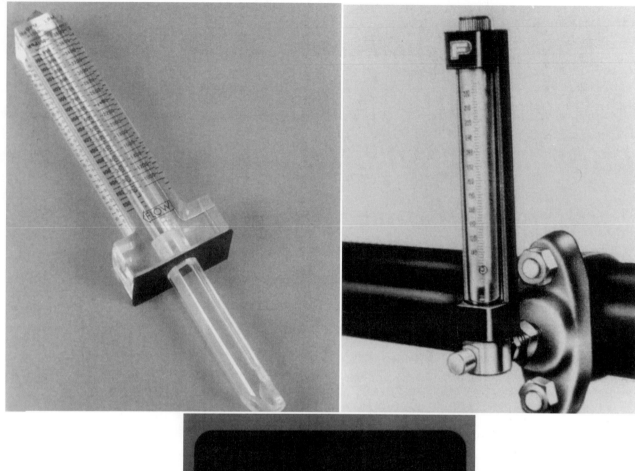

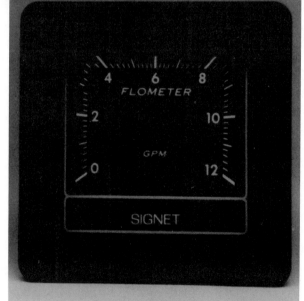

Fig. 4-14. **A,** Economy flow meter is inexpensive. **B,** Direct impact flow meter is very accurate and reliable. **C,** This flow meter is easy to read, accurate, and reliable. (Courtesy Brock Enterprises, Hamden, Conn.)

float valves. Regardless of the type, valves should be "exercised" by opening and closing them periodically. This helps keep the valves from sticking and scaling up and should be done especially for those valves that are seldom used.

Gauges usually measure pressure in pounds per square inch (psi). Pressure gauges monitor filtering efficiency by measuring pressure going into (influent) pressure filters and coming out of (effluent) filters. Vacuum filters use vacuum gauges.

Perhaps the most important reading in a filter room regarding circulation comes from the flow meter (Fig. 4-14). The location of the flow meter is extremely important. For accurate readings the flow meter should be placed on a long, straight, uninterrupted length of pipe, free of elbows, gauges, and other instruments. Flow meters should be selected on their ability to be read, removed, cleaned, and replaced. Flow meters are required in most municipalities and read in GPM.

Flow meters should be removed and cleaned with an acid solution periodically. Most flow meters require a rubber or Teflon gasket to prevent leakage. Once a flow meter is installed, it remains reliable provided it is kept clean. Additionally, if a flow meter is installed backwards, that is, the impact tube is not facing into the flow of water, no water will enter the tube; thus no flow will be indicated on the meter. If the flow meter is clean and installed properly and the reading is low, then the pump, filters, hair and lint strainer, and other components of the circulation system should be checked immediately. Like many other circulation components, a nonfunctioning flow meter may lead to closure of the pool.

Summary

Although the pump and the filter receive the most attention in a pool's circulation system, at least a dozen other components require daily attention. All circulation components must be continually monitored to ensure good water clarity and quality.

References

1. Mitchel K: *The proper management of pool and spa water*, BioLab, Inc., Decatur, Ga, 1988.

Bibliography

Gabrielson AM: *Swimming pools: a guide to their planning, design, and operation*, ed 4, Champaign, Ill, 1987, Human Kinetics.

Johnson R: *YMCA pool operations manual*, Champaign, Ill, 1989, YMCA.

Kowalsky L (ed): *Pool/spa operators handbook*, San Antonio, Tex, 1991, National Swimming Pool Foundation.

Mitchel K: *The proper management of pool and spa water*, Decatur, Ga, 1988, BioLab.

Pope J R Jr: *Public swimming pool management*, I and II, Alexandria, Va, 1991, National Recreation and Park Association.

Recreonics: *Buyers' guide and operations handbook*, Indianapolis, Ind, 1991, Catalog number 41.

Williams KG: *The aquatic facility operator's manual*, Hoffman Estates, Ill, 1991, National Recreation and Park Association, National Aquatic Section.

Review Questions

1. What exactly is a "turnover?"

2. What is the difference between a pool gutter and a skimmer?

3. What is a weir?

4. What is the function of a surge tank?

5. What pool component does the hair and lint strainer protect?

6. List three major types or categories of filters.

7. What water temperature is ideal for most special populations like senior citizens and disabled individuals?

8. What is the function of a heat exchanger?

9. What is an erosion feeder and how does it work?

10. What type of pump is most often used for swimming pool circulation?

11. What is the one working part of this pool pump?

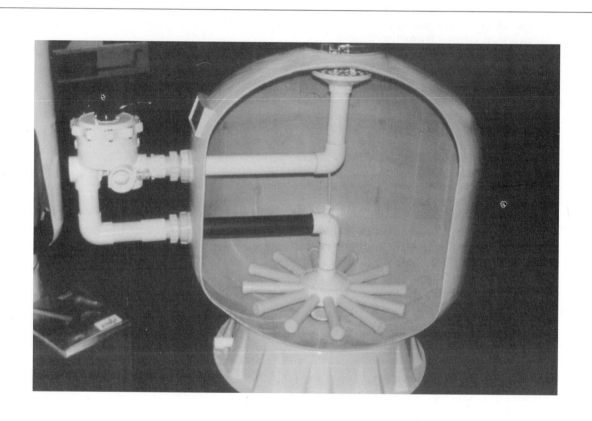

5

FILTRATION

A key to good filtration is the ability of the filter media to screen and trap dirt. Different filter medias have different entrapment capabilities. Before discussing each filter type specifically, a closer examination of filter media will now be undertaken. The following chart will help to illustrate how effectively diffent medias filter swimming pool water.

Grain of table salt:	90 to 100 microns*
Human hair:	70 microns

*1 micron is equal to .0000394 inches or 1 millionth of a meter.

Visible to the naked eye:	35 microns
Sand filtering capability:	20 to 25 microns
Talcum powder:	5 to 10 microns
Cartridge filtering capability:	5 to 10 microns
Red blood cells:	8 microns
Average bacteria:	2 microns
DE filtering capability:	1 to 3 microns

Filters, which do not allow particles of 15 microns or larger to pass through, produce outstanding water clarity. Water clarity results from a lack of turbidity. A nephelometer measures water clarity by assigning turbidity units. Good water clarity does not exceed 0.5 nephelometer turbidity units (NTUs). Remember, when the view of the pool bottom becomes obstructed because of poor water clarity, the pool shoud be closed.

Different filtration systems will be discussed in the following order: sand, diatomaceous earth, and cartridge (Fig. 5-1).

Sand Filtration

Although sand filters are perhaps the most widely used filters in the swimming pool industry, they are probably the least efficient when it comes to trapping dirt. The permanence of the sand as a media and the ease of backwashing are just two reasons for their popularity. When maintained properly, sand filters produce high water clarity.

Sand filters use a sand medium that seldom needs replacing, and they come in a variety of designs. Sand filters include pressure sand and gravel, pressure high rate sand, vacuum sand, and in rare instances, gravity sand.

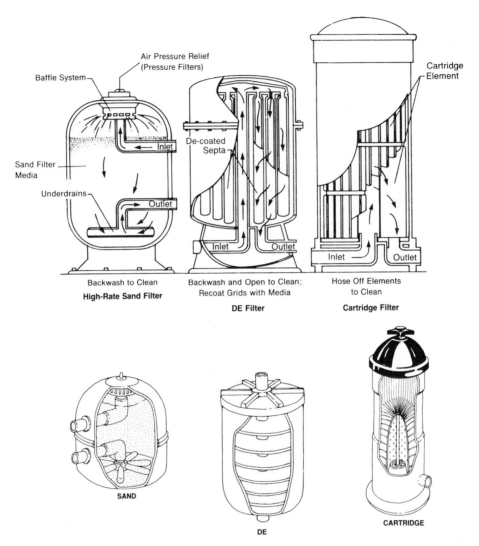

Fig. 5-1. Types of pool/spa filters. (From NSPI: *Basic pool and spa technology*, ed 2, Alexandria, Va, The Institute.)

Pressure sand and gravel

Between the 1920s and 1950s, large sand and gravel filters were used to filter the water in many swimming pools throughout this country. This filter system uses the layering of sand on top of differently sized gravel and stone. The filters themselves are extremely large, requiring large quantities of sand and gravel in the filters and a great deal of space in the filter room to store them.

Pressure sand and gravel filters are often called "rapid" sand filters, but compared with today's filtering rates, old sand and gravel filters are quite slow. The old "rapid" sand filters have filtering rates that vary between 1.5 to 5 GPM/sq ft of filter surface area,

whereas the popular high rate sand filter systems of today filter at a rate of between 12 to 20 GPM/sq ft of filter surface area. When speaking of a conventional sand and gravel filter, the term rapid should probably be avoided. Too many pool operators confuse rapid filters with high rate filters, thinking they are the same, when in fact, they are significantly different.

Sand and gravel filters are rarely installed in today's pools because they are too large, too costly to install, and require extensive amounts of time and water to backwash. Only older, larger pools still use pressure sand and gravel filters. In many cases sand and gravel filters in older pools have filter tanks that

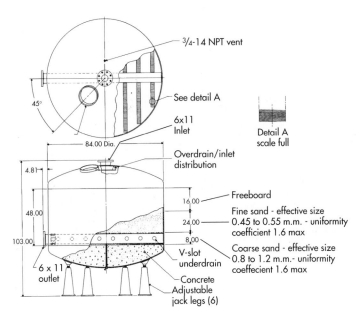

3/4-14 NPT vent

45°

See detail A

**Detail A
scale full**

**6x11
Inlet**

84.00 Dia.

**Overdrain/inlet
distribution**

4.81

16.00

Freeboard

48.00

24.00

**Fine sand - effective size
0.45 to 0.55 m.m. - uniformity
coefficient 1.6 max**

103.00

8.00

**Coarse sand - effective size
0.8 to 1.2 m.m.- uniformity
coeffecient 1.6 max**

**V-slot
underdrain**

**6 x 11
outlet**

**Concrete
Adjustable
jack legs (6)**

Fig. 5-2. Conventional sand and gravel (rapid rate) filter. (Courtesy Filtrex, Wayne,NJ.)

are taller and wider than the pool operator. For instance, a 180,000 gallon pool would require two sand and gravel filters, 11 feet in diameter.

The dynamics of the pressure sand and gravel filters are discussed in the following paragraphs. Sand and gravel systems are usually found in banks of between two and four filters with most pools having three filters. The filters may be positioned either vertically or horizontally (Fig. 5-2).

By definition, water enters a closed pressure tank containing sand and gravel. The water enters the top of the tank through a distributor or baffle. At this point the water is spread out evenly with a shower head plumbing arrangement, so that the incoming water does not disrupt or "channel" through the filter bed. The water then travels downward through the top layer of sand and then the gravel and stone. When the water finally arrives at the bottom of the tank, it is pushed out of the filter through perforated underdrains or "laterals," which collect the filtered water and return it to the pool. Before the filtered water is returned to the pool it is heated first, then treated. The top layer of sand is between 12 and 20 inches deep, but it is interesting to note that the majority of filtering is accomplished in the first 3 inches. The particle size of the sand shoud be between 0.4 and 0.6 mm, which is approximately a number 20 grade sand.

Filtering rates for pressure sand and gravel filters vary widely, but on the average, sand and gravel filters water at a rate of approximately 3 gpm per square foot of surface area. This is a relatively slow filtering rate.

Freeboard refers to the amount of air space between the top of the sand and the ceiling of the tank. This freeboard is necessary, because during the backwash cycle sand and water are forcefully displaced upward. When backwashing, this extra room is needed to allow the filter media to "expand."

Backwashing refers to cleaning pressure filter systems by reversing the flow of water in the filter tank and pushing the accumulated dirt out to waste. Backwashing should be performed just before filtering effectiveness becomes impaired. An extremely dirty filter will be accompanied by a significant pressure increase inside the tank and a drop in the filter flow rate. The manufacturer's recommendation should be followed for backwashing. When the pressure differnece between the water pressure going into the filter (influent) and the water pressure leaving the filter (effluent) reaches a predetermined point, the filters should be backwashed. Many filters are not backwashed until a pressure differential of at least 5 psi occurs. Backwashing every Saturday, for instance, is not a recommended practice unless the swimmer load is consistent. It should be remembered that a

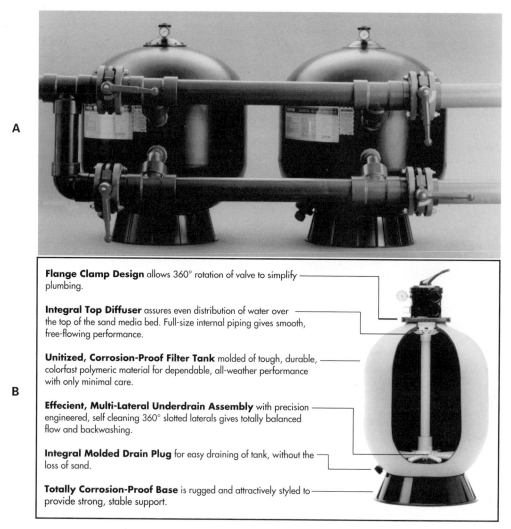

A

B

Flange Clamp Design allows 360° rotation of valve to simplify plumbing.

Integral Top Diffuser assures even distribution of water over the top of the sand media bed. Full-size internal piping gives smooth, free-flowing performance.

Unitized, Corrosion-Proof Filter Tank molded of tough, durable, colorfast polymeric material for dependable, all-weather performance with only minimal care.

Effecient, Multi-Lateral Underdrain Assembly with precision engineered, self cleaning 360° slotted laterals gives totally balanced flow and backwashing.

Integral Molded Drain Plug for easy draining of tank, without the loss of sand.

Totally Corrosion-Proof Base is rugged and attractively styled to provide strong, stable support.

Fig. 5-3. **A,** Commercial high rate sand filters. **B,** Residential pool high rate sand filters. (**A,** Courtesy Pac-Fab, Sanford, NC; **B,** Courtesy Hayward Pool Products, Elizabeth, NJ.)

dirty filter can often be an effective filter because dirt helps in filtering dirt.

One problem associated with backwashing a pressure sand and gravel system is that the backwashing flow rate must be about four times greater than the filtering flow rate. Backwashing flow rates must be maintained between 12 to 15 gpm to remove all the dirt from the filters. This is in contrast to the normal filtering flow rate of 3 gpm. To attain such high backwashing rates, each filter in this system must be backwashed individually and successively. This is accomplished by isolating each tank so that backwash water only travels through one tank at a time. Backwashing

all the filters in a sand and gravel system may last as long as 15 to 30 minutes.

Many pool operators keep the flow of water reversed until the backwash water, as viewed through a sight glass tube, becomes clear. Not surprisingly, backwashing sand and gravel filters is costly, both in terms of time and water.

Flocculants are sometimes added to the top of the sand and gravel filters to assist in the filtering process. Flocculants like Aluminum Sulfate create a gelatinous mass that floats on top of the filter and collects additional dirt. Flocculants are used only in conjunction with pressure sand and gravel filter systems.

The top layer of sand in a pressure sand and gravel sytem may encounter some problems. Most of these problems are caused by ineffective backwashing flow rates. *Mudballs* may form by a combination of hair, lint, and other organic materials. *Channeling* are holes in the sand bed that can result and lead to poor filtration. *Calcification* of the sand layer may also occur when the pool water is not balanced, particularly regarding high levels of calcium hardness and total alkalinity. To prevent these problems, the sand should be raked clean and inspected once a year. Maintaining balanced water and proper backwashing rates is sufficient to avoid these problems.

In summary, sand and gravel filters produce finely filtered water. They typically have long filter cycles, which means backwashing less frequently, and the sand media lasts at least 10 years. But as sand and gravel systems age, they are often replaced by newer, more advanced filtering systems that take up less room and are far less costly to purchase and install.

High rate sand

High rate sand filters became popular in the late 1950s and early 1960s primarily because of the reduction in both size and cost of the equipment (Fig 5-3). High rate sand systems filter and backwash at approximately the same rate, which is between 15 to 20 gallons per square foot of surface area. Because of these high filtering rates, less sand in smaller tanks is required, thus significant space is saved. Backwashing can also be accomplished in 2 to 3 minutes because all tanks are backwashed simultaneously.

High rate sand filters use *depth filtration*, that is, they use the entire sand bed to trap dirt. Cartridge and D.E. filters use only the surface of the media. Sand and gravel filters use the top 3 to 4 inches of sand.

Freeboard in a high rate sand filter can vary, but too much sand in the filter tank will find its way back to the pool through its inlets during the backwash cycle. An insufficient amount of sand will result in a filtering bed that is too small to trap sufficient amounts of dirt.

Mudballs, channeling, and calcification of the filter bed can also occur in high rate sand filters, but generally these problems are easier to correct because of the smaller size of the tank and the increased accessibility to the filter bed. High rate sand filters do require the sand replaced more often than other types of filters. This is because at high filtering rates, the individual sand granules in this system become smooth and lose their ability to trap dirt. The life in a high rate sand filter will vary from pool to pool but should last a minimum of 3 to 5 years.

It is not uncommon for some high rate sand filter systems to have oversized pumps. When this occurs channelling results and the powerful pool pump pushes the dirt right through the filter and back into the pool. If the pump size is in question, a local pool company or pump dealer should be contacted.

Backwashing should be performed whenever the flow of water becomes restricted through the filter because of an accumulation of dirt. This usually occurs when the pressure differential between the influent pressure gauge and the effluent pressure gauge on the filters reaches between 15 and 20 psi. The filter manufacturers recommendations should always be followed, however.

As mentioned previously, dirt in the filter helps trap dirt that comes from the pool. Backwashing too often will keep the sand too clean and allow dirt to pass through the filter bed. Not backwashing enough will cause the flow rate to drop and will result in cloudy water.

Some swimming pools, especially smaller pools like those found in private residences, have only one high rate sand filter tank. Many companies now manufacture a *multiport valve* that requires the owner/operator to simply turn a handle to control all circulation functions (Fig. 5-4).

The various functions controlled by the multiport valve are clearly marked on the top of the tank and include the following:

Filter

The circulation system is in the filter mode most of the time. The filtering cycle is used for normal filtration and in some pools is also used for vacuuming.

Backwash

Backwash is used for cleaning the dirty filter media as indicated by a rising pressure gauge reading on the tank. Some high rate sand filters are backwashed when the pressure in the tank increases by 6 to 8 PSI beyond the start-up pressure. When backwashing a multiport filter tank, the pump must be turned off first. The dial is then turned from "filter" to "backwash" and the pump is restarted. When the backwash water leaving the filter turns clear, as evidenced through the sight glass, the pump is turned off before the dial is reset.

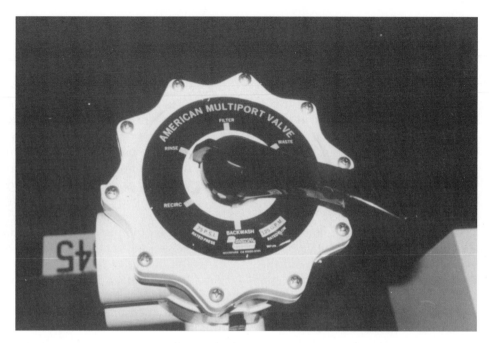

Fig. 5-4. Multiport valve.

Rinse

The rinse cycle is used following each backwash. Once the dial is positioned to the "rinse" cycle, the pump is restarted and the filter media is rinsed cleaned for 30 to 60 seconds.

Waste

The waste mode is used to by-pass the filter when draining or lowering the pool level and for vacuuming unusually heavy debris. During this cycle the water leaves the pool and goes directly to waste.

Recirculate

The recirculate cycle moves the water through the swimming pool system by by-passing the filter. This cycle is often used when adding chemicals.

Closed

When the filter is below the deck level, pool water may be lost if the filter is not closed when the pump is not running. This mode is used only when the pump is turned off.

Vacuuming

The vacuuming cycle is used for vacuuming directly back into the filter. Water is returned to the pool during vacuuming in this cycle.

Sometimes it may be wise to vacuum directly to waste, particular with heavy debris.

In some regions it may be possible to recycle back-wash for gardening, washing cars, or some other uses. Chlorine levels in backwashed water dissipates rapidly, particularly if it is sprayed out of the sytem. Health codes must be checked, however, before reusing treated swimming pool water.

Vacuum sand

The original vacuum sand filters used in the swimming pool industry, also know as gravity sand filters, filter water at very slow rates and required a lot of room. Today's vacuum sand systems are open, high-rate filter systems in which the filter media and water flowing through the filter can be viewed by the pool operator (Fig. 5-5). As mentioned previously, there is no hair and lint strainer in this arrangement, because the pump follows the filter.

Vacuum sand filter systems come in two configurations: "wet well/dry well" or "wet well only." The filter tank is a large, open rectangular tank, usually made of stainless steel to resist corrosion. The wet well houses the filtering sand, while the adjacent dry well contains all the required piping, gauges, valves, and controls. A collection manifold or lateral is located at the bottom of the sand.

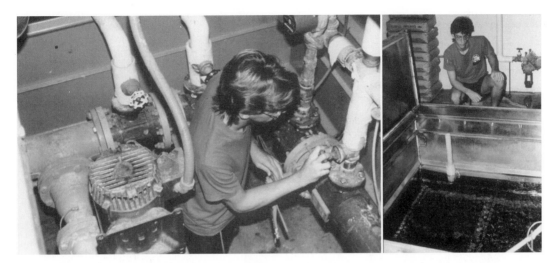

Fig. 5-5. Wet and dry wells for vacuum sand filters. (Courtesy Tim Gervinski.)

The sand in the vacuum filter tank is as much as 8 feet below the water level of the pool. To protect the surface of the filter bed, a water flow diversion screen is placed just above the sand bed. The filter tank provides ample space between the sand bed and the top of the filter tank. This extra space serves as a surge tank to store water when excessive bather loads are experienced. Water flows by gravity from the pool outlets to the wet well with sand media, and then is drawn by the pump through the sand and pushed back the the pool. The pump is located in the dry well adjacent to the sand in the wet well.

Vacuum sand filters can filter up to 20 gallons per minute per square foot of surface area. This filter also uses most of the filter bed for filtering. Backwashing can be accomplished in as little as 2 minutes.

The vacuum sand is a rugged, efficient, and low-maintenance system. It allows for easy inspection, access, and maintenance of the filter bed. One disadvantage of the vacuum system is the dry well, which houses the recirculation equipment. To access this equipment, the pool operator must use a ladder to climb down into the dry well. Once in the dry well, the operator has little room in which to work.

DE Filtration

DE filters use the fossilized skeletal remains of marine life sometimes referred to as "diatoms." DE is a white powder composed of billions of microscopic skeletons that are millions of years old. Under a microscope, DE resembles small sponges or snowflakes. Each diatom is actually 90% air space and only 10% fossil. DE filtration produces superior water clarity because of the ability of this irregular shaped filter media to screen out the smallest of particles. Unlike sand, DE filters dirt by trapping dirt *within* DE pores and holes, as well as between particles.

DE is a light, porous, white powder that clings to a fiber filter septum that allows water, but not dirt, to pass through the media before returning to the pool. The filter elements come in a variety of shapes and sizes. Tubes or cylinders are often used in pressure sytems, whereas retangular and circular leafs are common in vacuum systems. Most DE filters are designed to filter at the rate of one to 3 GPM per square foot of surface area.

Although DE produces great water clarity, its disadvantage is that DE as a medium is temporary, meaning it must be replaced often. Many DE filters require a new batch of DE after every backwashing. In addition, the filter septa to which the DE filter cake clings must be cleaned periodically. Disposing of old DE is becoming more of a problem in many municipalities throughout the country. Finally, when handling DE pool operators must wear protective masks so that the diatoms are not inhaled into the lungs.

The three types of DE filters discussed are the *pressure* system, using a closed, pressurized tank; the *regenerative* DE filter, which is also a pressure system and readjusts the DE in the tank to extend filter cycles; and the *vacuum* system, using an open tank

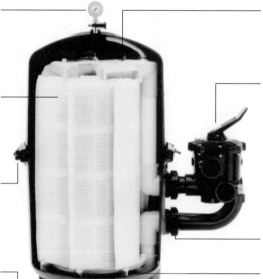

GAUGE/MANUAL AIR RELIEF VALVE provides manual release of air from system at start up. System design automatically purges entrapped air during filter operation. Pressure guage is located for easy access and readability.

FILTER ELEMENTS. Eight high impact grids custom fitted with monofilament polypropylene cloth which holds the D.E. filter powder on the outer surface. Elements are designed for up-flow filtration and top-down backwashing for maximum efficiency.

TAMPER-PROOF BOLTED CENTER FLANGE CLAMP. Provides extra strength and securely fastens tank top and bottom together. Allows for quick service access to all internal filter components without disturbing piping or connections.

DRAIN OUTLET. Full size 1½" integral drain provides fast, 100% clean out and easier flushing of tank.

HEAVY DUTY FILTER TANK. Injection molded of attractive, high strength Duralon™ for dependable, corrosion-free performance with only minimum care.

TOP MANIFOLD COLLECTOR assures secure uniform collection of clean, filtered water from the filter elements, plus provides efficient flow distribution for thorough cleaning of elements during backwashing.

6-POSITION VARI-FLO CONTROL VALVE with easy-to-use lever action handle to let you "dial" any of 6 valve/filter functions - Filter, Waste, Backwash, Rinse, Closed or Recirculate. Also available with optional Hayward 2-position slide valve for easy operation and simplified plumbing.

UNION LOCKNUTS make assembly or disassembly of the control valve easy.

FILTER ELEMENT LOCATOR securely locks elements in their designed spiral pattern to assure proper spacing and more efficient flow.

INLET DIFFUSER ELBOW distributes flow of incoming unfiltered water upward and evenly to all filter elements.

Fig. 5-6. Vertical grid pressure DE filter. (Courtesy Hayward Pool Products, Elizabeth, NJ.)

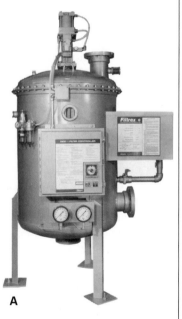

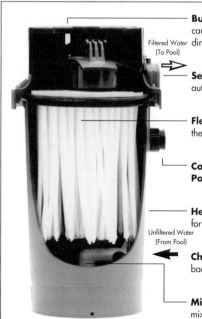

Bump Handle. An exclusive Perflex feature. It activates the mechanism causing the Flex-Tubes to instantly and uniformly clean themselves of dirt and filter powder.

Filtered Water (To Pool)

Self Venting. As filtered water is returned to the pool, Perflex filters automatically expel any air that may be present in the system.

Flex-Tubes. The proven patented filter elements that efficiently reuse the filter powder and dirt mixture forming a fresh filtering surface.

Combination Pressure Guage and Threaded Inspection/Service Port. Easy to read and remove when filter needs cleaning.

Heavy-Duty Filter Tank. Injection-molded of high-strength Duralon™ for dependable, corrosion-free performance.

Unfiltered Water (From Pool)

Check Valve. This integral valve automatically prevents system backflow whenever the pump is off.

Mixing Chamber. Engineered to produce a uniform, high velocity mixing of the filter powder and dirt that is removed from the Flex-Tubes by "Bumping".

Fig. 5-7. A, Large commercial regenerative DE filter. **B.** Extended (regenerative) cycle DE filters. (**A,** Courtesy Filtrex, Wayne, NJ; **B,** Courtesy Hayward Pool Products, Elizabeth, NJ.)

The filter septum to which the DE clings are composed of porous fabrics that come in a variety of shapes and sizes. It is important to note that DE leaves and discs filter on two sides instead of one. The DE filter septum holds the DE but allows filtered water to pass through it. Manifolds are attached between filter elements (septa) that allow the filtered water to return to the pool.

Pressure DE

DE is a temporary filtering medium, whereas sand is a permanent medium. This difference is highlighted during the backwashing cycle. Although the filtering process for pressure and regenerative DE filters is similar to pressure sand systems, the backwashing cycle is significantly different. Pressure DE filters reverse the flow of water for backwashing, but when this is done, the DE in the tank is flushed out to waste and must be replaced (Fig. 5-6). Thus new DE must be placed on the filter septa after each cleaning requiring additional work. This new coating of DE is called the "precoat" and must be accomplished slowly and evenly. The plumbing layout of pressure DE systems are almost identical to pressure sand systems because the hair and lint strainer and pump precede the filter. Both the sand and DE pressure filters are enclosed in tanks so the difference is somewhat suble to the untrained eye. Another problem associated with pressure DE systems is that the filter septa is difficult to inspect and to clean.

Before purchasing or installing a pressure DE system, easy access to the filter septum should be a requirement.

Regenerative DE

The newer regenerative DE filter systems add a feature that extends the filtering life of the DE in the pressure tank. It is important to note that because only the surface of the DE does the filtering, only 10% of the filtering capability is attained. By realigning and reusing existing DE in the filter tank, filter cycles can be extended (Fig. 5-7).

Under normal procedures, as DE filters accumulate dirt an increased resistance to flow through the media is experienced. When the pressure in the tank increases to approximately 10 PSI above the precoated pressure, the regenerative DE filter is "bumped."

"Bumping" shakes the dirty DE off the filter septa but does not allow it to escape from the tank. The individual diatoms then realign on the filter elements enabling clean sides and edges to face the dirty water. Bumping the filters in this fashion recycles the DE in the tank to extend the filter cycles before backwashing is required. This regenerating process returns filtration to near original flow rates (Fig. 5-8).

Regenerative DE filters may be bumped several times before backwashing. Therefore backwashing does not take place nearly as often as with the typical pressure DE system, thereby saving significant DE, water, time, and money.

Pool owners and operators should understand that many DE filters, including some older DE systems, are capable of being "bumped." By simply closing the valves to and from the pool and turning off the pump for three to five minutes, the DE will fall from the elements. When the pump is restarted, the DE will once again reattach itself to the filter elements producing excellent filtration with the same DE.

Vacuum DE systems

DE vacuum filters use open tanks with the pool pump following the filter tank (Fig. 5-9). No hair and lint strainer is required because the filter protects the pump. The major difference between the DE and sand vacuum systems comes when the filter elements must be cleaned. Concerning vacuum DE systems, when the filter media becomes dirty, it is manually hosed off the filter elements. Backwashing is not an accurate term to describe cleaning vacuum DE filters because the flow of swimming pool water is not reversed to clean the filter media.

An advantage of this system is that the filter elements as well as the DE filter cake can be easily inspected. As the white DE becomes dark brown, pool operators can get a better feel concerning when to backwash. Additionally, if there are any holes in the filter elements, allowing DE to pass back into the pool, this problem can be easily detected and repaired. Cleaning the filter septa also becomes easier because the filter elements are easier to remove.

Because DE is the only temporary filter medium discussed in this text, several unique features associated with DE use are now discussed.

Filter cake

Filtercake is the DE layer that clings to the filter septa or leaves and strains the dust, algae, oil, and other swimming pool debris. The filter cake catches just about everything that passes through it including some large bacteria, and as a result produces outstanding water clarity.

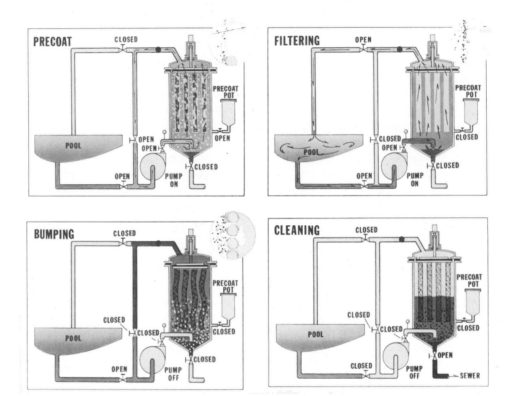

Fig. 5-8. Four cycles of regenerative DE filtration. (Courtesy Filtrex, Wayne, NJ.)

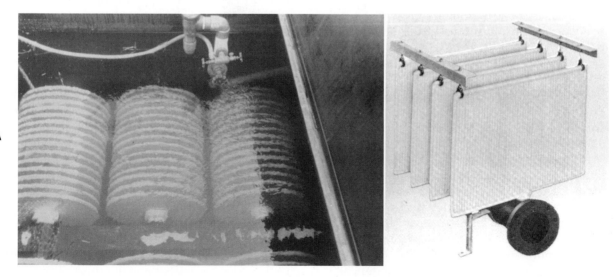

Fig. 5-9. **A,** Vacuum DE discs. **B,** Large, rectangular DE leaves. (Courtesy Brock Enterprises, Hamden, Conn.)

Precoat

Precoat refers to the layer of filtering DE placed on the filter septa to initiate the filtering process or after each backwashing or filter cleaning. *Precoating* filter cake should be between 1/16 and 1/8 of an inch thick. The amount of DE needed in any DE filter is measured by volume instead of weight. Although many formulas are available, a good rule of thumb is a 1 pound coffee can of DE for every 5 square feet of filter area. If a 40 square foot DE filter needs to be recharged, it would require approximately eight cans of DE. There are a variety of methods of precoating but most include simply recirculating the water within the tank without sending it back to the pool.

Slurry feeding

Slurry feeding is a procedure used to extend filter cycle on DE systems. During normal filtration the porous DE becomes saturated with dirt quickly and eventually becomes impervious. This occurs more quickly during heavy swimmer loads. By constantly adding small amounts of diluted DE, the new DE helps the older DE in catching dirt. Slurry feeding systems must be designed so that the mixing equipment does not damage the fragile DE. High speed agitators used to mix DE in water can pulverize the diatoms, rendering them less effective in filtering out dirt. Slurry mixers must be designed to dilute the DE in water slowly and gently.

A rough method of slurry feeding is to throw a coffee can or two of DE into the filtering tank periodically. When too much DE is added to the orginal precoat through slurry feeding, filtering water can be impeded. When excessive amounts of DE have been added so that the DE on one filter element touches the DE clinging to the adjacent filter septa, "bridging" has taken place and removal of all DE must commence. Regenerative DE filters accomplish what slurry feeds accomplish *without* adding DE.

Cleaning filter septa

Cleaning the filter septa is required periodically because scale, oils, and other organic materials eventually build up on the elements and must be removed with special cleaners. A strong cleaning agent called trisodium phosphate is often used to lift oil and grease from the septa fabric. After TSP is applied, muriatic acid is then used to remove scale build-up. If muriatic acid is used prior to TSP, oils and grease would be almost impossible to remove. Because of environmental concerns (it is not biodegradeable and is banned in some states), alternatives to TSP are now highly recommended to avoid the use of phosphates.

Additionally, whenever muriatic acid is used, strong vapors are released. Care must be taken not to breathe these fumes.

Handling DE

Because DE is a light powder, it often winds up all over the filter room. Caution must be exercised so that the fine powder is not inhaled. Protective masks covering the nose and mouth will help prevent breathing the DE. Some believe that breathing microscopic DE particles may cause silicosis of the lungs. The filter room floor should also have floor drains to permit the washing of DE from the floor.

In summary, although several disadvantages are associated with DE filters, DE still represents the most efficient filter medium. Although it requires some additional work and special handling, DE produces sparkling clear water. Recently, a biodegradable cellulose DE substitute has become available to operators and shows great promise. If water clarity is the most important consideration when designing a swimming pool, then DE filters should be considered. Some swimming pool experts claim they can actually tell when a DE filter is being used by the polished appearance of the water.

Cartridge filters

The latest technology in swimming pool filtration involves the use of cartridge filters. Cartridge filters have been used for many years in science and industry. Although the original cartridge filters were developed for residential pools during the 1950s, cartridge filters are now used in many different types of pools. The first generation of cartridge filtration used depth filtration, while the second generation (since 1970) moved to surface filtration. Cartridge filters utilize an artifical media. The filter element is composed of a pleated polyester cloth or other synthetic fabric that traps dirt. As the spaces and pores become clogged with dirt, the cartridge filter needs to be either cleaned or replaced. This usually occurs when the pressure rises to about 10 PSI above the starting pressure. Cartridge filters for pools somewhat resemble air filters that protect automobile carburetors (Fig. 5-10).

The advantages of cartridge filter systems include:

1. Cartridges are cleaned by hand and do not

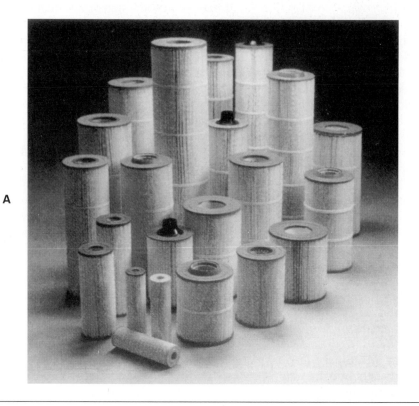

A

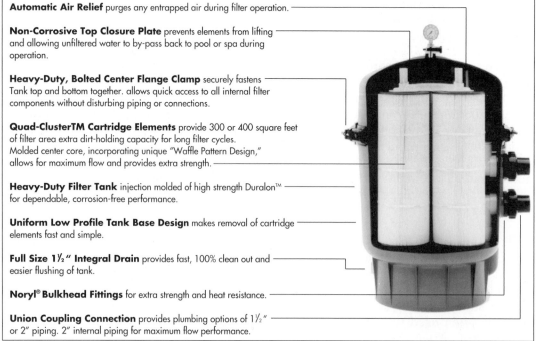

Automatic Air Relief purges any entrapped air during filter operation. ⎯⎯⎯

Non-Corrosive Top Closure Plate prevents elements from lifting ⎯⎯⎯
and allowing unfiltered water to by-pass back to pool or spa during
operation.

Heavy-Duty, Bolted Center Flange Clamp securely fastens ⎯⎯⎯
Tank top and bottom together. allows quick access to all internal filter
components without disturbing piping or connections.

Quad-ClusterTM Cartridge Elements provide 300 or 400 square feet
of filter area extra dirt-holding capacity for long filter cycles.
Molded center core, incorporating unique "Waffle Pattern Design,"
allows for maximum flow and provides extra strength. ⎯⎯⎯

B

Heavy-Duty Filter Tank injection molded of high strength Duralon™ ⎯⎯⎯
for dependable, corrosion-free performance.

Uniform Low Profile Tank Base Design makes removal of cartridge ⎯⎯⎯
elements fast and simple.

Full Size 1½" Integral Drain provides fast, 100% clean out and ⎯⎯⎯
easier flushing of tank.

Noryl® Bulkhead Fittings for extra strength and heat resistance. ⎯⎯⎯

Union Coupling Connection provides plumbing options of 1½" ⎯⎯⎯
or 2" piping. 2" internal piping for maximum flow performance.

Fig. 5-10. **A,** Pleated, cylindrical cartridge filters of various sizes. **B,** Cartridge filters. (**A,** Courtesy Brock Enterprises, Hamden, Conn; **B,** Courtesy Hayward Pool
Products, Elizabeth, NJ.)

require much water to clean; therefore they conserve water.

2. Cartridge filter systems are very simple to disassemble, analyze, repair, and replace. Most cartridge filter maintenance does not even require tools.

3. Cartridge filtration systems require little space and eliminate much of the valving and piping required by more traditional pool filters.

The disadvantages of cartridge filter systems include:

1. The filters are difficult to clean and some technicians claim that only 65% to 75% of the cartridge filtering capacity is recovered after each cleaning. New filters are required often.

2. Plastic lid covers that hold the cartridge filters in their pressure tank have been known to crack. The plastic lids should be checked often and replaced when necessary. When O rings and gaskets are used to secure the cover, they should be lubricated regularly.

Pool owners and operators utilizing cartridge filters recommend having plenty of extra filters on hand to replace the dirty cartridge being cleaned. Many dirty filters require soaking in trisodium phosphate (TSP) or a TSP substitute. Muriatic acid might also be needed after the oils are removed. Because a number of filters must be purchased during the swimming season, cartridge filtration becomes expensive in most applications. Cartridge filtration appears to be more popular with hot tubs.

Cartridge filters are designed to filter at a rate of between .375 and 1 GPM per square foot of surface area.

For example, a swimming pool with a flow rate of 475 GPMs would require a high rate sand filter bed with between 31 and 32 square feet of surface area. 475 GPMs divided by 15 GPM/FT^2 equals 31.66 square feet of filter surface area. When calculating the surface area for DE filters, it is important to remember that two sides of every DE filter element does the filtering; thus with DE filters the answer obtained with the above formula must be divided by 2.

Table 5-1.	Common Filter Types	
Filter Type	**Filter Media**	**Filter Rate**
Conventional sand and gravel	Permanent sand and gravel	3 GPM/ FT^2
High rate sand	Permanent sand	12-20 GPM/FT^2 (15 GPM/FT^2 average)
DE	Temporary DE	2 GPM/FT^2
Cartridge	Semi-permanent fibrous material	.375 GPM/FT^2

To determine how much surface area of a particular filter media is required, the following simple formula is used:

$$\frac{\text{Flow rate in GPMs}}{\text{GPM/FT}^2} = \text{Square feet of filter surface area}$$

Summary

When selecting a filtration system for a swimming pool, needs must be prioritized first. Filters that produce the best water clarity may also require the most work. Ease of operation and backwashing must be weighed against how clear the water must be. Although filter media must be cleaned regularly, it is possible to clean or backwash the filter too often.

In summary, three filtering factors determine water clarity in a swimming pool: the filtering rate, the amount of filtering media, and the effectiveness of the media. Table 5-1 includes typical characteristics of common filter types.

Bibliography

Gabrielson AM: *Swimming pools: a guide to their planning, design, and operation*, ed 4, Champaign, Ill, 1987, Human Kinetics.

Johnson R: *YMCA pool operations manual*, Champaign, Ill, 1989, YMCA.

Kowalsky L (ed): *Pool spa operators handbook*, San Antonio, Tex, 1991, National Swimming Pool Foundation.

Mitchel K: *The proper management of pool and spa water*, Decatur, Ga, 1988, BioLab.

Pool & Spa News, Los Angeles.

Pope JR Jr: *Public swimming Pool Management*. I and II. Alexandria, Va, 1991, National Recreation and Park Association.

Recreonics: *Buyers' guide and operations handbook*, 1991, Indianapolis, Ind, Catalog number 41.

Service Industry News, Torrance, California.

Taylor C: *Everything you always wanted to know about pool care*, Chino, Calif, 1989, Service Industry Publications.

Torney JA, Clayton RD: *Aquatic instruction, coaching and management*, Minneapolis, 1970, Burgess Publishing.

Washington Stage Public Health Association: *Swimming pool operations*, Seattle, 1988, The Association.

Williams KG: *The aquatic facility operator's manual*, Hoffman Estates, Ill, 1991, National Recreation and Park Association, National Aquatic Section.

Review Questions

1. List one distinct advantage and disadvantage for each type of filter.

2. Explain the difference between a pressure filtration system and a vacuum filtration system.

3. Define regenerative DE filtration.

4. What does slurry feeding pertain to?

5. What does "channeling" mean?

6. Can every type of filter be "backwashed"?

7. How do conventional pressure sand and gravel filters differ from high rate sand filters?

SECTION III
WATER CHEMISTRY

The next several chapters focus on the many different concepts concerning swimming pool water chemistry. Swimming pool water undergoes a variety of important chemical changes that take place continually. To promote safety and enjoyment in swimming pools, these chemical changes must be constantly monitored. Sparkling clear, clean water depends on good filtration, water balance, disinfection, and oxidation. The focus now is water balance, disinfection and oxidation.

In general, pH and chlorine levels receive much attention in the swimming world. pH and chlorine levels are important because they determine whether the pool water will be "people-friendly," that is, safe, comfortable, and enjoyable for swimmers. These levels are monitored on an hourly basis in most pools.

The Saturation Index, usually referred to as water balance, is also extremely important to pool patrons. Water balancing, which is often overlooked by pool personnel, is important in predicting if the swimming pool water is "plumbing-friendly." Unbalanced water is either aggressive (corrosive) or basic (scale forming). Aggressive pool water will corrode pipes, filters, heaters, valves, walls, floors, and whatever else it comes in contact with. Conversely, basic water clogs pipes filters, and heaters. Using the human body as an analogy for swimming pool chemistry, aggressive water is like cancer, while basic water is similar to bad cholesterol. Water balance, as measured by the Saturation Index, should be monitored anywhere between weekly and monthly depending on the pool characteristics.

Water chemistry as it applies to swimming pools not only helps to maintain crystal clear pool water but also the water bacteria free. Unfortunately, when it comes to swimming pool water, it is possible to have clear water that is not clean water. Understanding the concepts in this section aids the pool owner/operator in maintaining both clear and clean swimming pool water.

Specifically, the following chapters deal with chemicals used in swimming pool disinfection, oxidation, water balancing including total alkalinity, calcium hardness, pH, and temperature. A separate section is devoted to chlorination because it is the most common pool disinfectant and oxidizer.

Before beginning our discussion on pool chemistry, it is important to understand what a part per million (ppm) represents, since all pool chemical values, except for pH values, are expressed in ppm.

One ppm represents one part of something in a million equal parts of the same units. One ppm could be 1 pint in a million pints, 1 pound in a million pounds, or one tennis ball in a million tennis balls. This measure involves weight, so for swimming pool purposes, a part per million may be best expressed as 1 pound of chemical in a million pounds of pool water. A 120,000 gallon pool is just about a million pounds of water. So a pound of gas chlorine added to a 120,000 gallon pool is the equivalent of adding 1 ppm to this million pound pool. Readers should understand that gas chlorine is 100% effective chemical. Other forms of chlorine are not. So it would take 1½ pounds of calcium hypochlorite in a 120,000 gallon pool to increase 1 ppm in this pool because calcium hypochlorite is only 65% effective chemical.

6

DISINFECTION

Key Concept

- Iodine
- Ozone
- Ionization
- Enzymes
- Chlorine Generation
- UV/Hydrogen Peroxide
- Polymeric Biquanide

Swimming pool disinfection can be defined as the process of destroying living microorganisms and bacteria to prevent the transmission of disease (Sidebar 6-1). To provide efficient and continuous bacteria control, the disinfectant must have residual properties.

Residual properties mean maintaining minimal levels of active, available, chemical disinfectant in the swimming pool at all times.

Although the role of disinfection is extremely important, it is quite easily achieved. For instance, a chlorine residual of only 0.4 ppm of active available chlorine is all that is required to maintain a germ-free pool. Oxidation of organic debris, however, might require much higher levels of chemical disinfectant in pool water. Chemical compounds that do not have residual properties may not be used as primary swimming pool disinfectants or sanitizers.

The best way to ensure a germ-free pool is to have a weekly bacteria analysis conducted on pool water. Most states require this test for public pools. The analysis must be conducted under the direct supervision of a public health officer or certified laboratory. The absence of coliform indicates germ-free water.

The coliform count should not exceed two bacteria colonies per millimeter of pool water. The bacteria count should not be greater than 200 bacteria colonies per millimeter of pool water. These standards may vary among states, however.

Many swimming pools use some form of chlorine as a disinfectant. Chlorine is a member of Group VIIA of the periodic chart along with fluorine, bromine, iodine, and astatine, all of which are referred to as halogens. Of the halogens, only chlorine, bromine, and iodine are suitable for swimming pool disinfection. Chapter 7 is devoted to chlorination and bromination. Alternative disinfectants, some of which are old while others are more recent, are discussed. Included in the discussion are iodine, ozone, ultraviolet light, hydrogen peroxide, ionization, polymeric biquanide and electrolytic cells, and chlorine generation. Most of the alternative disinfectants are "chlorine-free" sanitizers.

Iodine

Iodine is a halogenlike chlorine and bromine that also can be used for swimming pool disinfection. although iodine was first investigated in the 1950s for use in swimming pools, its use has not become popular, although iodine showed much potential. When elemental iodine is dissolved in water, two active disinfectants are produced: diatomic iodine (I2) and hypoiodous acid (HOI). Pools using iodine for disinfection actually use potassium iodide, which is highly soluble in water. It is predissolved, then injected into the pool's recirculation system through a chemical feeder. Municipalities allowing the use of iodine usually require a higher residual than chlorine or bromine.

Some of the advantages of iodine use in swimming pools include: reduced pH dependence, increased

SIDEBAR 6-1

RISKING

INFECTION

Keeping adequate sanitizer levels in pool and spa water will prevent the build-up of any form of bacteria, but the *pathogenic bacteria* are really the only ones bathers need to worry about. And even among the pathogens, say the experts, there are only a few that pose any real hazard.

But if sanitization fails, there's the very real possibility that infection could occur—"not *will*," stresses Dave Knoop, pool chemical applications manager at Olin Corp in Cheshire, Conn., who adds that the presence of intestinal (*coliform*) bacteria in the water is a key indicator of the presence of pathogens.

Factors that influence the possibility of infection include the bacteria's strength (or *virulence*) and its mode of entrance. A person's mouth, for example, can by virtue of saliva and other means control the number and type of bacteria entering the body. By contrast, cuts and abrasions cannot."

If there are enough pathogens present and the person is susceptible, he or she might get sick," says Bob Speicher, an environmental health specialist for the Los Angeles County Health Department.

Beyond coliform contamination, says Paul Holmes, research microbiologist for Olin, the bacteria known as *Pseudomonas aeruginosa*, which causes swimmer's ear and a rash known as folliculitis, raises the most concern in pools and spas.

"If swimmer's ear is not treated right away," he says, "it could be serious. But it's so painful that you normally would have it treated right away."

Other potentially dangerous forms of bacteria include *staphylococcal bacteria*, which can infect the skin and cause boils. For people who have staph infections already, *streptococcus* will bring further irritation if it's present in the water."

If bacteria is in the water, there's always a chance of infection," Holmes remarks. "The nice thing is that a good level of sanitizer in the water is about all it takes to get rid of them."

From *Pool & Spa News*, March 22, 1993.

killing power for bacteria, and a longer lasting residual. Iodine does not combine with ammonia to produce iodamines, does not bleach hair or suits, and does not cause eye irritation.

But iodine's major function is to kill bacteria, not oxidize organic debris. As a result, oxidizers (usually chlorine) must be used in conjunction with iodine to control algae and destroy organics. Iodine is very expensive to use; some claim it is 20 times more expensive than chlorine. Iodine can also cause green pool water and does have a noticeable taste and smell. Iodine use in pools also has a reputation of discoloring jewelry. Based on these disadvantages, iodine is rarely used for swimming pool disinfection.

Ozone

Ozone has been a popular means of water disinfection in Europe since the early 1900s. Today most swimming pools and spas in Europe are treated with ozone. Although ozone disinfection has not been used much in the United States, it is rapidly gaining respectability as a sanitizing alternative to chlorine and bromine. Ozone's increased popularity in this country can probably be linked to environmentally conscious consumers who are concerned about the perceived dangers of using chemicals in swimming pools.

Ozone kills virtually all bacteria algae, mold, and viruses on contact. Ozone also produces an odorless,

SIDEBAR 6-2
ONE METHOD,
TWO
TECHNOLOGIES

There are two distinct methods of generating ozone for use in pools and spas: One uses corona discharge, the other ultraviolet radiation. According to ozone experts, the differences between these methods are quite dramatic.

• *Corona discharge* is the method used in all high-end applications, from treatment of public water supplies to ozonation of large swimming pools. Here, oxygen-containing gas is passed through an electrically charged chamber. What some describe as a miniature lightning storm is created within this chamber, electrolytically converting a portion of the oxygen into ozone.

Crucial to the economic generation of ozone by corona discharge is the use of dry air as the source of oxygen. When water is present, two bad things happen: First, the amount of ozone generated is greatly reduced; second, small quantities of nitrogen oxides are formed—quantities sufficient to form highly corrosive nitric acid.

To avoid these problems, ozone system manufactures employ air-drying systems or introduce pure oxygen to the reaction chamber.

From an application standpoint, corona-discharge systems generate far more ozone than do UV systems and are therefore the systems of choice for large bodies of water. On the downside, they are dramatically more expensive than UV systems—and certainly are not cost effective for use on spas unless that spa is coupled with an ozonated pool.

• *Ultraviolet* generation of ozone is achieved by moving air past a source of UV radiation, typically UV bulbs, and then mixing the resulting ozone gas with water. The ozone generated in this way comes at very low concentrations—anywhere from 10 to 1,000 times less than those produced by typical corona-discharge systems designed for pools.

As a result, UV/ozone systems are recommended only for use in residential spas, where they are truly cost effective—and, lest we forget, quite sufficent in terms of sanitizing capability.

With UV/ozone systems, however, experts caution that the bather load must be kept within reasonable limits and the circulation system must always be on when the spa is not in use for the systems to work effectively.

The experts add that the system should always be turned off when the spa is in use to prevent bather contact with undissolved ozone gas (see the sidebar on p. 62 for the rationale behind this recommendation).

From *Pool & Spa News*, March 8, 1993.

tasteless pool because chloramines are not produced during ozonation. Ozone has the unique ability to completely destroy urea introduced by swimmers, thereby eliminating the formation of obnoxious chloramines. Ozonation reduces the need for additional chemicals by 50% to 90%.

Proponents of ozone claim that when it is used for swimming pool disinfection there is no bleaching of hair and suits, no smell or eyeburn, and no build-up of total dissolved solids (TDS).

Basically, ozone is a form of oxygen that is produced when ultraviolet (UV) rays react with oxygen in the earth's atmosphere. During electrical storms, ozone is often produced when lightning moves through oxygen molecules. Some refer to ozone as "energetic oxygen." Ozone is a powerful disinfectant and oxidizer and in some respects is even more powerful than chlorine. Ozone is very effective in killing many types of bacteria and viruses. For instance, ozone kills the *E. coli* bacteria 25 times faster than hypochlorous acid, which is produced by chlorine.

Ozone is very unstable and as a result does not last long in pool water. Therefore ozone must be produced on-site and then added to the swimming pool circulation system. Ozone has a half-life of 22 minutes. This means that half the ozone produced will decompose and be rendered useless every 22 minutes. As a result ozone must be constantly produced and reintroduced to the pool. There are two basic methods of ozone production: corona discharge and UV generation (Sidebar 6-2).

Corona-discharge ozone generaton is the older of the two methods of producing ozone. It requires a continual supply of high-voltage electricity that produces large quantities of ozone at high concentrations. A special chamber is needed to house the corona-discharge equipment, which reacts with specially dehumidified air. What results in the chamber is similar to an electric storm in the atmosphere, and ozone is produced. Once the ozone is manufactured, it is introduced into the pool by utilizing either a venturi-suction system or an air compressor. The trend in ozone delivery appears to be away from compressors and more toward venturi injectors. In both cases ozone bubbles are mixed with swimming pool water that is returning to the pool. The cost of the corona-discharge equipment can be very expensive, and professional installation is a must because of the required combination of water and electricity.

UV ozone generation uses UV lamps, which produce low levels of ozone, which in turn attack oxygen molecules as air is passed in front of the lamps. Air dryers and compressors are sometimes added to the UV system to increase ozone production. UV lamps require little power, but they generate far less ozone than the older corona-discharge method.

European ozonation for pools is characterized by large corona-discharge chambers, followed by deozonation chambers using activated charcoal filters. Water purified by ozone must be "deozonated" before returning to the pool because it can reach dangerously high levels. Ozonation followed by activat-

---

SIDEBAR 6-2

WALKING THE LINE

As is noted prominently at several points in the accompanying article, the ionization systems used by the pool and spa industry have become something of a lightning rod for debate.

These disputes extend largely from the fact that there are no standards governing the manufacture or use of these devices. There is, for example, no established range of residual

From *Pool & Spa News*, May 3, 1993.

chlorine or bromine concentrations that should be used with ionizers. It's also unclear how much output an ionization system must have to be effective.

Indeed, even the precise bactericidal and algicidal properties and kill rates of copper and silver ions are still under study—and none of this in any way addresses the issues involved in the potential that both copper

and silver have to stain pool and spa surfaces.

Still, according to many who have come to believe in electrolytic mineral ionization as an effective means of sanitizing pool and spa water, the proof is in the clarity: You'll know when the system is working because the water will be crystal clear and chlorine and bromine costs will plummet at the same time.

ed charcoal rids the pool water of any obnoxious tastes and odors.

Most states mandate that ozone be used as a supplementary sanitizer only. Health codes require a minimum level of halogen residual to ensure water sanitation. Chlorine or bromine must also be added to ozonated pools because algae growth is actually encouraged in the presence of ozone. Only small residuals need to be maintained for the halogens in this case, but still, two forms of disinfectants are required when ozone is used as the primary disinfectant. Also, although ozone is safer on pool walls and floors than traditional disinfectants, it does corrode copper and some other metals. Because ozone is measured in parts per billion, a special test kit is required.

Ozonation systems are extremely expensive to install. As technology improves and the cost of installation decreases, ozone as a primary pool disinfectant in the United States should gain popularity. The 1984 Olympics held in Los Angeles used ozone in two out of three pools, while NASA plans to use ozonated drinking water in their proposed space station.*

Ionization

Ionization is an electrochemical process of converting electrically neutral (noncharged) atoms, molecules, or compounds into electrically charged ions. These ions, which are either positively (+) or negatively (-) charged, have disinfecting properties in pool water. In the swimming pool industry, ionization is usually accomplished by the use of copper and silver electrodes to produce copper and silver ions. Some also refer to the production of these ions as electrolysis. Both copper and silver serve as alacrities and bactericides.

The advantages of using an ionization disinfection system for swimming pools include reduced chemical usage, no effect on pH, and little maintenance or monitoring of disinfecting chemicals (Sidebar 6-3).

Ionization with copper and silver does not provide oxidation, however. As a result, an oxidizer is needed to deal with organic debris, and many health departments still require a halogen residual regardless of the disinfection system. Another drawback of ionization is green and black staining that may result from

* For further information concerning the use of ozone, contact the International Ozone Association, 83 Oakwood Avenue, Norwalk, CT 06850 (203-847-8169).

using copper and silver. Some states may also be concerned about dealing with discharge water that contains these metals. It appears that ionization is more appropriate for low usage private pools rather than high load public pools. Ionization systems were used to purify drinking water during NASA's Apollo misisons.

Chlorine Generation

Some pools disinfect their water by using electrical devices to actually produce chlorine from salts that have been predissolved in the pool water. Ordinary food grade salt or sodium chloride (NaCl) can be converted to sodium hypochlorite (NaOCl) through electrolysis made possible by electrodes in a separate salt-solution chamber.

This on-site production of sodium hypochlorite reacts with water to produce hypochlorous acid or active chlorine that provides effective sanitation. Chlorine generation commonly utilizes an electrolytic cell containing anode and cathode plates. The major advantage of this system is that disinfecting and sanitizing chemicals do not have to be purchased, stored, and handled.

Another distinct advantage of chlorine generation is regeneration. In this system combined chlorine is converted back to free available chlorine after it is used for disinfection. Although the future looks promising for chlorine generation, some disadvantages exist with its use. The system as it is used today is extremely expensive to install. Chlorine generation requires a swimming pool salt level to be approximately 2500 PPM, and as a result these swimming pools taste salty. Salt water can also be corrosive on a pool's plumbing.

Ultraviolet/Hydrogen Peroxide

A combination of ultraviolet (UV) light and hydrogen peroxide has worked well as a disinfectant but particularly for smaller pools, hot tubs, and spas. Concerning the UV light portion of this disinfection system, mercury vapor lights are used in a chamber through which swimming pool water passes. The lights radiate sufficient energy to sterilize water in the chamber or tube.

Two basic methods of UV disinfection are now being used for swimming pool disinfection: shell-side flow and tube-side flow. In the shell side flow, water flows over quartz sleeves housing a UV lamp. The tube side flow passes water through a UV transmittable material. In both cases the UV disinfection is a point source application without any residual disinfecting properties. In addition, UV radiation does not provide oxidation. If the water contains much organic debris and body wastes, the UV disinfecting process will be greatly hindered.

Because UV radiation fails to oxidize, hydrogen peroxide is used for this important function. Hydrogen peroxide is an effective oxidizer with a measurable residual, but it is a weak disinfectant. H_2O_2 levels should be maintained between 30 to 40 PPM.

Hydrogen peroxide does have some disadvantages because it is a strong oxidant, capable of causing combustion. It is expensive to buy, difficult to store and handle, and can be dangerous if spilled.

Polymeric Biquanide

Polymeric biquanide is a chlorine-free swimming pool disinfectant and algistat. As a polymer it aids in filtration by electrostatically clumping smaller particles together, making them easier to trap. This type of polymer is easily recognizable in the swimming pool industry as Bacquacil. Bacquacil is a broad-spectrum antimicrobial closely related to hospital antimicrobial scrubs that helps the filter physically remove impurities from the water while it sanitizes. Unlike halogen sanitizers, it is not affected by sunlight, temperature, or pH fluctuation. Bacquacil proponents claim that it last longer than other disinfectants and does not bleach or burn. Bacquacil is usually used only in private pools with water volume less than 50,000 gallons. Bacquacil requires the addition of hydrogen peroxide for oxidation in a biquanide pool. A special algacide is also recommended.

The disadvantages of Bacquacil are its incompatibility with many other pool chemicals, including the following:

- Any type of chlorine or bromine sanitizer
- Copper or silver ionizers
- Most household cleaners and detergents
- Water softeners
- Persulfate oxidizers

Bacquacil and other polymers may gain popularity as consumers continue to search for chlorine-free pool disinfections.

Enzymes

Enzymes are now being sold in the pool industry as the "natural" way of ridding the water of impurities. Enzymes digest organic wastes like body oils, dead skin, mucous, soap, deodorants, and many other contaminants that bathers add to the water. While enzymes cannot be used alone for pool disinfections, they significantly reduce the need for chemical sanitizers. Apparently, pool and spa enzymes are helpful in removing scum-lines of sides. Enzyme use has become particularly popular in spas and hot tubs.

Summary

Nonchlorine disinfectants are gaining popularity in the United States. Although chlorine still remains the primary swimming pool disinfectant in this country, its competitors are rapidly gaining ground. When selecting a pool disinfectant, cost, effectiveness, availability and ease of handling are primary concerns. Selecting a pool disinfectant without a local supplier can be frustrating. Before selecting an alternative sanitizer, it is recommended that those individuals already using the particular sanitizers be consulted for pros and cons. Just about every pool chemical has advantages and disadvantages. Whatever chemical is selected, safe storage and handling procedures must be followed.

Bibliography

Gabrielson AM: *Swimming pools: a guide to their planning, design, and operation*, ed 4, Champaign, Ill, 1987, Human Kinetics.

Johnson R: *YMCA pool operations manual*, Champaign, Ill, 1989, YMCA.

Kowalsy L (editor): *Pool/spa operators handbook*, San Antonio, Tex, 1991, National Swimming Pool Foundation.

Mitchel K: *The proper management of pool and spa water*, Decatur, Ga, 1988, BioLab.

Pool & Spa News, Los Angeles.

Pope JR Jr: *Public swimming pool management*. I and II. Alexandria, Va, 1991, National Recreation and Park Association.

Recreonics: *Buyers' guide and operations handbook*, Indianapolis, Ind, 1991, Catalog Number 41.

Service Industry News, Torrance, Calif.

Taylor C: *Everything you always wanted to know about pool care*, Chino, Calif, 1989, Service Industry Publications.

Torney, JA, Clayton, RD: *Aquatic instruction, coaching and management*, Minneapolis, 1970, Burgess Publishing.

Washington State Public Health Association: *Swimming pool operations*, Seattle, 1988, The Association.

Water quality and treatment: ed 3, 1971, The American Water Works Association.

Williams KG: *The aquatic facility operator's manual*, Hoffman Estates, Ill, 1991, National Recreation and Park Association, National Aquatic Section.

Review Questions

1. List an advantage and disadvantage for each of the following disinfectants: iodine, ozone, ionization, enzymes, chlorine generation, UV/hydrogen peroxide, and polymeric biquanide.

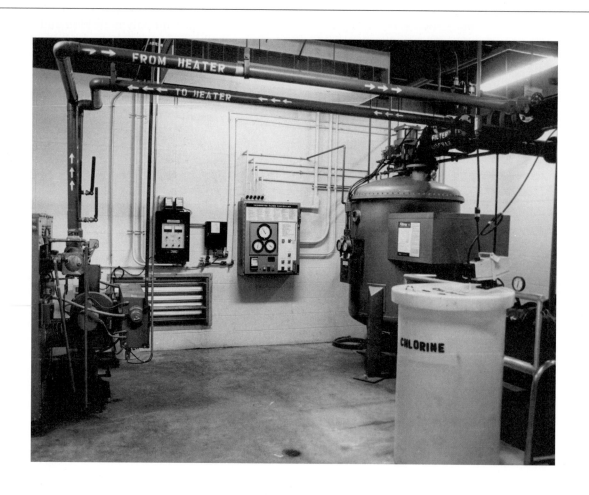

7

CHLORINATION AND BROMINATION

This chapter takes an in-depth look at chlorination, the most popular means of disinfecting and oxidizing swimming pool water (Sidebar 7-1). More than 90% of all pools in the United States use some type of chlorine. Although there is a strong movement away from chlorinated pools by experimenting with alternative sanitizers, chlorine still offers pool owners/operators an effective and economical way of keeping pool water clean and safe. A major advantage of chlorine is that it provides two functions: disinfection of bacteria, viruses, algae, and other pathogens and oxidation of organic debris and swimmer waste. Oxidation is an important function that assists the filtering process. Many alternative sanitizers offer disinfection without oxidation, necessitating the purchase of additional chemicals. Numerous forms of chlorine will be discussed, including the advantages and disadvantages of each. Bromine, another halogen similar to chlorine in many aspects, will also be addressed later in this chapter.

Disinfection and Oxidation

As mentioned previously, chlorination provides both disinfection and oxidation. *Disinfection* kills germs and algae to prevent the transmission of disease and other swimmer discomforts. *Oxidation* supplements the filtering process by "burning up" or bleaching out many organic impurities that are introduced to the pool by swimmers. Pool practitioners rightly say, "chlorine burns the trash and the filters remove the ash." Chlorine has the ability to burn up many smaller impurities that pass through filters. Killing bacteria is a relatively easy task for chlorine; only small amounts of free chlorine (0.4 ppm) will destroy most pathogens. On the other hand, a more difficult responsibility of chlorine is to destroy particulate organic matter. This often calls for higher chlorine levels because heavy swimmer loads create a larger amount of organic debris. For oxidation purposes, free chlorine levels can vary greatly but often fall somewhere between 2.0 ppm and 10.0 ppm. Dull-looking pool water is often blamed on poor filtration, when in reality, insufficient oxidation is the real culprit.

Hypochlorous Acid

Regardless of the type of chlorine used, hypochlorous acid (HOC1) is the primary chemical used for swimming pool disinfection. Chlorine reacts with water to produce hypochlorous acid, which in turn disinfects through a electrochemical process. Hypochlorous acid penetrates the cell walls of bacteria, killing them. Hypochlorous acid is very effective as a disinfectant, an algacide, and an oxidizer. Used at proper levels, hypochlorous acid does not taste, smell, or burn.

$$Cl_2 + H_2O = HOCl + HCl$$

SIDEBAR 7-1 **JUST THE FACTS**	The chlor-alkali industry in the United States is big — really big. Here are a few vital statistics to convey that fact, courtesy of the Chlorine Institute: • There are 53 chlorine plants in the United States

• U.S. chlorine and caustic soda production in 1990 consisted of 11.85 million tons of chlorine gas and 9.7 million tons of liquid chlorine — fifth in shipped volume among all individual products in the world

• Both chlorine and caustic soda rank in the top 10 of all chemicals made in the world
• Annual North American chlorine and caustic soda output equals three-and-a-half times the weight of the Great Pyramid in Egypt.

From *Pool & Spa News*, August 3, 1992.

HOCL is a mild acid that disinfects and oxidizes swimming pool water and is the active, killing agent produced by chlorine's reaction in water. Many pool experts refer to HOCl as free-available chlorine (FAC). HCl is hydrochloric acid, which is powerful acid.

It is important to note that as pH rises, HOCl breaks apart or disassociates (also referred to as ionization) in the following manner:

$$HOCl = H+ + OCl-$$

H^+ refers to the hydrogen ion and OCl- represents the hypochlorite ion. The hypochlorite's (OCl⁻) is not very active, and its killing power is insignificant. The higher the pH, the less HOCl available to disinfect and oxidize. At higher pH levels, more HOCl is required, plus bacteria and algae will take longer to kill. The likelihood of swimmer infections like swimmer's ear and sore throats may also increase. As pH levels decrease, the effectiveness of HOCl increases (Fig. 7-1). To prevent HOCl from losing its killing power, pH levels should be maintained between 7.2 and 7.8. Below a pH of 7.2 HOC1 becomes corrosive. pH is discussed in detail in the following chapter.

In Fig. 7-2, at a pH of 7.5, about 50% of the free-available chlorine is actually active HOCl. At the elevated pH 8.0, a mere 21% of the free-available chlorine is active HOCl.

Forms of Chlorine

Chlorine is available in three basic forms: gas, liquid, and solid. Within these three forms many varieties are commercially available.

Each is discussed now, beginning with the most popular of each of the three forms.

Gas Chlorine (Cl₂)

Of all the chlorines available for swimming pool use, gas chlorine is the most cost-effective because it consists of 100% available chemical. Pound for pound, gas chlorine is the cheapest and strongest of all chlorines, but perhaps not surprisingly, it is also the most potentially dangerous. Gas chlorine is extremely toxic and can be lethal. Those who use gas chlorine seldom want to part with it, yet those who use other disinfectants often fear gas chlorine. The Chlorine Institute, 2001 L Street, NW, Washington DC 20036, should be contacted for any information concerning gas chlorine usage.

Gas chlorine is a green-yellow gas that is 2.5 times heavier than air.

Gas chlorine is compressed into large metal cylinder, where it liquifies under pressure. As a liquid it is amber colored and is 1.5 times heavier than water. When released from the tank, the chlorine returns to the gaseous state. Chlorine gas cylinders normally weighs 150 pounds and must conform to standards established by the Chlorine Institute. For every pound of chlorine used, about a half pound of hydrochloric acid is produced, which in turns lowers the pH. As a result, for every pound of chlorine gas added to pool water, an additional pound of soda ash must be added to maintain the pH in the ideal range.

In addition to lowering the pH, the HOCl that chlorine gas produces dissipates quickly in sunlight. To combat this loss of chlorine outdoors, some pool operators stabilize their chlorine in sunlight by adding cyanuric acid (CYA). As one would expect,

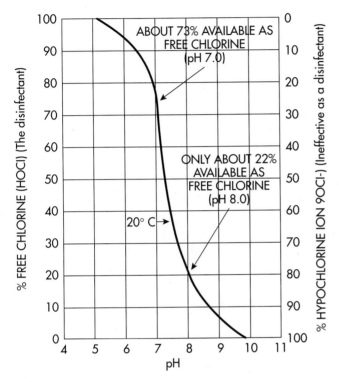

Fig. 7-1. Dissociation of HOCl at high pH. (From NSPI: *Basic pool and spa technology*, ed 2, Alexandria, Va, 1992, The Institute.)

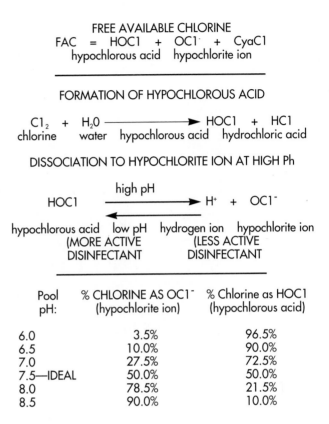

FREE AVAILABLE CHLORINE

$$FAC = \underset{\text{hypochlorous acid}}{HOCl} + \underset{\text{hypochlorite ion}}{OCl^-} + CyaCl$$

FORMATION OF HYPOCHLOROUS ACID

$$\underset{\text{chlorine}}{Cl_2} + \underset{\text{water}}{H_2O} \longrightarrow \underset{\text{hypochlorous acid}}{HOCl} + \underset{\text{hydrochloric acid}}{HCl}$$

DISSOCIATION TO HYPOCHLORITE ION AT HIGH Ph

$$\underset{\substack{\text{hypochlorous acid} \\ \text{(MORE ACTIVE} \\ \text{DISINFECTANT}}}{HOCl} \underset{\text{low pH}}{\overset{\text{high pH}}{\rightleftharpoons}} \underset{\text{hydrogen ion}}{H^+} + \underset{\substack{\text{hypochlorite ion} \\ \text{(LESS ACTIVE} \\ \text{DISINFECTANT}}}{OCl^-}$$

Pool pH:	% CHLORINE AS OCl⁻ (hypochlorite ion)	% Chlorine as HOCl (hypochlorous acid)
6.0	3.5%	96.5%
6.5	10.0%	90.0%
7.0	27.5%	72.5%
7.5—IDEAL	50.0%	50.0%
8.0	78.5%	21.5%
8.5	90.0%	10.0%

Fig. 7-2. The effect of pH on the killing power of chlorine. (From NSPI: *Basic pool and spa technology*, ed 2, Alexandria, Va, 1992, The Institute.)

there are also pros and cons of using CYA, which is discussed later.

Perhaps the greatest shortcoming of gas chlorine is the specialized equipment needed to prevent and escape a gas leak. The following gas chlorine equipment is required in most states:

1. A separate, fireproof room reserved for gas chlorine apparatus exclusively. The chlorine room should detached from the filter room.
2. Stored tanks, whether empty or full, must be chained to a wall and capped.
3. A fan and vent located near the floor (remember, chlorine gas is heavier than air) that can exchange the air in the room between 1 and 4 minutes. This fan should run continually.
4. A self-contained breathing apparatus (SCBA) located outside the room. Cannister gas masks are ineffective in high gas chlorine contents, (Fig. 7-3).
5. An emergency action plan to handle a gas leak.

One very important question must be answered before using gas chlorine: What is the role of the pool operator in the event of a gas leak? Is the primary responsibility of the pool operator to stop the leak, or to evacuate the facility and call for help? Where HazMat (Hazardous Materials) Teams exist, it is often wise to work with them in establishing emergency procedures. Pool operators should probably be trained to handle gas leaks only when HazMat personnel are not available.

6. Gas leaks should be checked daily by using ammonia hydroxide (household ammonia) in either a cloth or a misting spray bottle. If a leak exists when the ammonia is applied, a noticable white cloud will be produced.

It should be noted that the greatest chance for a gas chlorine leak is when tanks are being changed. For this reason SCBA should be worn whenever changing tanks. Perhaps the most common error during

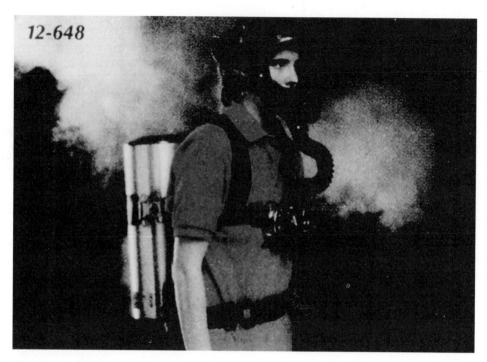

Fig. 7-3.   Self-contained breathing apparatus for gas chlorine applications. (Courtesy Recreonics, Louisville, Ky.)

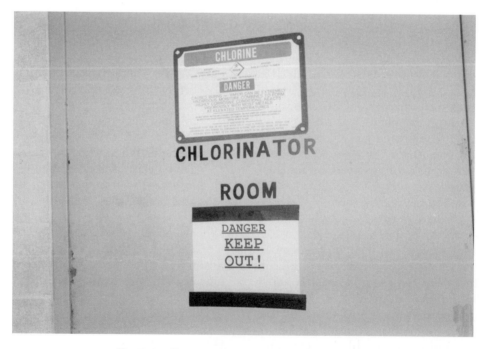

Fig. 7-4.   Separate, secure gas chlorine room.

this process is using a bad lead washer between the regulator and tank. A new lead washer should be used for every tank change. Old worn lead washers must be removed from the tank valve before placing a new washer in the valve. Old washers should be discarded so that they cannot be reused. Also, a good rule to follow is never enter a gas chlorine room alone; use the buddy system. Never change gas tanks when patrons are present in the facility (Fig. 7-4).

Finally, only mature, well-trained staff should handle gas chlorine. If younger, less experienced workers are responsible for chlorination, gas chlorine should probably be overlooked. During a chlorine emergency, the Chlorine Emergency Plan Team (CHLOREP) should be contacted at (800)-424-9300.

Residential pools should *not* use gas chlorine. When handled and managed properly, gas chlorine can provide the cheapest and best disinfection and oxidation to swimming pool water.

Sodium Hypochlorite (NaOCl)

The most popular liquid form of chlorine is sodium hypochlorite (NaOCl). Perhaps it's greatest advantage is found in its convenient and safe handling. Sodium hypochlorite (12% to 15% active chlorine) is only slightly more powerful than liquid bleach (5% to 6%). Sodium hypochlorite is most often referred to as either liquid chlorine, sodium "hypo," or simply, "bleach." Sodium hypochlorite is available in a clear, yellow liquid that is normally stored in large plastic drums. This type of liquid chlorine is introduced to the pool by a chemical feeder located in the filter room. Although sodium hypochlorite is more expensive than gas chlorine, it is usually much less expensive than other chlorines and could be the most popular form of chlorine used in the United States.

By far, sodium hypochlorite's greatest disadvantage however, is its short shelf-life. As storage temperatures increase, the percentage of available chlorine decreases caused by autodecomposition. Depending upon the environment in which it is stored, sodium hypochlorite usually does not maintain much strength beyond 30 days and could be less.

The chemical reaction taking place for liquid chlorine in swimming pool water is similar to that of gas chlorine:

$$NaOCl \ + \ H_2O \ = \ HOCl + NaOH$$

NaOCl represents sodium hypochlorite when mixed with water produces hypochlorous acid that disinfects and oxidizes. Another byproduct is NaOH,

which is sodium hydroxide, a very strong basic (alkaline) that raises pH. As a result whenever sodium hypochlorite is used for disinfection, an acid or CO_2 gas must be added to the pool water to decrease the pH. Muriatic acid (hydrochloric acid) is inexpensive and effective in lowering the pH for public pools. Residential pools and smaller swimming facilities seem to prefer sodium bisulfate, a safe, convenient, dry acid that is more expensive. A basic rule of thumb is to add 1 gallon of muriatic acid for for every 4 to 5 gallons of sodium hypochlorite. Acids used for lowering pH should be diluted before adding them to the pool water. Acids should be added to cool water in a clean, clear plastic container.

Although sodium hypochlorite is readily available and easy to handle, it does not come without pitfalls Sodium hypochlorite's biggest downfall is its short shelf life. It must be stored in a cool, dark room, which is often difficult to find at swimming pools. Because liquid chlorine decomposes so quickly, large quantities should not be stored for long periods of time.

Like gas chlorine, the HOCl produced by sodium hypochlorite is unstable, meaning that it loses its strength in sunlight. Again, it may be stabilized if the pool operator wishes to deal with cyanuric acid.

Another disadvantage includes the elevating effect sodium hypochlorite has on the pH of pool water. When sodium hypochlorite is used, a strong acid must also be added to maintain the pH within the ideal range. Another problem associated with the use of sodium hypochlorite is that it tends to clog chemical feeders pumping it into the pool. This occurs because of the scale produced by the high pH that sodium hypochlorite contains. When chemical feeders are used to inject sodium hypochlorite, they should be broken down and acid washed on a monthly basis to prevent clogging. Some pool operators will use the chemical feeder to pump fresh water, then pump muriatic acid for cleaning purposes. The manufacturers guidelines must be followed in this case, and care must be taken not to mix the liquid chlorine with acid, since dangerous gas is formed. Sodium hypochlorite also has a strong tendency to raise the Total Dissolved Solids (TDS) that can accumulate in pools. TDS will be discussed in detail later.

Sodium hypochlorite can be used effectively around the pool for cleaning decks, diving boards, and other areas. Because of its high pH, it is also an excellent way to superchlorinate the pool, particularly when gas chlorine is used as the primary sanitizer.

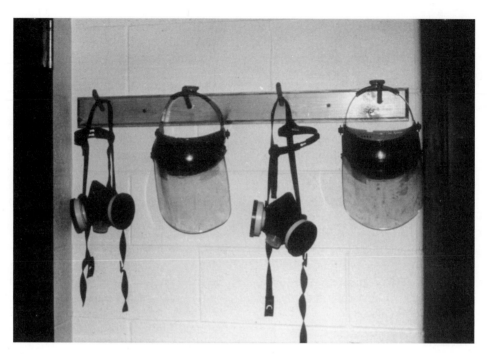

Fig. 7-5.   Protective equipment for safe handling of sodium hypochlorite.

Household bleach should never be substituted for sodium hypochlorite because it can clog a filter medium. It might be interesting to note that 1 gallon of sodium hypochlorite equals the strength of 1 pound of gas chlorine and 2 gallons of household bleach equals 1 gallons industrial liquid chlorine. Gloves and a face shield should be worn when working with sodium hypochlorite and also when working with the acids required to lower pH when liquid chlorine is used (Fig. 7-5). In summary, sodium hypochlorite is an effective disinfectant and oxidizer that is safe and easy to handle. Provided it is stored properly and pH levels are adjusted downward, pool operators can be very satisfied with sodium hypochlorite.

Calcium Hypochlorite (Ca(OCl)$_2$)

Calcium hypochlorite has been the leading solid form of chlorine in recent years. "Cal hypo" as it is sometimes referred to, is a white solid and is available in granular and tablet form. It contains 65% available chlorine, has a long shelf-life, and it is easily stored. Still, a cool, dark place and a tightly secured lid will extend the life of calcium hypochlorite. In larger pools the granular form is dissolved in water and then introduced to the pool in a liquid form through a chemical feeder. If this solution is not

allowed to settle for about 60 minutes, clogging of the feeder and clouding of the water may both result. In smaller operations, tablets are placed in erosion feeders or surface skimmers. Like liquid chlorine, calcium hypochlorite can be used for cleaning and disinfecting around the pool. It can also be broadcast over the pool for superchlorination, although when used in this fashion, it may cause cloudiness and leaves a slight residue on the pool bottom. Although this method of superchlorination is popular, many pool experts do not recommend it. Calcium hypochlorite should not be broadcast in a vinyl liner pool because undissolved granules may burn or bleach the liner. If cal hypo is used in this fashion, it should be predissolved for a vinyl-lined pool. The chemical reaction that takes place when calcium hypochlorite enters the pool water is as follows

$$Ca(OCl)_2 + H_2O = 2HOCl + Ca(OH)_2$$

Two molecules of HOCl are produced in this case and provide for the disinfection and oxidation. $Ca(OH)_2$ represents calcium hydroxide, a moderate alkaline by-product that is responsible for slightly increasing pH and calcium hardness.

Critics of calcium hypochlorite often claim it clouds the water and elevates the calcium hardness, but when cloudiness does occur, the water clears quickly. In most pools a higher calcium hardness is usually desirable so the second criticism is not always valid. Calcium hypochlorite has only a minimal effect on pH and may cause it to rise *slightly*.

Many pool owners/operators keep some calcium hypochlorite for a variety of pool-related purposes, most of which are related to cleaning. Because so many pools have calcium hypochlorite readily accessible, a risk of fire or explosion is present. Any organic material added to calcium hypochlorite can cause combustion. Soda, oil, sweat, paper, soap, other chemicals, and just about anything will cause a fire in this case. For this reason calcium hypochlorite should be stored separately to prevent other chemicals from being accidentally mixed with it. Chlorine drums must be also kept dry and up off the floor. Separate chemical scoops and buckets should be used for application of calcium hypochlorite. Trichlor, a stabilized chlorine, should never be mixed with calcium hypochlorite. Unfortunately, some pool operators have mistakenly placed both chlorines in the same chemical feeder, causing a violent explosion.

Calcium hypochlorite is also unstable and will dissipate in sunlight quickly. A little more than a pound and a half of calcium hypochlorite equals a pound of gas chlorine. Calcium hypochlorite is more often seen in residential pool applications rather than in public or commercial settings. Calcium hypochlorite also serves as an excellent algacide on pool decks and pool bottoms, particularly sloped areas.

Chlorine gas, sodium hypochlorite (liquid), and calcium hypochlorite (solid) have been referred to by some water chemists as "the big three" because they have been the most commonly used forms of chlorine to date. Each form of chlorine has pros and cons associated with its use. Other forms of chlorine are also valuable in swimming pool sanitation.

Lithium Hypochlorite

Lithium hypochlorite is a powdered chlorine that is extremely soluble in water. Lithium hypochlorite is approximately 35% effective. It dissolves quickly, making it ideal for superchlorination, particularly for vinyl-lined and painted pools, as well as hot tubs. Although lithium hypochlorite is intended to be used as a primary disinfectant, it is often used just for superchlorination because it is very expensive.

Lithium hypochlorite stores and handles well; it is not flammable. Some prefer lithium because it has no calcium in it, which may produce scale-forming

water. Lithium hypochlorite is usually dissolved in water first and then pumped into the recirculation system. Lithium hypochlorite will raise the pH slightly, and it is also an unstable chlorine, being lost rapidly in sunlight.

Stabilized Chlorines

All chlorine forms mentioned thus far have been of the unstabilized variety. This means these chemicals last longer in indoor pools than outdoor pools because the deteriorating UV rays of the sun dissipate chlorine. In an attempt to stretch chlorine in outdoor pools, cyanuric acid has been added to some chlorine compounds. It must be said that stabilized chlorine products represent the most controversial type of chlorination used today.

Chlorine can be stabilized in two ways: cyanuric acid can be added to a chlorinated pool or prestabilized chlorine can be purchased from pool suppliers in the form of chlorinated isocyanurates. Whether adding cyanuric acid to chlorinated pool water or using stabilized chlorinated isocyanurates, the process of protecting chlorine from the sun's UV rays is the same. Cyanuric acid is a ringlike molecule that latches onto HOCL molecules to form a more stable atomic structure. This combination of CYA and free chlorine delays chlorine loss but cannot stop it altogether. Some say that chlorine stabilized with CYA works as if it had sunscreen or it was time-released. So stabilized chlorine lasts longer than unstabilized chlorine in outdoor pools, but some experts question whether stabilized chlorine is as effective as its counterpart. Too much stabilizer can possibly "bind up" free chlorine, rendering it ineffective.

The main problem associated with the use of stabilized chlorine is that CYA levels in the water will increase as the stabilizer continues to be used. Most states prohibit CYA levels greater than 100 ppm. The greater the CYA, the less effective HOCl will be. Some say as you raise the CYA level you subtract the free chlorine level. Once the CYA level reaches 100 ppm, the only way of lowering cyanuric acid in the pool is by draining water from it. This is particularly a problem for Trichlor users because this stabilized chlorine is 50% CYA, and the 100 ppm limit is attained quickly in this case.

Many technicians recommend keeping the CYA levels between 30 to 40 ppm. At that range HOCl is being protected from the sun, but it still remains an effective killer. There are supporters of stabilized chlorine, however, who think the 100 ppm CYA limit

SIDEBARE 7-2

OPPORTUNITIES

UNTAPPED?

No supplier will deny it: When it comes to service professionals, there's a clear bias toward use of trichlor rather than sodium dichlor on the route.

Why is this so? For one thing, trichlor is more portable, offers a higher level of available chlorine and adequately delivers stabilizer to the water. Under those circumstances, why use any other product?

In effect, sodium dichlor has been relegated to a supporting role in pool service — at best a role player as the technician moves through a day's routines. And that, say manufacturers, is too bad, because

sodium dichlor offers certain benefits that could make a service technician's life easier.

"For example, I think they're really missing out on a great oppertunity to use dichlor products for shocking swimmings pools," explains Kirk Mitchell, director of technical services for BioLab Inc., Decatur, Ga.. "Because dichlor has a high level of solubility, you can easily and quickly increase your sanitizer level — and add stabilizer at the same time."

Indeed, Mitchell asserts that sodium dichlor stacks up quite well against shocking either with bleach or

calcium hypochlorite and adding stabilizer separately. "Cyanuric acid is not very soluble at all. Rather than going to the trouble of predissolving it or, worse, risk damaging the surface of the pool, a service technician can kill two birds with one stone by shocking pools with dichlor."

Mitchell advises technicians to watch stabilizer levels if they apply this strategy: "If the pool has a stabilizer level higher than 70 ppm, shock it with a non-stabilized product — especially if the pool is already running on trichlor."

From *Pool & Spa News*, October 5, 1992.

---

is an arbitrary figure. Some pool technicians would prefer to see a higher CYA limit and suggest CYA limits between 150 and 200 ppm.

Apparently, "locking up" free chlorine with CYA and reducing its effectiveness is not the only problem associated with stabilized chlorine. Some health officials believe that high cyanuric acid levels in the water may be hazardous to humans. Because swimming pool water can be swallowed and absorbed by the skin, this could be a real concern. High levels of cyanuric in the body may lead to liver and kidney damage, and that is why low levels of CYA are recommended by health officials. Conversely, some manufacturers state that CYA levels of 10,000 PPMS are not harmful, so it appears this debate will not be short-lived.

The two most popular types of commercially available stabilized chlorines are dichlor and trichlor.

Dichlor (sodium dichloro-s-triazinetrione) is a stabilized chlorine commercially produced by combining soda ash, cyanuric acid, and chlorine. This stabilized chlorine is sometimes referred to as sodium dichlor. Dichlor is 56% or 62% effective and is presently available in a granular form only. One

advantage of dichlor is that it has a neutral pH, so it has little effect on pH levels in pool water. If dichlor is used as a primary sanitizer, an unstabilized chlorine should be used for superchlorination because high levels of CYA will be reached quickly in this case. It is easily stored and handled, and it dissolves quickly. Dichlor is usually predissolved and introduced to the pool through a liquid chlorinator (Sidebar 7-2).

Trichlor (trichloro-s-triazine-trione) is another stabilized chlorine that is produced commercially and is available in tablets, sticks, and granules. Unlike dichlor, trichlor dissolves slowly and as a result can be introduced into pools through erosion feeders, floaters, and skimmers. Trichlor's popularity can probably be linked to this fact; homeowners can simply drop some trichlor tablets or sticks into a floater or feeder, and chlorine will be found in the pool regardless of the amount of sunlight. Erosion feeders and floaters are very inexpensive and easy to use. If introduced through a skimmer, however, it may damage the skimmer and the plumbing near the skimmer. When administered through a floater, children may be tempted to play with it, which is not

SIDEBAR 7-3

BROMINE

BACKGROUND

Bromine is one of five non-metallic chemical elements known collectively as halogens: The other four are flourine, chlorine, iodine and asatine. It is one of only two elements that ordinarily exists in a liquid state, mercury being the other.

Isolated in 1826 by French scientist Atoine-Jerome Balard, reddish-brown bromine is highly corrosive and easily volatilizes to form a gas extremely irritating to the eyes and mucous membranes. It's primary sources are seawater and potash mines.

Through the years, bromine has been used in photographic processing, as a dye, as an anti-knock additive to gasoline, as a disinfectant and, during World War I, as a poison gas. Because of its volatility, however, elemental bromine fell out of favor in most applications—until the 1950s, that is, when bromine was first combined with chlorine in tablet form and began to see use in swimming pools.

From *Pool & Spa News*, April 22. 1991

desirable. Trichlor is powerful, having an available chlorine content of almost 90%. Trichlor is highly acid and lowers the pH of swimming pool water.

The stabilized chlorines, dichlor, and trichlor are often called *organic* chlorines. *Inorganic* chlorines are those that are unstabilized and lost easily in sunlight. Stabilized chlorines should be used only in outdoor pools. Stabilized chlorines were developed to increase chlorine's longevity in sunlight. Because indoor pools have no deteriorating UV rays, stabilized chlorines are inappropriate indoors. Why worry about and test for CYA levels when UV rays are not present? As mentioned previously, although CYA does protect chlorine from the sunlight, it also reduce chlorine's ability to disinfect.

Perhaps the greatest benefactors of stabilized chlorine are the smaller pool owners, hotel/motel pools, and pool service companies, who have difficulty keeping chlorine levels up in a number of pools. These individuals would much rather use stabilized chlorine than risk closure of their pools by health officials for inadequate chlorine levels. In addition, the savings on chlorine is great. Although stabilizer is an additional cost, it saves significant sums of money by saving chlorine and reducing service calls.

But like any other disinfectant, stabilized chlorine has drawbacks. Constantly monitoring and controlling CYA levels is a major concern, requiring additional testing procedures. While easy to use and cost-effective, dichlor and trichlor are not good algacides. Again, stabilized chlorines should be used only outdoors. In summary, stabilized chlorines are both popular and controversial. All pros and cons must be studied before deciding to use stabilized chlorine. Local chemical suppliers should be contacted for details.

Bromination

Bromine, like chlorine, is a member of the halogen family, with excellent disinfection and oxidation properties. Elemental bromine is a difficult and dangerous liquid to handle. Elemental bromine reacts with water in the following fashion:

$$Br_2 \ + \ H_2O \ = \ HOBr \ + \ HBr$$

Rather than producing HOCl like chlorine, bromine produces two disinfecting agents. HOBr or hypobromous acid is the primary disinfectant, while HBr or hydrobromic acid reduces pH levels.

Elemental bromine is not available for swimming pool use in the United States. The primary source for bromine is seawater and potash mines, and bromine has also been used in photographic processing, dyes, gasoline, disinfectants, and as a poison gas in World War I (Sidebar 7-3).

While elemental bromine is used successfully in Europe, the United States has switched to sodium bromide salts in combination with other compounds to increase its effectiveness and ability to be handled. This two-part system includes an oxidizer that activates the bromine. Bromine in this form is available in sticks or tablets. The oxidizer is often chlorine or potassium monopersulfate, a non-halogen oxidizing agent, and in some cases, ozone. The bromine/potassium monopersulfate combination is usually reserved for small pools that can be hand-fed. The more popular combination is bromine/chlorine. The combination of bromine and chlorine produce hypobromous acid (HOBr) as the primary disinfectant and hypochlorous acid (HOCl), which serves as a regenerative catalyst and also assists with disinfection and oxidation.

The use of bromine has several advantages. Perhaps the greatest advantage is that combined bromine or bromamines does not irritate, burn, or smell the way combined chlorines or chloramines do.

Along those lines, chloramines must be "shocked" out of the water, whereas bromamines break down on their own.

Bromine is more stable at elevated temperature than chlorine. This explains why bromine is the preferred disinfectant in hot tubs and spas. Combined chlorines and bromines are produced quickly in hot water environments due to the relatively high swimmer load and the increased amounts of perspiration in the water due to the heat.

Bromamines are effective as disinfectants, whereas chloramines are not, giving bromine the advantage in hot water. Chloramines and bromamines will be explained fully in Chapter 8.

Being a strong oxidizer, bromine is combustible like chlorine and must be stored carefully. Bromine may also smell, turn the water green, and cause staining and sudsing if not maintained at appropriate levels. Generally, it is more expensive than chlorine. A chlorine test kit should not be used on a brominated pool; a special bromine test kit is needed. One major disadvantage of bromine is that it is unstable and will be lost rapidly in sunlight. Unfortunately, cyanuric acid cannot be used to stabilize bromine. Perhaps bromine's best application is in hot tubs and spas.

Summary

Chlorine is the most commonly used swimming pool disinfectant in the United States, but many different forms of chlorine are used in swimming pools. Once again, cost, effectiveness, availability, and ease of handling must be considering when selecting any type of chlorine. All chlorines must be handled with extreme care. Bromine is also a popular swimming pool disinfectant but is more commonly used in hot tubs and spas.

Bibliography

Gabrielson AM: *Swimming pools: a guide to their planning, design, and operation,* ed 4, Champaign, Ill, 1987, Human Kinetics.

Herman E: Sniffing out a sanitizing specialist, *Pool Spa News,* April 22, 1991.

Johnson R: *YMCA pool operations manual,* Champaign, Ill, 1989, YMCA.

Kowalsky L (editor): *Pool/spa operators handbook,* San Antonio, Tex, 1991, National Swimming Pool Foundation.

Mitchel K: *The proper management of pool and spa water,* Decatur, Ga, 1988, BioLab.

Pool & Spa News, Los Angeles.

Pope JR Jr: *Public swimming pool management.* I and II. Alexandria, Va, 1991, National Recreation and Park Association.

Recreonics: *Buyers' guide and operations handbook,* Indianapolis, Ind, 1991, Catalog Number 41.

Service Industry News, Torrance, Calif.

Taylor, C: *Everything you always wanted to know about pool care,* Chino, Calif, 1989, Service Industry Publications.

Torney, JA, Clayton RD: *Aquatic instruction, coaching and management,* Minneapolis, 1970, Burgess Publishing.

Washington State Public Health Association: *Swimming pool operations,* Seattle, 1988, The Association.

Water quality and treatment, ed 3, 1971, The American Water Works Association.

Williams KG: *The aquatic facility operator's manual,* Hoffman Estates, Ill, 1991, National Recreation and Park Association, National Aquatic Section.

Review Questions

1. List each chlorine type and the percentage of available chlorine and the effect on pH.
2. Which of the chlorines are stabilized?
3. Compare disinfection and oxidation.
4. List three additional precautions that must be taken when gas chlorine is used for swimming pool disinfection.
5. Does sodium hypochlorite have a long shelf-life?
6. When calcium hypochlorite is used for disinfection, is no special care needed when storing and handling this type of chlorine?
7. What is one major advantage of lithium hypochlorite?
8. What does cyanuric acid do when combined with chlorine in swimming pool disinfection?
9. What is the difference between organic and inorganic chlorine?
10. Does bromine need to be combined with an oxidizer to work effectively?
11. Do bromamines have the same effect as chloramines?

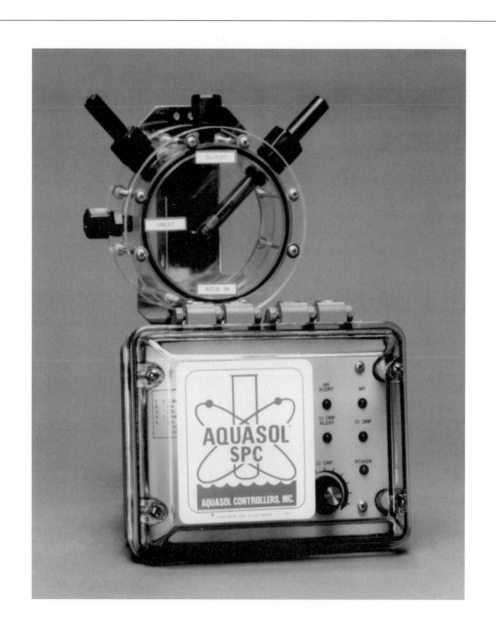

8

SUPERCHLORINATION

Before discussing the vital role superchlorination plays in the swimming pool industry, a discussion of combined chlorine or chloramines must take place. As mentioned in Chapter 7, hypochlorous acid (HOCl) is a by-product produced by adding chlorine to pool water. HOCl is an excellent disinfectant and oxidizer. HOCl is referred to as free-available chlorine (FAC).

Pool operations would indeed be simplified if the free HOCl produced remained free and active in the water, but unfortunately it does not. Free available chlorine combines with contaminates like algae, dust, pollen, urine, perspiration, and other ammonia-nitrogen compounds to form combined available chlorine (CAC). Chloramine is another term used to described combined available chlorine. Technically, there are three types of chloramines, monochloramines, di-chloramines, and tri-chloramines, but for the purposes of this text all three will be considered as simply chloramines. The obnoxious "chlorine odor" found at many pools is not free available chlorine but rather combined available chlorine or chloramines. Chloramines not only smell but also burn eyes and skin and cause cloudy water. Ironically, the very swimmers who complain about chlorine irritation and odor are the cause of it because of the ammonia compounds they naturally carry with them into the pool. It is also important to understand that

the chlorine smell is caused by too little, not too much chlorine. For instance, in a swimming pool that has been effectively superchlorinated, there will be no detectable "chlorine odor," even with high FAC levels (Fig. 8-1).

Chloramines are perhaps the number one problem facing chlorinated pools. As swimmer loads increase, so does the likelihood of chloramine formation. Chloramines are not effective disinfectants. The only way to rid a pool of its chloramines is by adding an amount of new chlorine that is *10 times greater* than the existing combined available chlorine count (CAC). Table 8-1 should help to explain this concept.

A DPD test kit is needed to determine the FAC and total available chlorine levels (TAC). Knowing these levels, FAC can be subtracted for TAC, resulting in a CAC count in ppm.

When using a DPD test kit, FAC is found first by adding five drops of the reagent no. 1 and five drops of reagent no. 2 (or a no. 1 DPD tablet) to the water sample. Using this FAC sample, another five drops of DPD no. 3 (or a no. 3 DPD tablet) is added to determine TAC. FAC is simply subtracted from TAC to find CAC.

Superchlorination, Breakpoint, and "Shocking"

Although there are subtle differences between superchlorination, breakpoint, and shocking, they are considered synonymous by many pool operators. It is important to clarify these concepts to help you operate your pool efficiently. Understanding how to destroy it is more important than knowing the exact terminology for CAC prevention and destruction.

Superchlorination usually refers the intentional elevation of FAC pool operators periodically maintain in the pool to prevent algae, odors, irritation, and

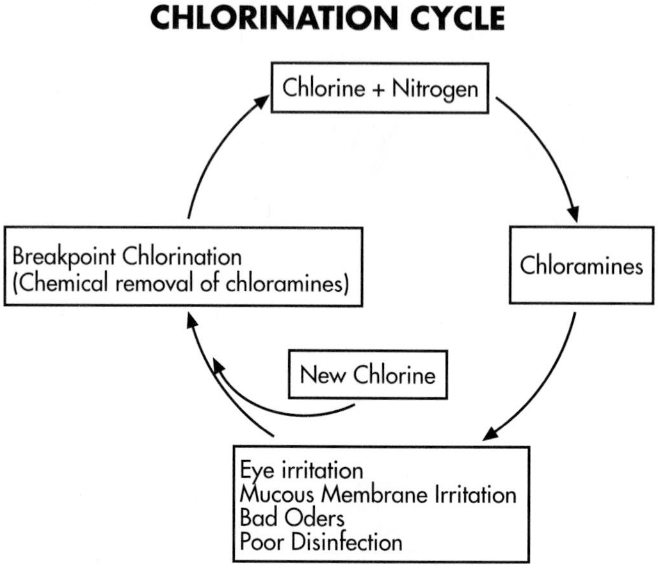

CHLORINATION CYCLE

Fig. 8-1. Chloramine cycle. (From NSPI: *Basic pool and spa technology*, ed 2, Alexandria, Va, The Institute.)

Table 8-1.	Determining CAC
Chlorine	**Amount**
TAC	1.8 ppm
FAC	-1.1 ppm
CAC	.7 ppm
FAC to be added	7.0 ppm

cloudiness. In this case FAC is often raised to between 3 and 10 ppm. Superchlorination is more of a preventive measure, keeping the water clear and comfortable by elevating FAC and not allowing problems to develop. Pool operators normally just estimate a level they think will work for them and increase the FAC if chloramines do develop.

Breakpoint, on the other hand, refers to a very specific and measurable point at which all organic impurities are oxidized. The point at which this occurs (FAC approximately 10 times greater than the CAC count), can be measured with a test kit. Maintaining breakpoint chlorination is slightly different and refers to keeping FAC levels sufficiently high so that ammonia and nitrogen compounds are "burned out" as they are introduced into the pool. In this case, organics are immediately oxidized, and therefore chloramines are

unable to develop. Maintaining breakpoint requires maintaining a 10:1 ratio of FAC to ammonia compounds. The level of FAC needed to ensure a chloramine-free pool will vary; low usage pools will require lower FACs, whereas heavy volume pools require relatively high FACs.

Shocking usually refers to a corrective measure that must be performed because a pool problem has arisen because of algae or chloramines. Shocking means attaining breakpoint through superchlorination. The point of this discussion, however, is to illustrate the importance of eliminating CAC in swimming pools, regardless of how that is accomplished. Knowing the difference between superchlorination, breakpoint, and shocking is a matter of semantics.

When should a pool be shocked? When a test kit reveals a CAC level of between .2 ppm and .4 ppm, the pool should probably be shocked to 10 times the CAC count. Usually at .4 ppm CAC, eye irritation and "chlorine" odors become offensive. If the CAC levels are at .4 ppm, then 4.0 ppm of FAC should be added to the pool to kill all ammonia compounds. It is important to note that if the amount of new chlorine is *less* than 10 times the CAC level, even more chloramines will be found in the pool, compounding the existing problem. When shocking a pool, it is always better to overchlorinate rather than under-chlorinate.

As the new chlorine attacks chloramines, it converts the chloramines to nitrogen, which leaves the pool as a harmless gas. For this reason outdoor pools are much easier to superchlorinate than indoor pools because indoors pools may not allow the gas to escape, making breakpoint difficult to attain. Likewise, shocking should not be performed on a pool that is covered. When shocking an indoor pool, doors and windows should be opened to allow sufficient ventilation for the nitrogen gas to escape.

Once breakpoint is accomplished, the pool should remain closed until the FAC levels drop to an acceptable level (3.0 to 5.0 ppm). Also, the addition of Sodium Thiosulfate may be used to neutralize excessively high amounts of FAC. In general, superchlorination should probably be performed more frequently in many pools around the country. This is probably because many pool operators fear high levels of chlorine in the water. These individuals must realize that it is CAC that causes problems, not FAC. Many European pools that still use chlorine often maintain FAC levels between 8 to 10 ppm. The "burning out" of contaminants and chloramines is a routine practice that is highly recommended.

Dosages

How much chlorine is required to shock a pool? The answer to this question depends on many variables, but once the CAC level is established a simple formula may be followed. To rid the chloramines from a pool, 10 times the amount of CAC in new FAC must be added to the pool. Realizing that a 120,000 gallon pool weighs approximately 1 million pounds, then it follows that 1 pound of gas chlorine will raise the FAC 1 ppm in a 120,000 gallon pool. One gallon of sodium hypochlorite and 1.6 pounds of calcium hypochlorite are equivalent to 1 pound of gas.

EXAMPLE 1

For example, if a CAC of .4 ppm is found in a 80,000 gallon pool, how much chlorine must be added to successfully shock this pool?

1. Find the total amount of chlorine needed to burn out the chloramines. 10 X .4 ppm CAC = 4.0 ppm FAC must be added to 80,000 gallons for shocking.

2. Find the "pool factor" by dividing 80,000 gallons by 120,000 gallons 80,000 gallons divided by 120,000 gallons = a pool factor of .66.

3. Multiply FAC of 4.0 X pool factor of .66 X 1 pound of gas, *OR* 1 gallon of liquid, *OR* 1.6 pounds of cal hypo.

ANSWER

4.0 X .66 X 1 pound = 2.64 pounds of gas chlorine

4.0 X .66 X 1 gallon = 2.64 gallons of sodium hypochlorite

4.0 X .66 X 1.6 pounds = 4.22 pounds of calcium hypo

NOTE: For practical purposes and to ensure that breakpoint chlorination is achieved, the above figures should be rounded up to 3 pounds of gas, 3 gallons of liquid, and 5 pounds of calcium hypochlorite.

EXAMPLE 2

CAC levels in a 240,000 gallon pool are found to be .5 ppm. How much chlorine is needed to shock this pool successfully?

1. 10 x .5 ppm = 5.0 ppm FAC must be added

2. Pool factor = 240,000 ÷ 120,000 = pf of 2

3. 5.0 ppm X 2 X 1 pound of gas, *OR* 1 gallon of liquid, *OR* 1.6 pounds of calcium hypochlorite

ANSWER

10 pounds of gas

10 gallons of sodium hypochlorite (liquid)

16 pounds of calcium hypochlorite

Perhaps an even easier way of determining how much chlorine should be added to a pool is to figure how much FAC must be added and then simply refer to a chart furnished by many pool chemical companies. Adjustments might be required for very large pools containing a larger volume of water than is found on the chart. One example found below is furnished by Taylor Technologies (Table 8-2).

Gas chlorine is not a practical form of chlorine to shock with because it takes time to inject the chlorine into the pool, and many chlorine regulators are not capable of delivering sufficiently high dosages. Chlorine gas levels may climb slowly and even dissipate while being added. The advantage of shocking with sodium and calcium hypochlorite is that they can both be broadcast directly into the pool and therefore reach breakpoint more rapidly. Calcium hypochlorite used for shocking may cause temporary cloudiness. Another advantage of using sodium hypochlorite to shock, particularly when gas is the

Table 8-2. Amount of chlorine compound to introduce 1 ppm chlorine

Available chlorine (%)†	Volume of water*						
	250 gals / 946 L	400 gals / 1,514 L	1,000 gals / 3,785 L	5,000 gals / 18,927 L	20,000 gals / 77,708 L	50,000 gals / 189,271 L	100,000 gals / 378,541 L
5	3.90 tsp / 18.9 mL†	2.00 TBS† / 30.2 mL†	2.60 oz / 75.6 mL†	1.60 cups† / 378 mL†	3.20 pts / 1.51 L†	4.00 qts / 3.78 L†	2.00 gals† / 7.56 L†
10	1.90 tsp / 9.45 mL†	1.00TBS* / 15.1 mL†	1.30 oz / 37.8 mL†	.80 cups† / 189 mL†	1.60 pts / 756 mL*	2.00 qts / 1.89 L†	1.00 gals* / 3.78 L†
12	1.60 tsp / 7.88 mL†	.83 TBS / 12.6 mL†	1.10 oz / 31.5 mL†	.67 cups† / 158 mL†	1.33 pts / 630 mL†	1.67 qts† / 1.58 L†	.83 gal / 3.15 L†
35	.088 oz / 2.71 g	.15 oz / 4.33 g	.38 oz / 10.8 g	1.91 oz / 54.1 g†	7.62 oz / 216 g	1.19 lbs / 541 g	2.38 lbs / 1.08 kg
60	.056 oz / 1.58 g	.088 oz / 2.53 g	.22 oz / 6.32 g	1.11 oz / 31.6 g	4.40 oz / 126 g	11.10 oz / 316 g	1.39 lbs / 632 g
65	.052 oz / 1.46 g	.082 oz / 2.33 g	.21 oz / 5.82 g	1.03 oz / 29.1 g	4.12 oz / 116 g	10.30 oz / 291 g	1.29 lbs / 582 g
90	.037 oz / 1.05 g	.059 oz / 1.68 g	.15 oz / 4.20 g	.74 oz / 21.0 g	3.00 oz / 84.0 g	7.40 oz / 210 g	14.8 oz / 420 g
100	.033 oz / .95 g	.053 oz / 1.51 g	.13 oz / 3.78 g	.67 oz / 18.9 g	2.67 oz / 75.6 g	6.67 oz / 189 g	13.3 oz / 378 g

Courtesy Taylor Technologies, Sparks, Md.

*If there is not a column which corresponds exactly to the pool/spa size, the correct amount can be calculated from existing columns. For instance, to recieve treatment amounts for a 30,000 gallon pool, the value for 20,000 plus 2 times the 5,000 gallon value will give approximately the amount of chemical to add. Alternatively, the 20,000 gallon value plus .5 times the 20,000 gallon value will give a result.

†To add chlorine products as prescribed the following products can be used:

Chlorine Product	Available Chlorine
chlorine gas	100%
trichlorisocyanurate	80%-90%
calcium hypochlorite	65%
dichlorisocyanurate	55%-65%
lithium hypochlorite	30%
sodium hypochlorite	5%-15%

primary disinfectant, is that sodium hypochlorite elevates the pH while shocking so that pH adjustments are usually not needed. Because of its fast solubility in water, lithium hypochlorite is also becoming popular for superchlorination.

Monopersulfate-based oxidation

An alternative to superchlorination is a nonchlorine shocking agent called monopersulfate. Monopersulfate is also known as potassium peroxymonosulfate or monopotassium persulfate. Monopersulfate is an oxygen-based shocking chemical that oxidizes like chlorine but without the disadvantages associated with superchlorination. Some of the drawbacks of shocking with chlorine include closing the pools for 8 to 10 hours, bleaching of vinyl liners and similar equipment, and misjudging breakpoint, therefore adding too much, or worse yet, too little chlorine.

Monopersulfate destroys all chloramines and organic wastes without having to climb to a predetermined "breakpoint." One pound of monopersulfate per 10,000 gallons is the recommended dosage. This dosage may vary, however, because monopersulfate comes in both 42% and 32% active ingredient. Overdosing does not result in high levels of chlorine and underdosing does not result in additional chloramine formation. Underdosing with monopersulfate simply kills some but not all of the chloramines. But perhaps the greatest advantage of monopersulfate is

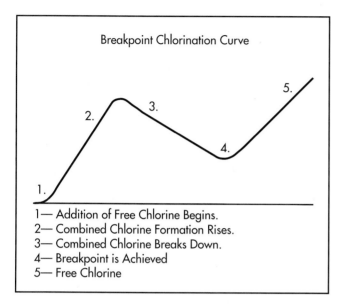

Fig. 8-2. Breakpoint chlorination curve. (From *Service Industry News*, Torrance, Calif, 1993.)

that swimmers can return to the water within 15 minutes of shocking. This advantage of nonchlorine shocking agents becomes even more important during large swimming events, when shocking may be required but closing the pool is not possible. Nonchlorine shocking agents like monopersulfate are quite expensive, however, and as a result are recommended for pools having less than 100,000 gallons.

Summary

Good pool chemistry requires constant monitoring of TAC and FAC to determine the presence of combined available chlorine (CAC). As chloramines develop, the pool should be shocked. Preventing chloramines through periodic superchlorination and maintaining breakpoint is much more desirable than burning out chloramines through shocking.

To best review superchlorination, it would be helpful to examine the chlorine cycle that takes place in swimming pools (Fig. 8-2).

Bibliography

Gabrielson AM: *Swimming pools: a guide to their planning, design, and operation*, ed 4, Champaign, Ill, 1987, Human Kinetics.

Johnson R: *YMCA pool operations manual*, Champaign, Ill, 1989, YMCA.

Kowalsky L (ed): *Pool/spa operators handbook*, San Antonio, Tex, 1991, National Swimming Pool Foundation.

Knoop DF: Redd R: Shocking news: analyzing the options, *Aquatics* March/April 1991.

Mitchel K: *The proper management of pool and spa water*, Decatur, Ga, 1988, BioLab.

Pool and Spa News, Los Angeles.

Service Industry News, Torrance, Calif.

Taylor C: *Everything you always wanted to know about pool care*, Chino, Calif, 1989, Service Industry Publications.

Taylor Technologies: *Pool and spa water chemistry, testing and treatment guide with tables*, Sparks, Md.

Williams KG: *The aquatic facility operator's manual*, Hoffman Estates, Ill, 1991, National Recreation and Park Association, National Aquatic Section.

Review Questions

1. What exactly causes the "chlorine odor" around swimming pools?
2. How much FAC must be added to a pool to rid it of all chloramines?
3. Name a nonchlorine shocking agent.
4. If a 75,000 gallon pool contains .6 ppm of CAC, how much sodium hypochlorite must be added to the pool to achieve breakpoint?
5. If a 200,000 gallon pool has a CAC level of .4 ppm, how much calcium hypochlorite must be added to achieve breakpoint?
6. If a 120,000 gallon pool has 2.0 ppm TAC and 1.0 ppm FAC, how many pounds of gas chlorine must be added to achieve breakpoint?

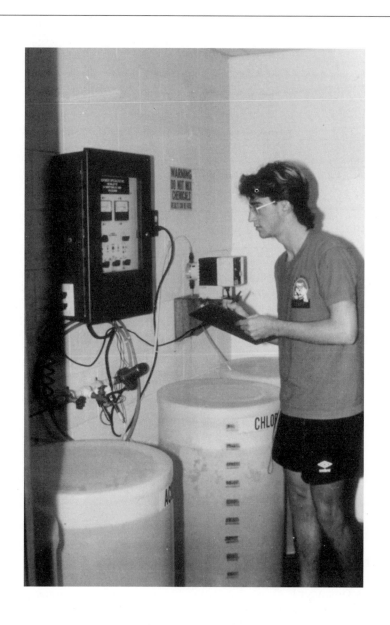

9

pH AND WATER BALANCE

KEY CONCEPTS

- *Unbalanced Water*
- *Total Alkalinity*
- *Scaling Water*
- *Calcium Hardness*
- *Corrosive Water*
- *Langelier Index*
- *TDS*
- *Hamilton Index*
- *pH*

Swimming pool water may come from one of several sources including municipal water companies, private wells, and surface run-off. Sources like lakes and reservoirs are the most common supplies. This source water used to fill swimming pools is usually called "make-up" water. Make-up water may not provide perfectly balanced water and may in fact have components that are not compatible with pools. In addition, the environment may introduce many forms of debris into the pool water to affect its balance.

Water balance refers to water that is neither corrosive nor scale-forming. The factors that determine the balance of water are pH, total alkalinity, calcium hardness, total dissolved solids, and temperature. For swimming pool equipment to function effectively, balanced water is a must. Unbalanced water can destroy a pool shell and its plumbing in a matter of a few years. pH plays two major roles in water chemistry: it buffers acidic disinfectants added to swimming pool water, thus enhancing bather comfort, and second, pH is the most significant determinate in water balancing.

It must be emphasized that most health depart-

ments regulating public pools are only concerned with pH and chlorine readings. Health officials care little about other components of water balance like total alkalinity and calcium hardness, because they do not affect the health and well-being of pool patrons. The importance of all elements of water balance, however, cannot be overlooked by the pool owner/operator. In the New York City area, for example, water generally has a pH of approximately 6.5 and a total alkalinity of about 10 ppm. This extremely aggressive water would destroy a swimming pool and its components quickly, if left unbalanced.

pH

Many pool experts agree that pH is the most important element in swimming pool water chemistry. Every chemical produced or introduced into the pool is either affected by or has an effect on pH. pH not only buffers disinfectants but also determines the water balance in the pool. Swimmers are comfortable in water that is slightly basic, usually between 7.2 and 7.8 (Fig. 9-1).

Simplified, pH is a numerical value that indicates whether water is acidic or basic. Water dissociates much like hypochlorous acid to form hydroxide (OH^-) ions and hydrogen (H^+) ions. The concentration of hydrogen ions determines the pH of water. "pH" actually means potential of hydrogen ions. The greater the hydrogen concentration, the lower the pH. The lower the pH, the more acidic and the less basic the pool water. When the hydrogen ion concentration is equal to the hydroxide ion concentration, the water is said to be neutral. Neutral water has a pH of 7. Distilled water is neutral. The pH scale extends from 0 to 14 with values below 7 being acidic and values above 7 being basic. The smaller the pH

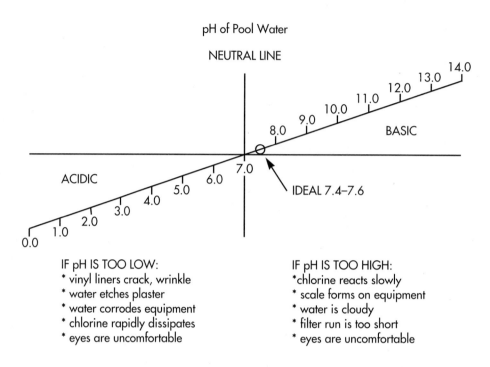

Fig. 9-1. The pH of pool water. (From NSPI: *Basic pool and spa technology*, ed 2, Alexandria, Va, 1992, The Institute.)

value, the more acidic the water. The larger the pH value, the more basic the water.

Acidic water is corrosive, whereas basic water is scale-forming. Acidic water can corrode metal surfaces including filter tanks, valves, pipes, heaters, and other pool plumbing. Corrosive water can also burn skin and eyes and even erode tooth enamel. Scale, on the other hand, is a white precipitate that builds up on pipes, pumps, and other pool equipment making them either less effective or nonfunctional. Basic water can also cause cloudiness and skin irritation. The higher the pH, the less effective the disinfectant.

The pH scale is a logarithmic concept that is important to understand yet somewhat complicated. When looking at the pH scale it is important to realize that each unit division represents a tenfold increase or decrease in acidity. Each division on the scale is a multiple of 10. For instance, beginning at the neutral value of 7, a pH of 6 is ten times more acidic than a pH of 7, a pH of 5 is 100 times more acidic than a pH of 7, and a pH of 4 is a 1000 times more acidic than a pH of 7. Going in the other direction, a pH of 8 is 10 times more basic than a pH of 7, while a pH of 9 is 100 times more basic and a pH of 10 is a 1000 times more basic than a pH of 7. A movement of just 0.5 on

the pH scale will result in a 280% increase or decrease in acidity depending on which direction the pH changes. Hopefully, this discussion illustrates just how significant relatively small pH changes affect water balance. The pH values of most swimming pools should be maintained between 7.2 and 7.8. As the pH climbs closer to 7.8, bather comfort may increase, but more chlorine will be required at this elevated pH. As the pH lowers towards 7.2, less chlorine is needed but bather comfort is reduced. A pH of 7.5 is considered ideal by many.

Raising pH

To raise pH, basic or alkaline compounds are used. Soda ash (sodium carbonate) is the most common substance used to increase pH. Soda ash is a fine white powder that is usually mixed with water first and then injected by a chemical feeder pump into the pool water. Soda ash feeders are notorious for becoming clogged, particularly around the ball check valves and the injector. Soda ash feeders must be cleaned on a regular basis. Running muriatic acid periodically through the feeder often prevents clogging. Soda ash can also be added directly into the pool, but it should be mixed with water first.

In some pools sodium hydroxide (caustic soda) is used instead of soda ash. Sodium hydroxide is a liquid that is extremely effective in raising pH and less expensive than soda ash, but it is difficult to handle and freezes between 50° and 60° F. Although sodium bicarbonate does raise the pH, it is not intended for that purpose. Sodium bicarbonate should only be used to raise total alkalinity.

Gas chlorine significantly lowers the pH, so when gas chlorine is used, soda ash is also added to raise the pH. Testing and adjusting for pH will be thoroughly discussed in Chapters 10 and 11.

Lowering pH

When the pH needs to be lowered, an acid must be introduced into the pool. The most common acid used for this purpose, particularly in large, public pools is muriatic acid(hydrochloric acid). Muriatic acid is a corrosive acid that is relatively inexpensive, but it must be handled carefully. If muriatic acid container lids do not fit snugly, muriatic fumes escaping from the container can cause severe damage to electrical equipment like telephones and automatic chemical controllers. Rubber gloves and safety goggles should always be worn when working with muriatic acid.

A safer alternative to muriatic acid is sodium bisulfate, which is often referred to as dry acid because it comes in a white granule. Sodium bisulfate is much easier to handle, but it is quite expensive. Many residential and smaller pools use sodium bisulfate or dry acid.

CO_2 gas is a relatively new method of lowering pH in swimming pools. This gas is inherently safe to use, as evidenced by its use in restaurants to produce the carbonation in soft drinks. CO_2 also raises the total alkalinity as it lowers the pH, another big advantage for pools with low total alkalinity. This gas is also kind to metals and does not emit corrosive gases. CO_2 can be used in the equipment room very safely and conveniently. CO_2 mixed with water forms carbonic acid, which in turn liberates hydrogen ions, which lowers pH. To use CO_2 successfully at a pool, an expert must install the system, a local supplier must be available, and it should be delivered in bulk. Some claim when CO_2 is used, an increase in algae growth may be noticed. A pool using sodium hypochlorite will experience a continual and significant rise in pH, therefore either muriatic acid, sodium bisulfate, or CO_2 must be added in this case.

pH levels are determined with a test kit. Phenol Red is perhaps the most common pH test reagent. pH reagents should be replaced every 6 months. pH levels should be checked with chlorine levels on an hourly basis in most pools.

Total Alkalinity

Total alkalinity is a measure of the resistance of water to changes in pH and is measured in ppms. The higher the total alkalinity, the more difficult it is to change pH with either acid or soda ash. The lower the total alkalinity the more likely pH is to change; even slight changes in chemicals, swimmer loads, and weather can have a significant effect on pH or cause "pH" bounce. Pool operators experiencing difficulties either adjusting pH levels or maintaining a target pH should analyze the total alkalinity.

More specifically, total alkalinity is a measurement of alkaline components in the water. These components include carbonate (CO_3^{-2}), bicarbonate (HCO_3^{-1}), and hydroxide (OH^{-1}) with some other alkaline materials making minor contributions. In the ideal pH range for pools (7.2 to 7.6), the bicarbonates make the greatest contribution.

pH and total alkalinity in swimming pools are closely related. When pool water has a low pH, all carbonate ions are converted to bicarbonates and no calcium carbonates are formed. As a result, without calcium carbonate available, the water becomes corrosive to the shell, equipment, and plumbing. Conversely, when pool water has a high pH, calcium precipitates out of the water and causes cloudiness.

Most pools should maintain the total alkalinity levels between 100 to 150 ppm. It should be noted that most health departments do not dictate ideal ranges for total alkalinity because they only effect pool plumbing and not people's health. Vinyl liner and fiberglass pools may need a slightly higher total alkalinity (125 to 175 ppm). Total alkalinity should not drop below 100 ppm, except in regions that have very high calcium hardness levels. In this case, when the calcium hardness in a pool is greater than 500 ppm, the total alkalinity may be allowed to drop to no less than 80 ppm.

When in doubt about the recommended total alkalinity level for a particular pool, the pool builder or local pool company should be consulted. It should be noted that when cyanuric acid is added to pool water to stabilize chlorine, it artificially elevates the total alkalinity level. When the total alkalinity is low (less

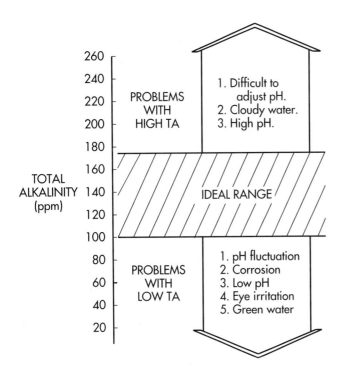

Fig. 9-2. Problems when TA is not in proper range. (From NSPI: *Basic pool and spa technology*, ed 2, Alexandria, Va, 1992, The Institute.)

than 80 PPM), and the CYA level is high (more than 60 PPM), one third of the CYA reading should be subtracted from the total alkalinity level for a true total alkalinity level.

Raising total alkalinity

A low total alkalinity not only makes it difficult to maintain the ideal pH but may also eventually lead to highly corrosive water, which could damage filters, pool shell, heaters, and other equipment. Low alkalinity is also associated with green water and the etching of plaster. Very low total alkalinity (below 50 PPM) can also be linked to eyeburn.

Sodium bicarbonate ($NaHCO_3$) should be added to raise total alkalinity. Sodium bicarbonate is also known as baking soda, bicarb, and bicarbonate of soda. Sodium bicarbonate only slightly affects the pH. Although soda ash also tends to raise the total alkalinity, sodium bicarbonate is the recommended chemical for this purpose. Specific instructions regarding total alkalinity adjustments will be discussed in Chapter 11.

Lowering total alkalinity

High total alkalinity causes the pH to stick at a certain level, making it difficult to change. Much time and money can be spent on moving the pH even slightly. Additionally, high total alkalinity leads to scale build-up and may cause cloudy water.

To lower total alkalinity, an acid must be used. Muriatic acid (liquid) and sodium bisulfate (powder) are two acids commonly used for this purpose. Muriatic acid is more commonly used in public pools. Special instructions for adding these acids will be discussed in Chapter 11. Total alkalinity should be adjusted prior to adjusting other chemicals, particularly pH and calcium hardness (Fig. 9-2).

Calcium Hardness

"Hardness" is a term often used to refer to the mineral content of water. All water supplies have varying amounts of calcium and magnesium that make water "hard." In swimming pools calcium accounts for nearly 95% of the hardness. The hardness of water is created by water moving over soil, rocks, and other solids. Although calcium and magnesium are the major contributors to hardness, other elements like carbonates, chlorides, nitrates, sulfates, and other mineral salts all help to make water hard.

Although many households prefer "soft" water, this type of water can be disastrous in swimming pools. Pool water must have a high degree of hardness or the pool itself and its equipment will deteriorate. Although the U.S. Geological Survey considers water having more than 180 PPM of calcium hardness "very hard," this level is actually too "soft" for most swimming pools.

Soft water foams, whereas very hard water does not. Hot tubs that foam may need the calcium hardness adjusted. Swimming pools with less than 200 PPM calcium hardness are considered "hungry" for calcium and as a result will dissolve any source of hardness, but particularly plaster and grout. Low hardness will also adversely affect the water balance in the pool.

As measured in swimming pools in parts per million, calcium hardness (CH) indicates calcium (Ca^{+2}) content of the water. The recommended range for calcium hardness is between 200 and 400 ppm (Fig. 9-3). This text does not examine total hardness, which is the sum of two types of hardness: carbonate and noncarbonate. These types of hardness are also referred to as temporary and permanent.

Typically, low calcium hardness is more of a problem to swimming pools than high calcium hardness. Low calcium hardness combined with a low pH and

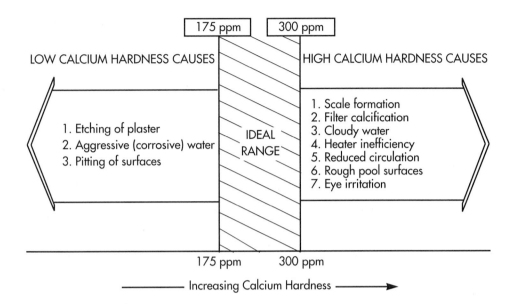

Fig. 9-3. Problems when calcium hardness is not in proper range. (From NSPI: *Basic pool and spa technology*, ed 2, Alexandria, Va, 1992, The Institute.)

low total alkalinity will significantly increase the corrosiveness and aggressiveness of the water. Water that is low in calcium hardness will result in surface etching and pitting of the pool shell. As the aggressiveness of the water increases, the solubility of calcium carbonate also increases. This means that plaster and marsite pool finishes will deteriorate quickly because calcium carbonate is a major component of both plaster and marsite. The dissolving or breakdown of these pool finishes is called etching.

Low calcium hardness also leads to corrosion of metal components in the pool plant, particularly in heat exchanges. Calcium carbonate usually provides a protective film on the surface of copper heat exchangers and heat sinks. This thin layer prevents much water to metal interaction but does not adversely affect the heating process. Without this protective layer caused by low calcium hardness, heat exchangers and associated parts can be destroyed prematurely. Strangely enough, as water temperature increases, solubility of calcium carbonate decreases. The recommended range for most pools is between 200 and 400 ppm. Calcium hardness should be tested bimonthly in most pools.

Raising calcium hardness

If calcium hardness needs to be raised, calcium chloride dehydrate should be added to the pool.

Calcium chloride should be predissolved before it is added to the pool. Specific instructions for adding calcium chloride are discussed in Chapter 11.

Lowering Calcium Hardness

In rare instances the calcium hardness may be too high in a swimming pool. High calcium hardness causes a host of pool problems including:

1. Scale formation
2. Filter calcification
3. Heater inefficiency
4. Rough pool surfaces
5. Eye irritation

Perhaps the only practical way of removing calcium hardness from the water is to drain varying amounts of water from the pool, depending of course on how high the calcium level is. This may also be accomplished by simply prolonging the backwash cycle. If source (make-up) water has exceedingly high calcium hardness, the pH and total alkalinity levels may have to be lowered. However, the pH should never be allowed to drop below 7.2, nor should the total alkalinity be allowed to fall below 80 ppm.

If after draining water and adjusting pH and total alkalinity levels, high calcium hardness still causes unbalanced, overly basic pool water, a water softener

Table 9-1. To Increase Calcium Hardness Using Calcium Chloride Dihydrate (CaCl$_2$-2H$_2$O)

Desired calcium increase	Gallons of water			
	1000	5000	10,000	25,000
10 ppm	2 oz	10 oz	1.25 lbs	6.25 lbs
25 ppm	5 oz	1.6 lbs	3.12 lbs	15.6 lbs
50 ppm	10 oz	3.2 lbs	6.24 lbs	31.2 lbs

16 oz equals 1 lb; 1 oz equals 28.35 g.

may be required to reduce the calcium hardness level. Sodium phosphate water softeners are not recommended for pool use, but sodium zeolite softeners are. Some sequestering agents may also be used to prevent calcium carbonate scale formation in water with high calcium hardness.

It must be pointed out that as temperatures climb and evaporation rates increase, water leaves the pool but the minerals remain; thus calcium hardness increases. Also, if calcium hypochlorite is used as the primary disinfectant, calcium hardness levels will tend to rise (Table 9-1).

Total Dissolved Solids (TDS)

Total dissolved solids can be best described as the sum total of all solids dissolved in water. If all the water in a swimming pool was allowed to evaporate, TDS would be accumulated on the bottom of the pool much in the same way white deposits are left in a boiling pot after all the water has evaporated. Some of this dissolved material includes hardness, alkalinity, cyanuric acid, chlorides, bromides, and algacides. TDS also includes bather wastes such as perspiration, urine, body oil, suntan lotion, and others.

TDS levels are a general indicator of pool or spa water quality. Pools with less than 1000 ppm TDS usually have good water quality, whereas pools with more than 3000 ppm may have poor water clarity, but this does not hold true in every case. One of the first signs of high TDS is a dull or cloudy appearance of the water.

TDS accumulates over time. The more chemicals and people added to pool water, the faster the TDS levels will increase. In general, "new" water in recently filled pools will have low TDS levels, whereas

"old" water that has been in a pool or spa for a long period of time will have a high TDS level. A rough rule of thumb is that the TDS level will double during the first year after a pool is filled. Most make-up water has less than 400 ppm TDS. By comparison, salt water in the ocean has a TDS level of approximately 35,000 ppm. Not surprisingly, when pool water has excessively high TDS levels the water will actually taste salty.

High TDS values can lead to some pools problems (Fig 9-4). These include a reduced chlorine efficiency, algae growth, corrosive water, and worst of all, cloudiness. Hot tubs and spas have a more significant problem with TDS levels than pools because the swimmer load is relatively higher, more chemicals are added for superchlorination and sudsing, and as water temperature increases, calcium carbonate becomes less soluble. Increased corrosion is due to the increased electrical conductance that a high TDS pool promotes, resulting in electrolysis or "galvanic" corrosion.

To reduce the TDS level in a pool simply requires replacing some or all of the water with fresh water that has normal TDS levels. Hot tubs should probably be "dumped" on a weekly basis. Many pools, however, can keep TDS levels in control by simply adding fresh water on a daily basis. Emptying a pool should not be a seasonal or annual occurrence unless the TDS elevate above so high that the water becomes cloudy.

TDS has only a small effect on the Langelier Saturation Index, which will be discussed next. Because corrosiveness increases as TDS increases it is a good practice to subtract a tenth (.1) from the Saturation Index for every 1000 ppm TDS above 1000.[1]

Measuring TDS requires a portable electronic ana-

TOTAL DISSOLVED SOLIDS

Potable Water	200-600 ppm
Brackish Water	3,000-5,000 ppm
Sea Water	35,000 ppm
Great Salt Lakes	260,000 ppm

Total Dissolved Solids are introduced into the pool water by:

INCREASED TDS CAN

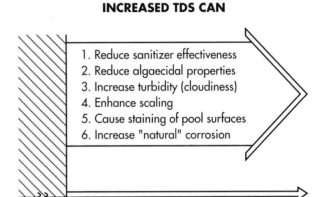

1. Reduce sanitizer effectiveness
2. Reduce algaecidal properties
3. Increase turbidity (cloudiness)
4. Enhance scaling
5. Cause staining of pool surfaces
6. Increase "natural" corrosion

0   2,000 ppm   INCREASING TDS

DISINFECTANTS
CALCIUM HARDNESS
BALANCE CHEMICALS
ALGAECIDES
WIND BLOWN DUST & DIRT
SOURCE WATER
BATHERS
TOTAL ALKALINITY
BODY OILS
EVAPORATION

Fig. 9-4. Problems when TDS is not in proper range. (From NSPI: *Basic pool and spa technology*, ed 2, Alexandria, Va, 1992, The Institute.)

lyzer. Every hot water pool should consider this TDS analyzer a standard piece of equipment, but it may not be required for most public pools. If high TDS is suspected at larger public pools, a local pool supplier may be called to analyze the water.

Temperature

As temperature increases, calcium carbonate becomes less soluble, causing it to precipitate out of solution at higher temperatures. Additionally, temperature is one of five important factors considered in the Langelier Saturation Index. The Saturation Index determines whether a pool is corrosive or scale-forming. The Saturation Index compares different values of pH, CH, and TA for water of varying temperatures. As temperature increases, the water balance tends to become more basic and scale-producing. However, as temperature drops, water becomes more corrosive.

In addition to helping determine water balance, temperature will also affect algae growth (as temperature increases so does algae growth), chlorination, and evaporation.

Water Balance and The Langelier Saturation Index

In 1936 a scale was developed by Langelier of the University of California to determine water balance. Perfectly balanced water is usually defined as water that is neither corrosive nor scale-forming. The corrosiveness or scaling properties of water can be determined by the use of Langelier's Index. This complicated scale was originally developed to better understand hot water chemistry so that boilers and heat exchangers would operate more efficiently. The main purpose of this index was to predict if the water analyzed will keep calcium carbonate in solution or will it precipitate out.

The original index has been simplified for swimming pool use. Pool owners and operators should note that chlorine and other disinfecting chemicals are not are part of water balance. Before examining the specifics of this index it would be wise to review two basic properties of water balance, corrosiveness and scaling.

Corrosive Water

Corrosive water is "hungry" water that attempts to "eat" everything it comes in contact with. Corrosive water aggressively dissolves metals, particularly copper and iron. Corrosive water also dissolves and etches plaster. A swimming pool plant with corrosive water in it is being "eaten away" and destroyed by the water. A saturation index with a minus (-) value indicates corrosive water.

Scaling Water

Scaling water does not corrode but causes another problem by precipitating scale, cloudiness, or residue. Unlike "hungry" aggressive water, scaling water may be considered overfed or overstuffed, containing too many components. Scaling water will clog pipes and valves and calcify filter mediums. Basic water that is only slightly scaling may produce a beneficial protective coating on all pool parts. A saturation index with a plus (+) value indicates basic or scale-forming water.

Equilibrium

Perfectly balanced water is said to be in equilibrium with calcium carbonate. Zero (0) on the saturation index indicates water in the state of equilibrium that will neither precipitate calcium carbonate in the form of scale nor dissolve the pool shell and equipment in an attempt to increase calcium carbonate.

Although the Langelier Saturation Index has been criticized over the years, it still has value in swimming pool applications. It is simple to use and should be conducted on a bimonthly basis for most pools. The following factors are needed to determine water balance:

1. pH
2. Total Alkalinity (TA)
3. Calcium Hardness (CH)
4. Temperature
5. Total Dissolved Solids (TDS)

Only pH, TA, and CH are normally adjusted to achieve water balance. Pool water will often be balanced if pH, TA, and CH are kept within the recommended ranges.

The Saturation Index

To use the saturation index (SI), pH is used as measured with phenol red. Readings for total alkalinity (TA), calcium hardness (CH), and temperature are

---

Table 9-2 The Langelier SI Table					
Table 1 (TF) **temperature**		**Table 2 (CF)** **calcium hardness**		**Table 3 (AF)** **total alkalinity**	
Degrees F	TF	CH(ppm)	CF	TA(ppm)	AF
32	0.1	5	.3	5	.7
37	0.1	25	1.0	25	1.4
46	0.2	50	1.3	50	1.7
53	0.3	75	1.5	75	1.9
60	0.4	100	1.6	100	2.0
66	0.5	150	1.8	150	2.2
76	0.6	200	1.9	200	2.3
84	0.7	300	2.1	300	2.5
94	0.8	400	2.2	400	2.6
105	0.9	800	2.5	800	2.9
128	1.0	1000	2.6	1000	3.0
SI = ph + TF + CF + AF + -12.1					

taken with a standard pool test kit and a thermometer. Once true values are found they are converted to the factors found in the SI table listed below. Once TA, CH, and temperature are converted to AF, CF, and TF, they are totaled and a constant of -12.1 is added to the sum (Table 9-2).

The Formula
SI = pH + TF + CF + AF + -12.1

An index of -0.5 and +0.5 is acceptable pool water

An index of more than +0.5 is scale-forming

An index below -0.5 is corrosive

EXAMPLE 1

A pool has a pH of 8.0, a total alkalinity of 150 PPM, a calcium hardness of 400 PPM, and a temperature of 86° F. Is the pool water corrosive, scaling, or neutral?

SI = pH + TF + AF + CF + -12.1

SI = 8.0 + 0.7 + 2.2 + 2.2 + -12.1 = +1.0

The saturation index indicates that the pool contains water that is too basic, and as a result it is scale-forming. This water would precipitate residue, cloudiness, or scale. The easiest adjustment to make for water balance would be to reduce the pH by adding an acid like muriatic acid. By reducing the pH to 7.3, which is within the ideal range, the SI would be changed to +0.3, which is acceptable.

If, however, a more balanced pool was desired, the total alkalinity could be reduced to 80 ppm, which when combined with a 7.3 pH would result in a SI of +0.1.

SI = pH + TF + AF + CF + -12.1

SI = 7.4 + 0.7 + 1.9 + 2. 2 + - 12.1 = + 0.1

The example above demonstrates an important point concerning the saturation index and water balance. There is a one-to-one relationship between pH and the SI, so therefore pH has the greatest effect on changing water balance. Also, the acid used to lower pH will also lower total alkalinity.

EXAMPLE 2

If a pool has a pH of 6.8, a total alkalinity of 50 PPM, calcium hardness of 30 PPM and a temperature of 78° F, is the pool corrosive, scaling, or balanced?

S I = pH + TF + AF + CF + -12.1

SI = 6.8 + 0.6 + 1.7 + 1.0 + -12.1 = -2.0

The pool in this example is extremely corrosive. Several changes must be made to the water chemistry to protect the pool. Using the saturation index once again, a pH of 7.5, CH of 400 PPM, and a TA of 80 ppm would result in a SI of +0.1.

SI = pH + TF + AF + CF + -12.1

SI = 7.5 + 0.6 + 1.9 + 2.2 + -12.1 = +0.1

By reviewing the ideal ranges recommended for swimming pools, it could be quickly determined that in both examples the water would be out of balance without running a saturation index, because most parameters were well above or below what they should be. In example 1, high pH, TA, and CH levels indicated that this pool was basic. On the other hand, low pH, TA, and CH levels in example 2 predict the aggressiveness of the pool water.

Many swimming pool suppliers offer simple calculators and slide rules that figure the saturation index for the user without having the user work with the math in the saturation index. The pool owner/operator simply uses the actual values for pH, TA, CH, and temperature found with a standard test kit and manipulates the calculator for the saturation index. These devices are accurate, easy to use, inexpensive, and becoming quite popular (Fig. 9-5).

Most pools cannot remain balanced for long periods of time because they are in a state of "dynamic equilibrium." Significant changes in the water take place daily. Also, make-up water in general tends to be either aggressive or scaling. When adding chemicals to balance a pool, it is often a good idea to compensate for the tendencies of a particular pool to "drift" towards the minus or plus side of the Langelier saturation index. As a result many experienced pool owners and operators will move their "target" SI to the other side of zero from the SI usually found.[2] Chemical adjustments will be covered in the next chapter.

As mentioned previously, it must also be remembered that pH has the most significant effect on water balance. Conversely, the temperature of pool water has about one tenth as much effect on water balance as pH. Further, total dissolved solids have even less effect on water balance than either pH or temperature. A change of 1000 ppm TDS has the same effect as changing the pH by 0.1.

To sum up the effects that different components have on the saturation index, the following comparison is offered by Williams[1]:

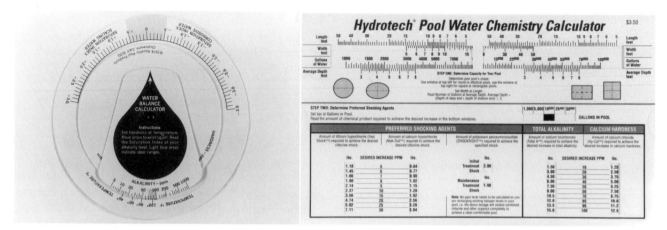

Fig. 9-5. Pool calculators can solve many problems. **A**, watergram. (Courtesy Taylor Technologies, Sparks, Md.) **B**, Water chemistry calculator. (Courtesy BioLab, Decatur, Ga.)

To change the SI by .1:

1. Change the pH by .1
2. Change the water temperature by 8° F
3. Change the total alkalinity by 30 PPM
4. Change the calcium hardness by 50 PPM
5. Change the total dissolved solids by 1000

It is important to note that the Langelier SI provides a basic starting point from which owners and operators may begin to balance their pool water. The Langelier Index examines water balance through a wide angle lens, but many pool operators need a telephoto lens to perfectly balance their water. The Langelier Saturation was developed for closed loop water systems, not dynamic, open water systems like swimming pools.

Jock Hamilton, president of the United Chemical Corporation, developed a water balancing scale that is similar to the saturation index but uses only three factors instead of the five factors needed to calculate Langelier's scale. He also recommends maintaining a higher pH range (7.8 to 8.2). The Hamilton Index uses total hardness, total alkalinity, and pH. Whether or not this method of water balance is more accurate than the Langelier Index has yet to be determined. The Hamilton Index is even easier to use than the Langelier Index.

Summary

pH is one of the most important pool factors and should be checked hourly in most pools. pH is the

most important ingredient for balanced water that is neither corrosive nor scaling. The pool and all its associated parts will last longer and work more efficiently if the water is balanced. The recommended ranges for pH, total alkalinity, calcium hardness, and total dissolved solids is found below (Table 9-3).

References

1. Williams KG: *The aquatic facility operator's manual*, Hoffman Estates, Ill, 1991, National Recreation and Park Association, National Aquatic Section.
2. Olin Corporation: *The complete pool care book*, 1992, Stamford, Conn.

Bibliography

Gabrielson AM: *Swimming pools: a guide to their planning, design, and operation*, ed 4, Champaign, Ill, 1987, Human Kinetics.

Johnson R: *YMCA pool operations manual*, Champaign, Ill, 1989, YMCA.

Kowalsky L (editor): *Pool/spa operators handbook*, San Antonio, Tex, 1991, National Swimming Pool Foundation.

Mitchel K: *The proper management of pool and spa water*, Decatur, Ga, 1988, BioLab.

Pool & Spa News, Los Angeles.

Pope JR Jr: *Public swimming pool management*. I and II. Alexandria, Va, 1991, National Recreation and Park Association.

Service Industry News: Torrance, Calif.

Taylor C: *Everything you always wanted to know about pool care*, Chino, Calif, 1989, Service Industry Publications.

Taylor Technologies: *Pool and spa water chemistry, testing and treatment guide with tables*, Sparks, Md.

Table 9-3. Chemical Operational Guidelines Commercial Application*

	Minimum	Ideal	Maximum	Comments
Disinfectant Levels				
Free Chlorine				Chlorine should be maintained at this level continually; super chlorinate as needed; depends on balanced pH for effectiveness.
Pools	1.0	2.0-3.0	5.0	
Spas	2.0	3.0-4.0	6.0	
Combined chlorine (ppm)	None	None	0.2	If combined chlorine is too high you may have: •Sharp chlorinous odors •Eye burn •Algae growth •Bacterial growth (*Combined chlorine is eliminated by super chlorination).
Bromine (PPM)				Accepted by most Health Departments, often preferred in hot water applications over 95° F.
Pools	1.0	3.0-4.0	5.0	
Spas	2.0	4.0-5.0	6.0	
Ozone				An effective oxidizer to be used with chlorine or bromine sanitizer; short residual life; must be controlled to avoid excess.
Chemical Values				
pH	7.2	7.4-7.6	7.8	If pH is: TOO LOW: •Rapid dissipation of chlorine •Plaster/concrete etching •Eye discomfort •Corrosion of metals / TOO HIGH •Lower chlorine efficiency •Scale formation •Cloudy water •Increased chemical demand •Eye discomfort
Total alkalinity (ppm as $CaCO_3$)	80	100-150	200	If total alkalinity is: TOO LOW •pH bounce •Corrosion tendency •Low pH / TOO HIGH •Cloudy water •Increased scaling potential •pH maintained too high

From Aquasol Controllers, Houston, Tex.
From Aquasol Controllers, Houston, Tex.
*Chemical treatment alone will not produce sanitary pool water. A filtration system in proper operational condition is also required to attain sparking clear, polished sanitary pool water. Remember, it is essential that every spa or pool have proper circulation and filtration to maintain a chemical balance, and clear, sparkling water.

Continued.

Table 9-3.   Chemical Operational Guidelines Commercial Application—cont'd

	Minimum	Ideal	Maximum	Comments
Cyanuric acid	10	30-50	100	Controls chlorine from UV dissipation; used in outdoor and indoor pools; controls stability of chlorine, especially sodium hypochlorite (liquid bleach).
Dissolved solids (ppm TDS)	300	1000-2000	3000	If disolved solids are: TOO LOW: •Total alkalinity may be too low •Aggressive water TOO HIGH: •Chlorine may be less effective •Scaling may occur •Fresh water should be adding to reduce solids •Salty taste •Dull water •Chemical balance difficult to maintain
Hardness (ppm as $CaCO_3$)	150	200-400	800	If hardness is: TOO LOW •Plaster or concrete etching may occur •Corrosion TOO HIGH: •Scaling may occur •Water has bad "feel" •Short filter runs
Copper (ppm)	None	None	0.3	If copper content is TOO HIGH: •Staining may occur •Water may discolor •Chlorine dissipates rapidly by decomposition •Filter may plug •May indicate pH too low, corrosion, etc.
Iron (ppm)	None	None	0.2	If iron is TOO HIGH: •Staining may occur •Water may discolor •Chlorine dissipates rapidly •Filter may plug

Continued.

Table 9-3. Chemical Operational Guidelines Commercial Application—cont'd

	Minimum	Ideal	Maximum	Comments
Biological Values				
Algae	None	None	None	If algae are observed: •Shock treat pool. •Supplement with brushing and vacuuming. •Maintain adequate disinfectant residual. •Use approved algicide according to label directions.
Bacteria	None	None	Refer to local code	If bacteria count exceeds local health department requirements: •Superchlorinate and follow proper maintenance procedures •Maintain proper disinfectant residual

Tepas JJ: Putting Langelier in perspective, *Pool and Spa News*, June 19, 1989.

Washington State Public Health Association: *Swimming pool operations*, Seattle, 1988, The Association.

Water quality and treatment: ed 3, 1971, The American Water Works Association.

Williams KG: *The aquatic facility operator's manual*, Hoffman Estates, Ill, 1991, National Recreation and Park Association, National Aquatic Section.

Review Questions

1. Unbalanced water may be either _____ or _____?
2. To raise pH, what do you add?
3. To lower pH, what do you add?
4. Most pools should maintain the total alkalintiy (TA) somewhere between what ppm?
5. To raise TA, what do you add?
6. To lower TA, what do you add?
7. How will low levels of calcium hardness (CH) affect swimming pools?
8. To raise CH, what do you add?
9. How are high levels of TDS in a swimming pool lowered?
10. List five factors needed to calculate the Langelier Saturation Index.

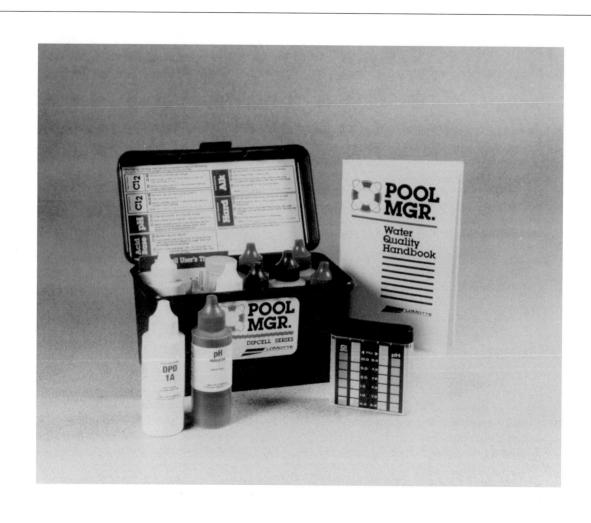

10

WATER TESTING

Just because swimming pool water looks good does not necessarily mean that it is balanced and bacteria-free. Although clear and sparkling pool water is important, it must be monitored frequently to keep good water quality and also detect shifts in water chemistry and balance. A vigilant water testing program will permit pool operators to prevent pool problems before most patrons notice them in the water. Proper use of a swimming pool test kit is a must for all pool owners and operators. For test results to be accurate and reliable, several guidelines must be adhered to. Perhaps the two greatest problems with water testing are testing that is too infrequent and use of test reagents that are too old to produce accurate results.

Types of Tests

Several different types and methods of pool tests can be conducted to analyze water conditions (Fig. 10-1). The following tests have been commonly associated with analyzing pool water and are described as follows:

Colorimetric

These tests utilize the theory that the more you have of a chemical substance in the water, the darker the sample color will become. By adding a chemical indicator or reagent to a sample of pool water, a certain color will be produced. Comparing the color of the test sample with color standards provided with the test kit will determine the level of chemical in the water. Proper lighting is important when conducting a colorimetric test, and the manufacturer's guidelines should be followed closely in this regard. Although this may sound sexist, some test kit companies contend that females are genetically equipped to determine different shades and hues required by colorimetric tests, more so than males. Testing for pH with phenol red is a good example of a colorimetric test.

Titrimetric

During this test a reagent is added or titrated to a prepared test sample until a dramatic change in color takes place. The number of drops needed for this color change is counted to determine ppms. Both total alkalinity and calcium hardness are usually measured in this manner.

Turbidimetric

This test is used to produce a precipitate until a black dot is obscured on the bottom of a vial that is filled with a test sample. This test is usually reserved for measuring cyanuric acid. Melamine is the reagent added to the water sample in this case.

Sampling Techniques

To achieve accurate test results, it is important that the pool water sample is collected and treated properly so that the water is not contaminated (Fig. 10-2). The following guidelines should be followed:

- Hands should be washed with soap and water before collecting a sample.
- Vials used to collect the sample should be rinsed several times in the water that is to be tested. Vials

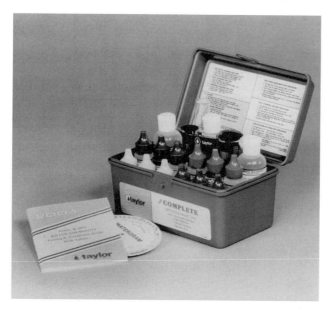

Fig. 10-1. A complete pool water testing kit with instructions and calculator. (Courtesy Taylor Technologies, Sparks, Md.)

used as test cells should also be washed with a detergent periodically and rinsed with distilled water.

• The water collected must be a "representative" sample, that is, it should not be collected from the surface where contaminates collect or in front of an inlet where water with high chemical concentrations is found. Every attempt should be made to collect water samples from 12 to 18 inches below the surface and from several different locations around the pool.

• When attempting to collect the appropriate amount of water in the test cell for a particular test, the bottom of the meniscus curve should lay on top of the test line provided on the vial or test cell. The meniscus curve is the curved surface of a water sample placed in a tube or chamber.

Test Kit Procedures

Many different test kits are available to pool owners and operators (Fig. 10-3). Although prices vary, test kits are generally inexpensive. A commercial grade test kit with a variety of different water tests

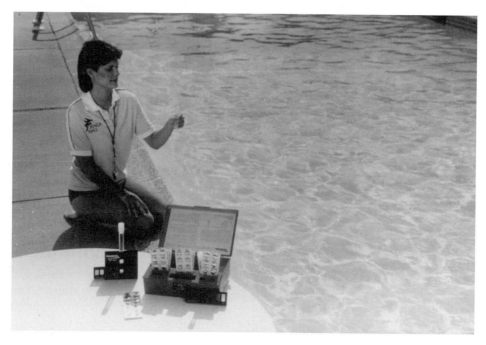

Fig. 10-2. Proper sampling techniques. (Courtesy La Motte, Chestertown, Md.)

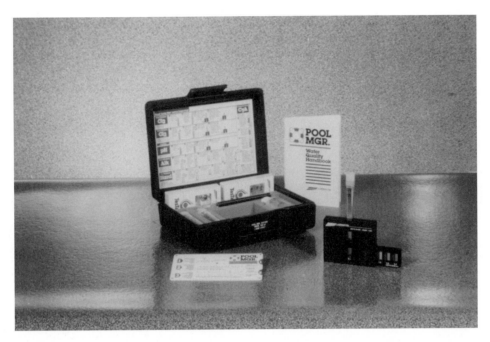

Fig. 10-3. A commercial grade test kit. (Courtesy La Motte, Chestertown, Md.)

and a wide range in readings is recommended. When using a test kit, the following rules should apply:

- Read and follow the directions carefully.
- Only use reagents that are specified by the test kit manufacturer. Do not interchange test kits and reagents. Even different test kit models from the same manufacturer often require different reagents.
- Reagents have a short shelf life and should probably be replaced every 6 months or at the beginning of the season.
- All reagents should be marked with the date of purchase. Whenever possible, reagents should be purchased directly from the manufacturer to ensure freshness.
- When mixing reagents with the water sample in the test cell, use the cover or caps provided. If fingers are used to cover the sample, it could become contaminated. When mixing reagents with a sample, the sample should not be shaken vigorously because this may bruise the sample and cause a false reading. Swirl the sample slowly, or carefully invert the sample to mix it with the reagent.
- Store the test kit and reagents in a cool, dark, dry area away from other chemicals. Do not store the test kit and reagents outside in the sun or near the water. KEEP OUT OF REACH OF CHILDREN.

- Reagents are easily contaminated. Do not allow chemical droppers or reagent bottles to come in contact with foreign substances. Tightly replace the lids after each use. STORE OUT OF CHILDREN'S REACH.
- When dropping reagents into the test cell, hold the reagent dropper vertically. Do not allow the reagent to drip down the inside walls of the vial.
- Use separate test vials for different tests.
- Read the sample by holding at eye level. Use a white card as a background. Do not read in direct sunlight.
- After completing a water test, do not throw the used sample with reagents back into the pool. Dispose of the reagents by placing them into a deck drain or other waste receptacle.

pH Testing

Swimming pool water should be maintained between 7.2 and 7.6 on the pH scale. Testing for pH is one of the simplest and most standardized of all pool tests. This is a colorimetric test using phenolsulfonephthalein, more commonly known as phenol red. Phenol red comes mostly in a liquid, although tablets are available. Phenol red is a very effective indicator of pH between the values of 6.8 and 8.2. When testing

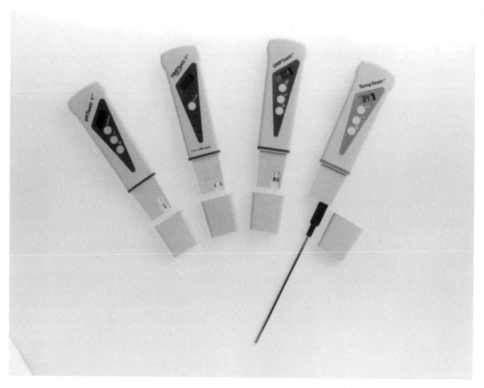

Fig. 10-4.   A pH meter (*far left*) alongside of TDS, ORP, and temperature meters. (Courtesy La Motte, Chestertown, Md.)

for pH usually either five drops of phenol red or one tablet is added to a water sample. The sample will turn darker shades of red in the presence of higher pH levels. The color of the water sample must be compared to the color comparater provided with the test kit. At lower levels of pH, phenol red will turn yellow and then orange at slightly higher levels. Shades of red indicate proper pH levels; dark red often indicates excessively high levels of pH.

Whenever high levels of sanitizer are present, the reagent in the test cell may be bleached yellow or may turn dark purple. If this occurs, two to four drops of sodium thiosulfate (chlorine neutralizer) can be added to a new sample, before phenol red is added. The temperature of the test sample should be between 60° and 80° F.

It is important to remember that phenol red will only remain effective for 6 months. Other pH reagents that can be used are bromothymol blue (pH 6.0 to 7.6) or cresol red (7.2 to 8.8).

Electrochemical pH meters can also be used to determine pH levels in a pool. pH meters include a submersible electrode and electrical circuitry to quickly monitor and display pH readings. Although

pH meters can be extremely accurate, they are also prone to operator and calibration error. pH meters should be calibrated with distilled water often (Fig. 10-4).

If pH is found to be low, a base demand test using a base demand reagent (BDR) should be conducted to determine how much soda ash or caustic soda ash must be added to raise the pH to the desired level. Likewise, when pH is high, an acid demand test should be conducted utilizing an acid demand reagent (ADR) to determine how much muriatic acid or sodium bisulfate should be added to return the pH to recommended levels. In both cases, the number of drops required to change the color of the existing pH test sample to a color within the appropriate range determines the amount of chemical to be added.

Chlorine/Bromine Testing

The DPD Method

The most common method of testing for chlorine is the Palin or DPD colorimetric testing technique. DPD

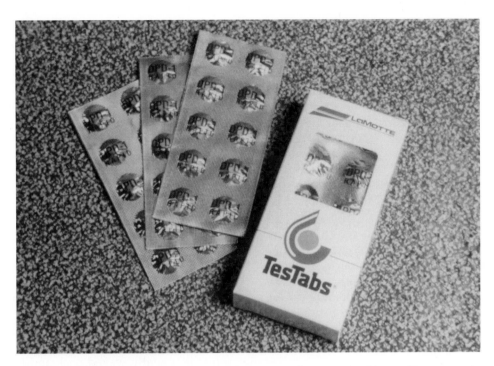

Fig. 10-5. DPD tablets wrapped in cellophone. (Courtesy La Motte, Chestertown, Md.)

is short for a technique using diethyl-p-phenylenediamine. DPD testing determines two types of chlorine residuals: free-available chlorine (FAC) and total available chlorine (TAC). Once these levels are found, combined available chlorine (CAC) can be calculated by subtracting FAC from TAC. Although required FAC levels vary from state to state, most pools should probably maintain their FAC levels between 1.0 and 3.0 ppm. CAC levels should not exceed .3 ppm.

Orhtotolidine or (OTO), which once was the standard test for total chlorine, is no longer recommended. The OTO method cannot detect chloramine levels, is prone to errors, and is a carcinogen.

DPD is available in both liquid and tablets and in addition to the colorimetric procedure, DPD also is available in titrant or drop testing (Fig, 10-5). Although DPD tablets have a longer shelf life, some individuals have a problem with managing and disposing of the foil and cellophane packets containing the tablets, which tend to make a mess.

The advantage of the DPD system is that it distinguishes between free available chlorine and combined available chlorine.

TAC = FAC + CAC

When using the DPD tablet system, DPD no. 1 is used to determine the FAC level. Once the FAC level is found, DPD no. 3 is added to the water sample containing DPD no. 1 to find the TAC level. The first reading (FAC) is subtracted from the second reading (TAC) to find the combined available chlorine level (CAC). If there is no color change from the first test (FAC) and the second test (TAC), then no chloramines exist in the pool. A summary is found below:

DESIRED TEST DPD	REAGENT REQUIRED
FAC	DPD no. 1*
TAC	DPD no. 1 + DPD no. 3
Total bromine†	DPD no. 1

$$\begin{array}{r} \text{TAC} \\ \underline{-\text{FAC}} \\ \text{CAC} \end{array}$$

*When using liquid reagents, DPD no. 1 and no. 2 are used to determine FAC.

† Bromamines are effective sanitizers, so there is no need to differentiate between free and combined bromine.

As with the pH colorimetric test, when the color caused by the DPD reagents turns darker shades of red, higher levels of chlorine are indicated. Bromine may be measured with a standard chlorine test, but the level found on the chlorine indicator must be multiplied by 2.25 to find the bromine level because bromine is 2.25 times heavier than chlorine.

A word of caution is in order when high levels of sanitizers are suspected. When chlorine and bromine levels are exceedingly high (at least 10 ppm and 22 ppm, respectively), the sanitizer will bleach the reagent immediately as it enters the test tube. This false reading indicates that there is no chlorine/bromine in the pool or there is a very low level. The result may be a completely opposite and incorrect reaction from the pool operator; the introduction of more sanitizer. When high levels of sanitizers are expected, the water sample should be diluted 50/50 with distilled water and the results doubled. In the case of extremely high chlorine levels, the

dilution may need to be one third pool water and two thirds distilled water, in which case the results should be tripled.

Ozone, iodine, and oxidized manganese can also lead to faulty DPD readings. It is also very important to allow hot tub water to cool before testing. At high temperatures, a high CAC reading will actually appear to be a high *FAC* reading.

DPD should not be touched with bare hands because Aniline, which is found in DPD, is toxic when absorbed through the skin.

Test Strips

FACTS is an acronym for "free available chlorine test strip." FACTS is a test strip composed of two chlorine indicators, syringaldazine and vanillinazine. These test strips are best utilized as a quick check for the presence of chlorine only (Fig. 10-6). Typically, the test strip is placed in pool water for 30 seconds while it is gently waved back and forth. The strip is then removed from the water, and the color of the test strip is compared to a color chart supplied with the strips. Newer test strips even give readings for calcium hardness, total alkalinity, and pH (Fig. 10-7). The accuracy of test strips, however, has been questioned.

Oxygen-Reduction Potential Testing

Perhaps the most sophisticated instrument available to pool personnel for measuring the amount of disinfectant in the water is the oxygen-reduction potential (ORP) analyzer (Figs. 10-8 and 10-9). This ORP method of chemical analysis is also known as the redox method. ORP is a measure of the oxidizing capability or "work value" of any sanitizer used in water. ORP is a qualitative measure, whereas standard test kit procedures offer a quantitative measure of a sanitizer in the water. Rather than measuring sanitizers in ppm, the ORP analyzer measures in millivolts (mV). This electrochemical measurement uses silver and silver chloride electrodes to determine the electrical potential of sanitizers in the water. Apparently, ORP levels predict the killing rate of *E. Coli* organisms much more accurately than traditional chlorine readings. Pathogens cannot survive in water measuring more than 650 mV. As a result, the World

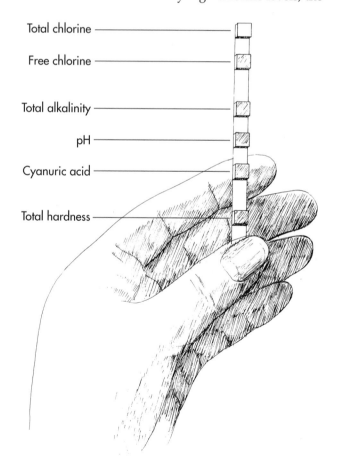

Total chlorine

Free chlorine

Total alkalinity

pH

Cyanuric acid

Total hardness

Fig. 10-6. Quick, easy hand-held test strips. (Illustrator, Nancy Bauer.)

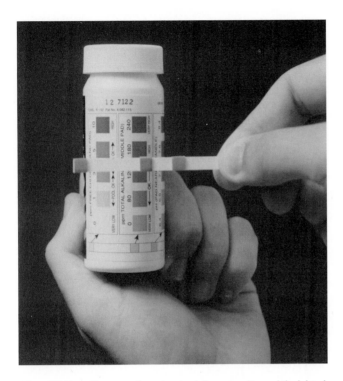

Fig. 10-7. Comparing test strip results with ideal ranges. (Courtesy AquaChek, Elkhart, Ind.)

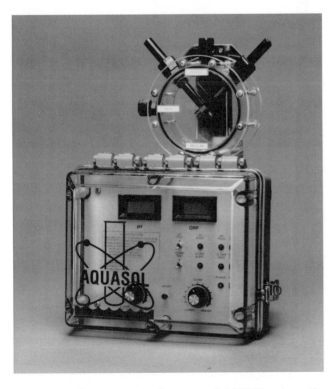

Fig. 10-8. Oxygen-reduction potential (ORP) automatic control system. (Courtesy Aquasol, Houston, Tex.)

Health Organization (WHO) recognizes 650 mV as the minimum ORP level for drinking water, while Germany and other European countries have adopted 750 mV as the minimum ORP level for public pools and spas. When used with chlorine, ORP measures the level of hypochlorous acid as it disassociates according to pH levels.

Perhaps the greatest advantage of the ORP system is that the pool water is being monitored continually (Fig. 10-10). In addition to continual monitoring, many ORP systems have been expanded to include the ability to make chemical adjustments. Some ORP systems come with a digital read-out for chlorine and pH levels, whereas others have a print out. There are even ORP controllers now that report in English, through a speech synthesizer, the chemical balance of the pool water. To receive a chemical report of pool conditions, users simply dial the controller's phone number. Handheld models are also becoming popular.

One of the disadvantages of the ORP system is that the sensors need to be cleaned and replaced periodically. It must be mentioned that this is not a major drawback. Also, all ORP analyzers must be calibrated with manual means of testing sanitizers. Despite these concerns, ORP testing appears to be the most accurate, reliable, and sophisticated method of analyzing water sanitation.

Total Alkalinity Testing

Total alkalinity should be tested weekly or bimonthly depending on the pool load. Total alkalinity readings are required to determine the saturation index and will also aid in controlling the pH of the water. Total alkalinity readings should be between 80 to 150 ppm. Total alkalinity is measured by means of a titration test. A predetermined volume of water is taken from the pool, and this sample is titrated with an acid until the sample color changes dramatically. The sample must be prepared with an indicator before reagents are dropped into it. The indicator commonly used for total alkalinity tests is green/methyl red. As one of two common titrants (hydrochloric acid or sulfuric acid) is added to the sample, it will turn color from green to pink.

To determine the exact amount of total alkalinity in the water, the reagent is slowly dropped into the prepared sample and the number of drops needed to change the color of the sample is counted. Many test

Table I	
pH ELECTRODE READINGS	
pH SCALE	mV
0 (HIGHLY ACIDIC)	+420
7.0 (NEUTRAL)	0
7.5 (IDEAL)	-30
8.0 (BASIC)	-60
14 (HIGHLY BASIC)	-420

TABLE II	
ORP ELECTRODE READINGS	
mV	CONDITIONS
BELOW 650	UNSANITARY WATER (Germs, Bacteria)
654	MINIMUM LEVEL
700 to750	IDEAL LEVEL

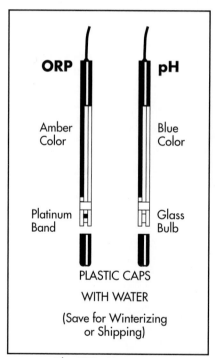

The ORP pH sensors.

Fig. 10-9. Examples of chemical sensors—pH and ORP sensors. (From NSPI: *Basic pool and spa technology*, ed 2, Alexandria, Va, 1992, The Institute.)

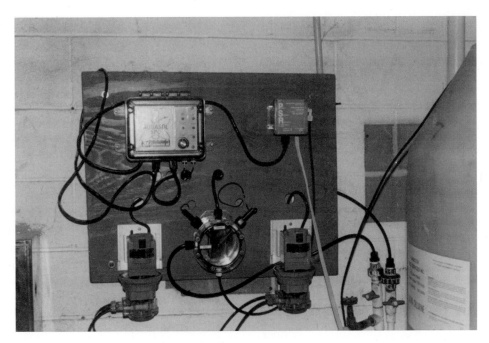

Fig. 10-10. ORP automatic controllers located above pool disinfectant pumps. (Courtesy Aquasol, Houston, Tex.)

kits use 10 ppm per drop to calculate ppm of total alkalinity. Therefore, if it takes 10 drops to change the green sample to pink, there would be 100 ppm of total alkalinity in the pool. When high disinfectant levels are found in the pool, the color change will be from blue to yellow rather than green to pink. Tablets are also available for this test but may not be as accurate as the drop test.

Calcium Hardness Testing

Calcium hardness levels should be maintained between 200 and 500 ppm. If below 200 ppm, pool water may be too corrosive; if above 500 ppm, the calcium hardness may produce scale. The calcium hardness test is another titration technique whereby a specified volume of water is titrated with a standard calcium hardness titrant.

After a predetermined volume of water is collected as a sample, a pH increasing reagent is added to assist in the color change. Then a titrant called EDTA (ethylenediamine) is slowly dropped into the sample and the drops are counted. The sample will turn from red to blue during titration, but this change takes place slowly and subtly. The number of drops

required to change the sample from red to blue should be recorded and then often multiplied by 10 ppm per drop.

Cyanuric Acid Testing

Cyanuric acid (CYA) is used for stabilizing chlorine against the damaging UV rays of the sun. Most states do not allow CYA levels above 100 ppm in swimming pools. If CYA levels drop below 30 ppm, its chlorine stabilizing ability is greatly reduced. CYA should only be used in outdoor pools.

A turbidometric test is used to determine CYA levels. In this case a reagent called Melamine is added to a water sample to create a white precipitate that clouds the water in proportion to the amount of CYA in the water. A common method of CYA testing requires the tester to add drops of melamine until a dot on the bottom of a test tube becomes obscured. Basically, the sooner the dot disappears, the more CYA in the water. The tube is graded so that the water in the column can be read in ppm.

This is not the only means of testing for CYA, however. One test kit utilizes a rod and vial to measure CYA rather than a dot at the bottom of a test tube.

There are also electronic test meters and quick test strips that require only 30 seconds of submersion for a color change.

CYA levels should not be allowed to exceed 100 ppm. Not only do most states dictate this ceiling, but chlorine's effectiveness is reduced at this level and in addition, ORP readings will be reduced. The only practical way of reducing CYA is to drain off some of the pool water. Because cartridge filters are cleaned without being backwashed, pools employing both CYA and cartridge filters may experience a more rapid rise in CYA.

Testing for CYA in warmer water becomes tricky. The water sample should be allowed to cool to 70° F or less. Higher temperatures restrict the production of turbidity, leading to inaccurately low readings.

Copper and Iron Testing

If pool water turns green or orange, tests for copper and iron may have to be conducted. If these metals are causing a problem, they are either at high levels in the make-up water, or highly acidic, unbalanced pool water is removing surface layers from copper and iron plumbing components and depositing them in the pool.

Simple colorimetric tests, similar to those described above, are available. If a copper or iron problem is suspected, the source water should be tested as well as the pool water. Sequestering agents may be used to prevent both copper and iron from precipitating out of solution, while maintaining proper pH levels will prevent the etching of circulation components.

Testing for copper and iron is not usually conducted until a metals problem in the pool is suspected.

Bacteriological Testing

To ensure that diseases will not be transmitted through swimming pool water, bacteriological tests are required of most public pools. This is one type of test that is normally not conducted at poolside. Rather, samples must be collected and sent to a laboratory, where an environmental health agency supervises the test (see box on page 136). Total plate counts and coliform counts are the most common bacteriological tests of swimming pool water. The total count should not exceed 200 bacterial colonies per millimeter, and the coliform count indicating fecal matter should be zero. Most states require weekly bacteriological testing of swimming pools.

Potable Water Laboratory

Office of Physical Plant

PADER Approval No.14-058

Date sample collected ——————————— Time sample collected ———————————

Facility name ———————————

Location (check one) ☐ fountain ☐ restrooms ☐ sink ☐ well ☐ pool ☐ spring

☐ other

Chlorine residual (mg/l) ———————————

Collected by ———————————

Date received in laboratory ——————————— Time received in laboratory ———————————

Date analysis begun ——————————— Time analysis begun ———————————

Examined by ———————————

Total coliforms per 100 ml ———————————

Fecal coliforms per 100 ml ———————————

Total count per 1 ml ———————————

Remarks:

When pool disinfectants are kept at acceptable levels, bacteria proliferation is not a problem.

Sterilized bottles are used for this testing procedure, and great care must be taken not to contaminate the top, cap, neck, or inside of the bottle. Some labs require the sample to be refrigerated. The sample must be sent to a state-certified lab quickly. (Often within 24 hours).

Summary

Pool water testing, if performed properly and regularly, will help to keep the water sparkling clear, clean, and free of germs. Test kits must be stored properly and the reagents used must always be fresh. Testing should be conducted often, during the same time of the day, from several different sites around the pool. All water testing records should be kept for 5 years. Before purchasing a test kit, several kits should be analyzed at a local pool store or dealer.

Bibliography

The pool book: Decatur, Ga, 1981, BioGuard Lab.

Johnson R: *YMCA pool operations manual*, Champaign, Ill, 1989, YMCA.

Kowalsky L (editor): *Pool/spa operators handbook*, San Antonio, Tex, 1991, National Swimming Pool Foundation.

Mitchel K: *The proper management of pool and spa water*, Decatur, Ga, 1988, BioLab.

Pool & Spa News, Los Angeles.

Service Industry News, Torrance, Calif.

Steininger J: Clean up with ORP, *AQUA*, June 1990.

Taylor C: *Everything you always wanted to know about pool care*, , Chino Calif, 1989, Service Industry Publications.

Taylor Technologies: *Pool and spa water chemistry, testing and treatment guide with tables*, Sparks, Md.

Washington State Public Health Association: *Swimming pool operations*, Seattle, 1988, The Association.

Water quality and treatment: ed 3, 1971, The American Water Works Association.

Williams KG: *The aquatic facility operator's manual*, Hoffman Estates, Ill, 1991, National Recreation and Park Association, National Aquatic Section.

Review Questions

1. What is used to test for pH levels in pool water?

2. Which is the preferred method for chlorine tesing?

3. What do ORP analyzers actually measure?

4. Describe one advantage of the ORP method of testing for disinfectant levels.

5. How often should total alkalinity be tested?

6. Is the TA test a colorimetric, titrimetric, or turbidometric test?

7. CYA should not exceed how many PPM?

8. How often should bacteriological tests be conducted?

11

CHEMICAL ADJUSTMENTS AND POOL CALCULATIONS

KEY CONCEPTS

- *Chemical Safety*
- *Ideal Ranges*
- *Chlorine*
- *pH*
- *Calcium Hardness*
- *CYA*
- *Total Alkalinity*
- *Pool Volumes*

Because the chemical condition of pool water is in a constant state of flux, the addition of chemicals must be done periodically. When performing chemical adjustments, safety is an important consideration for both the pool patron and the person handling the chemicals. Second, adding the right amount of chemical to the pool is also important because miscalculations can cost valuable time and money to get the pool water back within appropriate chemical parameters.

Because safety is of the utmost concern and because most chemical adjustments are done manually, a discussion of chemical safety will now take place.

Safe Chemical Handling

The following tips should be followed to help make chemical adjustments safely.

- Chemicals should be stored properly. This includes keeping all chemicals locked in a separate storage facility that is dry, dark, cool, and has adequate ventilation. All chemicals must be in sealed containers and kept away from heat sources.

- Gloves and goggles should always be worn when handling chemicals. Separate clean, dry scoops and buckets must be used for each chemical. Scoops and buckets should be marked for the chemical for which they are intended.
- All chemical instructions must be read, understood, and followed.
- A water hose should be nearby to assist in the clean-up of chemical spills.
- Chemicals must be kept well away from pool patrons. Swimmers should not be present when major chemical adjustments are being made.
- When mixing chemicals, ALWAYS ADD CHEMICALS TO WATER. NEVER ADD WATER TO CHEMICALS.

Suggested Chemical Ranges

Before discussing how specific chemical adjustments should be made, it would be wise to review once again the suggested chemical ranges for swimming pools and spas. Found below is a listing available through the National Spa and Pool Institute (NSPI).[1] It must be remembered that the figures from NSPI are suggested standards only. Local and state health codes may differ and should be consulted on an annual basis (Tables 11-1 and 11-2).

Specific Chemical Adjustments
Increasing chlorine

Superchlorination is recommended for most pools on a regular basis. Not only does superchlorination destroy chloramines, a persistent pool problem, but it also kills algae and oxidizes organic debris which in turn "polishes" the water. Chloramines can be destroyed completely only when 10 times the CAC level is added in new FAC. Because there are so

Table 11-1. NSPI suggested chemical standards for swimming pools

	Minimum	Ideal	Maximum
Free chlorine (ppm)	1.0	1.0-3.0	3.0
Combined chlorine (ppm)	None	None	0.2
Bromine (ppm)	2.0	2.0-4.0	4.0
pH	7.2	7.4-7.6	7.8
Total alkalinity (ppm)	60	80-100* 100-120†	180
TDS (ppm)	300	1000-2000	3000
Calcium hardness (ppm)	150	200-400	500-1000+
Cyanuric acid (ppm)	10	30-50	150‡

From ANSI/NSPI-1: Standard for public swimming pools, Alexandria, Va, 1991, The Institute.

* For Liquid chlorine, calcium hypochlorite, and lithium hypochlorite.

† For gas chlorine, dichlor, trichlor, and bromine compounds.

‡ Except where limited by health departments requirement, often to 100 PPM.

Table 11-2. NSPI suggested chemical standards for spa

	Minimum	Ideal	Maximum
Free chlorine (ppm)	1.0	3.0-5.0	10.0
Combined chlorine (ppm)	None	None	0.2
Bromine (ppm)	2.0	3.0-5.0	10.0
pH	7.2	7.4-7.6	7.8
Total alkalinity (ppm)	60	80-100* 100-120†	180
TDS (ppm)	300	1000-2000	3000
Calcium hardness (ppm)	150	200-400	500-1000+
Cyanuric acid (ppm)	10	30-50	150‡

From ANSI/NSPI-1: Standard for public swimming pools, Alexandria, Va, 1991, The Institute.

* For liquid chlorine, calcium hypochlorite, and lithium hypochlorite.

† For gas chlorine, dichlor, trichlor, and bromine compounds.

‡ Except where limited by health departments requirement, often to 100 PPM.

many different forms of chlorine used in swimming pools today, superchlorination can become confusing. The following information should clarify how to superchlorinate any swimming pool, regardless of type or size. This information will also be helpful to those attempting to simply raise chlorine without superchlorinating.

When making chemical adjustments, the first question that needs to be answered is "... how many parts per million must be added to the pool for the desired change?" In the case of superchlorination, the question would be how many PPM chlorine must be added to achieve breakpoint? In Chapters 8 and 10, the important relationship of CAC equals TAC minus FAC is discussed. A test kit is used to find both TAC and FAC. Then FAC is simply subtracted from TAC to find CAC. Once the chloramine level is computed, this number is then multiplied by 10 to find how much FAC should be added to the pool. For example, a pool with 0.4 PPM of CAC would require 4.0 PPM FAC to burn off all CAC. A pool with 0.8 PPM CAC would need a FAC level of 8.0 ppm to destroy all chloramines and so on.

Since a 120,000 gallon pool (which is a fairly standard sized public pool) weighs approximately 1 million pounds, a pound of gas chlorine added to this million pound pool would add one part per million.[2] Using the example in the preceding paragraph, 4 pounds and 8 pounds of gas, respectively, would oxidize 0.4 ppm and 0.8 ppm CAC levels.

It is important to note that 1 gallon of sodium hypochlorite (liquid) is equal to 1 pound of gas, and 1.6 pounds of calcium hypochlorite (dry) is also equivalent to 1 pound of gas. Although gas chlorine is an excellent primary sanitizer, sodium and calcium hypochlorite are often preferred as superchlorinators.

To introduce high chlorine concentrations into a particular pool, the size of that pool also becomes important because not every pool is 120,000 gallons. A "pool factor" must be created by dividing a particular pool's gallonage by 120,000 gallons before multiplying by the amount of chemical. For instance, if a 60,000 gallon pool had a CAC level of 0.5 PPM, how much chlorine would have to be added to burn out all chloramines? To kill all chloramines, 10 times 0.5 ppm CAC or 5.0 ppm FAC is needed.

EXAMPLE 1

5 lbs gas or
5 gal liquid or X $\dfrac{60,000}{120,000}$ = ?
8 lbs cal hypo

5 lbs gas   = 2.5 pounds gas
5 gal   = 2.5 gallons
sod hypo   X   .5 pool   liquid
8 lbs   factor (pf)   = 4 pounds
cal hypo   calcium hypo

EXAMPLE 2

In a 190,000 gallon pool a CAC level of .6 ppm is found. How many ppm of FAC must be added and how much chlorine must be added to achieve this?

To rid a pool of .6 ppm CAC, 6.0 ppm must be added to the pool. In a 190,000 gallon pool, the following calculations are necessary.

6 lbs gas
6 gal sod
hypo   X $\dfrac{190,000}{120,000}$ = ?
9.6 lbs
cal hypo

6 lbs   9.48 pounds
gas   gas
6 gal   9.48 gallons
sod hypo   X   1.58 (pf) =   sodium hypo
9.6 lbs   15.16 pounds
cal hypo   calcium hypo

EXAMPLE 3

In a 250,000 gallon pool a CAC level of 0.8 is found. How many ppm of FAC is needed to burn out all chloramines? How much chlorine will be needed to accomplish this?

An FAC level of 10 times greater than the CAC level is needed to rid the pool of all chloramines. In this case 8.0 ppm FAC must be added to the pool.

8 lbs gas
8 gal
sod hypo   X $\dfrac{250,000}{120,000}$ = ?
12.8 lbs
cal hypo

8 lbs gas   16.64 pounds
                                       gas
8 gal   16.64 gallons
sod hypo   X   2.08 (pf)   =   sod hypo
12.8 lbs   26.62 pounds
cal hypo   cal hypo

When attempting to reach breakpoint chlorination, it is important to increase the FAC by *at least* 10 times the CAC levels. For that reason all values found in the answers to the problems above should be rounded up. Falling short of breakpoint will waste much chlorine and only add to chloramine development.

For those individuals who do not wish to make calculations, numerous charts and tables, are available that have a wide variety of chlorine levels and pool sizes, (Tables 11-3 and 11-4).

Also, it must be emphasized when breakpoint is the goal, the chemical addition must be made as quickly as possible. Broadcasting calcium hypochlorite around the pool or "walking" sodium hypochlorite along the perimeter are two common procedures. Pool patrons should not be present when this is taking place. Close attention must also be paid to pH levels while superchlorination is taking place.

Superchlorination is not limited to the three agents listed above. Many options are available for shocking including nonchlorine shocking agents. Dosages for some alternative shocking agents are found below.

Lowering Chlorine

If chlorine levels need to be lowered, the addition of sodium thiosulfate is recommended. A good rule of thumb when adding sodium thiosulfate is 1 pound per 100,000 gallons of water to reduce the chlorine level by 1 ppm. If the size of a particular pool to be treated is different than 100,000 gallons, it should be divided by 100,000 gallons to find the pool factor. For

Table 11-3. Amount of chlorinating agent per gallons in pool to introduce 1 ppm FAC

Breakpoint chlorinating agent	Gallons in pool			
	1000	5000	10,000	25,000
	Amount			
Sodium hypochlorite*	1.6 oz	8 oz	16 oz	40 oz
Lithium hypochlorite	0.024 lbs	0.12 lbs	0.24 lbs	0.60 lbs
Calcium hypochlorite	0.012 lbs	0.06 lbs	0.12 lbs	0.312 lbs

Courtesy Biolab, Decatur, Ga.
* Volume measurement: 16 oz equals 1 pt.

Table 11-4. Amount of persulfate required to oxidize the designed chloramine level*

Chloramine concentration (PPM)	Gallons in pool			
	1000	5000	10,000	25,000
	Amount (gm)	Amount (lb)	Amount (lb)	Amount (lb)
0.20	9	0.1	0.2	0.50
0.40	18	0.2	0.4	1.0
0.60	27	0.3	0.6	1.5
0.80	36	0.4	0.8	2.0
1.0	45	0.5	1.0	2.5

Courtesy Biolab, Decatur, Gas.
* Persulfate amounts based on peroxymonosulfate active strength of 42.8%. Corrections will be required when using peroxymonosulfate oxidizers that contain less than 42.8% active ingredient. For example, if a product contains 32.3% as peroxymonosulfate, a multiplier of 1.32 (42.8 ÷ 32.3 = 1.32) will be required.

instance, if a pool is 150,000 gallons and has a FAC of 10.0 ppm that must be lowered to 2.0 ppm, how much sodium thiosulfate must be added to this pool to reduce the chlorine level by 8.0 ppm?

$$8 \text{ lbs sodium thiosulfate } \times \frac{150,000}{100,000} = ?$$

$$8 \text{ lbs} \times 1.5 \text{ (pf)} = 12 \text{ lbs sodium thiosulfate}$$

When using sodium thiosulfate, caution must be exercised. If too much sodium thiosulfate is added to the pool, it will be extremely difficult to get any chlorine readings, resulting in a waste of time, chlorine, and money. Unlike chlorine, sodium thiosulfate should be added a little at a time. Sodium thiosulfate is normally used after superchlorination only when chlorine readings are exceedingly high. It should be noted that in some regions, sodium sulfite or sodium bisulfite is used instead of sodium thiosulfate. Some prefer sodium sulfite because its chemistry is more predictable, and less is required to lower chlorine/bromine.

Increasing pH

When using gas chlorine the pH of the pool water will drop dramatically. As a result, for every pound of gas chlorine added to the pool, a corresponding 1.5 pounds of soda ash should be added.

If the pH must be raised for any reason, particularly when gas chlorine is not in use, the following table may be used (Table 11-5). A base demand reagent (BDR) from a test kit is needed in this case to determine how much soda ash or caustic soda must be added to raise the pH to the desired level.

Table 11-5. To raise pH employing the taylor base demand procedure*

Taylor base demand reagent (drops)†	Volume of water						
	250 gals / 946 L	400 gals / 1,514 L	1,000 gals / 3,785 L	5,000 gals / 18,927 L	20,000 gals / 75,708 L	50,000 gals / 189,271 L	100,000 gals / 378,541 L
1	.13 oz / 3.6 g	.21 oz / 5.8 g	.52 oz / 14.4 g	2.6 oz / 72.0 g	10.4 oz / 288 g	1.63 lbs / 720 g	3.25 lbs / 1.44 kg
2	.26 oz / 7.2 g	.42 oz / 11.6 g	1.04 oz / 28.8 g	5.2 oz / 144 g	1.30 lbs / 576 g	3.25 lbs / 1.44 kg	6.50 lbs / 2.88 kg
3	.39 oz / 10.8 g	.62 oz / 17.4 g	1.56 oz / 43.2 g	7.8 oz / 216 g	1.95 lbs / 864 g	4.88 lbs / 2.16 kg	9.75 lbs / 4.32 kg
4	.52 oz / 14.4 g	.83 oz / 23.2 g	2.08 oz / 57.6 g	10.4 oz / 288 g	2.60 lbs / 1.15 kg	6.50 lbs / 2.88 kg	13.0 lbs / 5.76 kg
5	.65 oz / 18.0 g	1.04 oz / 28.8 g	2.6 oz / 72.0 g	13.0 oz / 360 g	3.25 lbs / 1.44 kg	8.13 lbs / 3.60 kg	16.3 lbs / 7.20 kg
6	.78 oz / 21.6 g	1.25 oz / 34.8 g	3.12 oz / 86.4 g	15.6 oz / 432 g	3.90 lbs / 1.73 kg	9.75 lbs / 4.32 kg	19.5 lbs / 8.64 kg
7	.91 oz / 25.2 g	1.46 oz / 40.6 g	3.64 oz / 101 g	1.14 lbs / 504 g	4.55 lbs / 2.02 g	11.4 lbs / 5.04 kg	22.8 lbs / 10.1 kg
8	1.04 oz / 28.8 g	1.66 oz / 46.4 g	4.16 oz / 115 g	1.30 lbs / 576 g	5.20 lbs / 2.30 kg	13.0 lbs / 5.76 kg	26.0 lbs / 11.5 kg
9	1.17 oz / 32.4 g	1.87 oz / 52.2 g	4.68 oz / 130 g	1.46 lbs / 648 g	5.85 lbs / 2.59 kg	14.6 lbs / 6.48 kg	29.2 lbs / 13.0 kg
10	1.30 oz / 36.0 g	2.08 oz / 58.0 g	5.2 oz / 144 g	1.63 lbs / 720 g	6.50 lbs / 2.88 kg	16.3 lbs / 7.20 kg	32.5 lbs / 14.4 kg

Courtesy Taylor Technologies, Sparks, Md.

* Adjustment compound used in soda ash (sodium carbonate).

† With Taylor 2000 Test Block, use Taylor #R-0006, or with #4024 Lucite test cell use Taylor #R-0862 Base Demand Reagent.

Lowering pH

When pH climbs out of the ideal range and must be lowered, either muriatic acid or sodium bisulfate may be used reduce pH. Likewise, an acid demand reagent (ADR) is required to determine the amount of acid needed to lower the pH to the desired level. In addition, it is important to predissolve or dilute these acids before adding them to the pool water. If added directly to the pool without dilution, muriatic acid or sodium bisulfate may reduce the total alkalinity without any appreciable effect on pH (Table 11-6 and 11-7).

Increasing total alkalinity

Total alkalinity must be maintained between 100 to 150 ppm to keep pool water balanced. When total alkalinity must be increased, sodium bicarbonate (baking soda) is added to the pool. A good rule for this chemical adjustment is 15 lbs. of sodium bicarbonate for each 10 ppm increase in total alkalinity in 100,000 gallons of water. It must be remembered that when using this formula, the pool being adjusted must be divided by 100,000 gallons to determine the pool factor. In addition, Table 11-8 may be used rather than making these calculations.

It should be mentioned that the ideal range of 100 to 150 ppm for total alkalinity is an approximate one. In geographical areas with very hard source water, the total alkalinity may be lowered to 80 ppm. Conversely, in the case of fiberglass or vinyl-lined pools, the total alkalinity may need to be elevated to 125 to 175 ppm.

Decreasing total alkalinity

When total alkalinity becomes excessively high, a strong acid like muriatic acid or sodium bisulfate must be added to the pool water. When adding muriatic acid to reduce total alkalinity, it should be added

Table 11-6.   To lower pH employing the taylor acid demand procedure*

Taylor acid demand reagent (drops)†	Volume of water						
	250 gals / 946 L	400 gals / 1,514 L	1,000 gals / 3,785 L	5,000 gals / 18,927 L	20,000 gals / 75,708 L	50,000 gals / 189,271 L	100,000 gals / 378,541 L
1	1.00 tsp / 4.9 mL	1.6 tsp / 7.8 mL	1.33 tbsp / 19.6 mL	3.33 oz / 98.0 mL	1.67 cups / 390 mL	1.04 qts / 980 mL	2.08 qts / 1.96 L
2	2.00 tsp / 9.8 mL	1.07 tbsp / 15.6 mL	1.33 oz / 39.2 mL	6.66 oz / 196 mL	1.67 pts / 780 L	2.08 qts / 1.96 L	1.04 gals / 3.92 L
3	1.00 tbsp / 14.7 mL	1.60 tbsp / 23.4 mL	2.00 oz / 58.8 mL	1.25 cups / 294 mL	1.25 qts / 1.18 L	3.12 qts / 2.94 L	1.56 gals / 5.88 L
4	1.33 tbsp / 19.6 mL	1.07 oz / 31.2 mL	2.66 oz / 78.4 mL	1.67 cups / 392 mL	1.67 qts / 1.57 L	1.04 gals / 3.92 L	2.08 gals / 7.84 L
5	1.67 tbsp / 24.5 mL	1.34 oz / 39.0 mL	3.33 oz / 98.0 mL	1.04 pts / 490 mL	2.08 qts / 1.96 L	1.30 gals / 4.90 L	2.60 gals / 9.80 L
6	1.00 oz / 29.4 mL	1.60 oz / 46.8 mL	3.99 oz / 118 mL	1.25 pts / 588 mL	2.50 qts / 2.35 L	1.56 gals / 5.88 L	3.12 gals / 11.8 L
7	1.17 oz / 34.3 mL	1.87 oz / 54.6 mL	4.66 oz / 137 mL	1.46 pts / 686 L	2.92 qts / 2.74 L	1.82 gals / 6.86 L	3.64 gals / 13.7 L
8	1.34 oz / 39.2 mL	2.14 oz / 62.4 mL	5.32 oz / 157 mL	1.67 pts / 784 mL	3.34 qts / 3.14 L	2.08 gals / 7.84 L	4.16 gals / 15.7 L
9	1.50 oz / 44.1 mL	2.40 oz / 70.6 mL	5.99 oz / 176 mL	1.87 pts / 882 mL	3.76 qts / 3.53 L	2.34 gals / 8.82 L	4.68 gals / 17.6 L
10	1.67 oz / 49.0 mL	2.67 oz / 78.0 mL	6.65 oz / 196 mL	1.04 qts / 980 mL	1.04 gals / 3.90 L	2.60 gals / 9.80 L	5.20 gals / 19.6 L

Courtesy Taylor Technologies, Sparks, Md.

* Adjustment compound used in muriatic acid (Hydrochloric Acid-20° Baumé).

† With Taylor 2000 Test Block, use Taylor #R-0005, or with #4024 Lucite test cell use Taylor #R-0853 Acid Demand Reagent.

to the pool full strength, undiluted. This should be done in the deep end of the pool. The pool operator should pour the acid into one spot. When done in this fashion, a very low pH is achieved, resulting in the conversion of carbonate alkalinity to carbon dioxide that is released from the water. This procedure may be repeated in several areas over several days until the desired level of total alkalinity is achieved.

Sodium bisulfate (dry acid) should be mixed in cool water then introduced to the pool in the same manner as muriatic acid. Broadcasting either acid diluted over the pool is not recommended. The total alkalinity is not effectively reduced by broadcasting, particularly when diluted acids are used (Table 11-9).

Increasing calcium hardness

Calcium chloride is the chemical that must be added when calcium hardness needs to be raised. When added to water, calcium chloride produces a significant amount of heat. As a result, after the total amount of calcium chloride to be added is determined, this amount should be halved and then applied to the pool in two equal doses. When dissolving chemicals, add chemicals to water. *NEVER ADD WATER TO CHEMICALS* (Tables 11-10 and 11-11).

Decreasing calcium hardness

As mentioned previously, lowering calcium hardness is both rare and difficult to do. Draining water from the pool and adding new water with a lower calcium hardness level is one way to lower calcium hardness. Another technique is the addition of a water softener but this is very expensive. Before adding a water softener, pool experts should be consulted because some water softeners are not recommended for pool use.

Increasing stabilizer (CYA)

The addition of cyanuric acid (CYA) will protect unstabilized chlorine like gas, sodium hypochlorite,

Table 11-7. To lower pH employing the Taylor acid demand procedure*

Taylor acid demand reagent (drops)[†]	Volume of water						
	250 gals / 946 L	400 gals / 1,514 L	1,000 gals / 3,785 L	5,000 gals / 18,927 L	20,000 gals / 75,708 L	50,000 gals / 189,271 L	100,000 gals / 378,541 L
1	.26 oz / 7.26 g	.42 oz / 11.6 g	1.04 oz / 29.0 g	5.2 oz / 145 g	1.30 lbs / 581 g	3.25 lbs / 1.45 kg	6.50 lbs / 2.90 kg
2	.52 oz / 14.5 g	.83 oz / 23.2 g	2.08 oz / 58.1 g	10.4 oz / 290 g	2.60 lbs / 1.16 kg	6.50 lbs / 2.90 kg	13.0 lbs / 5.81 kg
3	.78 oz / 21.8 g	1.25 oz / 34.8 g	3.12 oz / 87.1 g	15.6 oz / 436 g	3.90 lbs / 1.74 kg	9.75 lbs / 4.36 kg	19.5 lbs / 8.71 kg
4	1.04 oz / 29.0 g	1.66 oz / 46.5 g	4.16 oz / 116 g	1.30 oz / 581 g	5.20 lbs / 2.52 kg	13.0 lbs / 5.81 kg	26.0 lbs / 11.6 kg
5	1.30 oz / 36.3 g	2.08 oz / 58.1 g	5.20 oz / 145 g	1.63 oz / 726 g	6.50 lbs / 2.90 kg	16.3 lbs / 7.26 kg	32.5 lbs / 14.5 kg
6	1.56 oz / 43.6 g	2.50 oz / 69.7 g	6.24 oz / 174 g	1.95 oz / 872 g	7.80 lbs / 3.48 kg	19.5 lbs / 8.71 kg	39.0 lbs / 17.4 kg
7	1.82 oz / 50.8 g	2.91 oz / 81.3 g	7.28 oz / 203 g	2.28 lbs / 1.02 kg	9.10 lbs / 4.07 kg	22.8 lbs / 10.2 kg	45.5 lbs / 20.3 kg
8	2.08 oz / 58.1 g	3.33 oz / 92.9 g	8.32 oz / 232 g	2.60 lbs / 1.16 kg	10.4 lbs / 4.65 kg	26.0 lbs / 11.6 kg	52.0 lbs / 23.2 kg
9	2.34 oz / 65.3 g	3.74 oz / 105 g	9.36 oz / 261 g	2.93 lbs / 1.31 kg	11.7 lbs / 5.23 kg	29.3 lbs / 13.1 kg	58.5 lbs / 26.1 kg
10	2.60 oz / 72.6 g	4.16 oz / 116 g	10.4 oz / 290 g	3.25 lbs / 1.45 kg	13.0 lbs / 5.81 kg	32.5 lbs / 14.5 kg	65.0 lbs / 29.0 kg

Courtesy Taylor Technologies, Sparks, Md.

* Adjustment compound used in Dry Acid (Sodium Bisulfate).

† With Taylor 2000 Test Block, use Taylor #R-0005, or with #4024 Lucite test cell use Taylor #R-0853 Acid Demand Reagent.

and calcium hypochlorite from the UV rays of the sun. The combination of CYA and FAC is a dynamic process that allows additional chlorine to be released while some FAC is being consumed. CYA only protects chlorine in sunlight and has no disinfecting properties. The optimum CYA level is probably between 30 and 50 ppm. When first adding CYA to a pool, the target level should be about 50 ppm. The table below describes how much CYA should be added for the level desired. Again, CYA should be added to outdoor pools ONLY (Table 11-12).

Decreasing stabilizer (CYA)

Although a controversial limit, most states require pools to maintain CYA levels below 100 ppm. When the stabilized chlorines (dichlor and trichlor) are used, the CYA levels can increase rapidly. Some pool operators also complain of increased algae growth and cloudiness when CYA levels go above 100 ppm.

As CYA levels approach 70 ppm the effectiveness of chlorine is greatly reduced. The only way to reduce CYA levels is to drain off some of the pool water.

Pool Volume Calculations

Much of the preceding discussion dealing with chemical adjustments assumes that the pool owners/operators knows the volume or gallons contained in their pool. This is not always the case, however. If the pool volume (pool capacity) is not known, the total gallonage is simple to compute. For the purposes of this text, pool volume and pool capacity are synonymous and are expressed in gallons.

Knowing the pool capacity is a must if chemical adjustments are to be made correctly. The following formulas are used to calculate pool capacity in gallons:

Table 11-8. To raise total alkalinity using sodium bicarbonate

Desired increase in ppm	Volume of water						
	250 gals / 946 L	400 gals / 1,514 L	1,000 gals / 3,785 L	5,000 gals / 18,927 L	20,000 gals / 75,708 L	50,000 gals / 189,271 L	100,000 gals / 378,541 L
10	.60 oz / 17.0 g	.96 oz / 27.2 g	2.40 oz / 68.1 g	12.0 lbs / 341 g	3.00 lbs / 1.36 kg	7.50 lbs / 3.41 kg	15.0 lbs / 6.81 kg
20	1.20 oz / 34.1 g	1.92 oz / 54.5 g	4.80 oz / 136 g	1.50 lbs / 680 g	6.00 lbs / 2.72 kg	15.0 lbs / 6.81 kg	30.0 lbs / 13.6 kg
30	1.80 oz / 51.1 g	2.88 oz / 81.7 g	7.20 oz / 204 g	2.25 lbs / 1.02 kg	9.00 lbs / 4.10 kg	22.5 lbs / 10.2 kg	45.0 lbs / 20.4 kg
40	2.40 oz / 68.1 g	3.84 oz / 109 g	9.60 oz / 272 g	3.00 lbs / 1.36 kg	12.0 lbs / 5.45 kg	30.0 lbs / 13.6 kg	60.0 lbs / 27.2 kg
50	3.00 oz / 85.1 g	4.80 oz / 136 g	12.0 oz / 341 g	3.75 lbs / 1.70 kg	15.0 lbs / 6.81 kg	37.5 lbs / 17.0 kg	75.0 lbs / 34.1 kg
60	3.60 oz / 102 g	5.76 oz / 163 g	14.4 oz / 409 g	4.50 lbs / 2.04 kg	18.0 lbs / 8.17 kg	45.0 lbs / 20.4 kg	90.0 lbs / 40.9 kg
70	4.20 oz / 119 g	6.72 oz / 190 g	1.05 lbs / 477 g	5.25 lbs / 2.38 kg	21.0 lbs / 9.53 kg	52.5 lbs / 23.8 kg	405 lbs / 47.7 kg
80	4.80 oz / 136 g	7.68 oz / 218 g	1.20 lbs / 545 g	6.00 lbs / 2.72 kg	24.0 lbs / 10.9 kg	60.0 lbs / 27.2 kg	120 lbs / 54.5 kg
90	5.40 oz / 153 g	8.64 oz / 245 g	1.35 lbs / 613 g	6.75 lbs / 3.06 kg	27.0 lbs / 12.3 kg	67.5 lbs / 30.6 kg	135 lbs / 61.3 kg
100	6.00 oz / 170 g	9.60 oz / 272 g	1.50 lbs / 680 g	7.50 lbs / 3.41 kg	30.0 lbs / 13.6 kg	75.0 lbs / 34.1 kg	150 lbs / 68.0 kg

Courtesy Taylor Technologies, Sparks, Md.

Table 11-9. Amount of muriatic acid/sodium bisulfate required to lower alkalinity

Desired Decrease (ppm)	Gallons in pool			
	1000	5000	10,000	25,000
	Amount (muriatic acid/sodium bisulfate)			
10	2 oz/0.16 lbs	10 oz/0.80 lbs	1.3 pts/1.60 lbs	6.5 pts/8.00 lbs
20	4 oz/0.32 lbs	20 oz/1.60 lbs	2.6 pts/3.20 lbs	1.6 gal/16.0 lbs
30	6 oz/0.48 lbs	1.9 pts/2.40 lbs	3.9 pts/4.80 lbs	2.4 gal/24.0 lbs
40	8 oz/0.64 lbs	2.5 pts/3.20 lbs	5.2 pts/6.4 lbs	3.2 gal/32.0 lbs
50	10 oz/0.80 lbs	3.1 pts/4.00 lbs	6.5 pts/8.00 lbs	4.0 gal/40.0 lbs

Courtesy BioLab, Decatur, Ga.

Table 11-10. Amount of chlorinating agent per gallons in pool to introduce 1 ppm FAC

Desired calcium increase (ppm)	Gallons in pool			
	1000	5000	10,000	25,000
	Amount			
10	2 oz	10 oz	1.25 lbs	6.25 lbs
25	5 oz	1.6 lbs	3.12 lbs	15.6 lbs
50	10 oz	3.2 lbs	6.24 lbs	31.2 lbs

Courtesy BioLab, Decatur, Ga.
16 oz equals 1 lb; 1 oz equals 28.35 g.

Table 11-11.   To increase calcium hardness using calcium chloride dihydrate*

Desired increase in ppm	Volume of water						
	250 gals / 946 L	400 gals / 1,514 L	1,000 gals / 3,785 L	5,000 gals / 18,927 L	20,000 gals / 75,708 L	50,000 gals / 189,271 L	100,000 gals / 378,541 L
10	.49 oz / 13.9 g	.78 oz / 22.2 g	1.96 oz / 55.6 g	9.80 lbs / 278 g	2.45 lbs / 1.11 kg	6.12 lbs / 2.78 kg	12.2 lbs / 5.56 kg
20	.98 oz / 27.8 g	1.57 oz / 44.4 g	3.92 oz / 111 g	1.22 lbs / 555 g	4.90 lbs / 2.22 kg	12.2 lbs / 5.55 kg	24.5 lbs / 11.1 kg
30	1.47 oz / 41.7 g	2.35 oz / 66.8 g	5.88 oz / 167 g	1.84 lbs / 835 g	7.35 lbs / 3.34 kg	18.4 lbs / 8.35 kg	36.7 lbs / 1.67 kg
40	1.96 oz / 55.5 g	3.14 oz / 88.8 g	7.84 oz / 222 g	2.45 lbs / 1.11 kg	9.80 lbs / 4.44 kg	24.5 lbs / 11.1 kg	49.0 lbs / 22.2 kg
50	2.45 oz / 69.5 g	3.92 oz / 111 g	9.80 oz / 278 g	3.06 lbs / 1.39 kg	12.2 lbs / 5.56 kg	30.6 lbs / 13.9 kg	61.2 lbs / 27.8 kg
60	2.95 oz / 83.5 g	4.72 oz / 134 g	11.8 oz / 334 g	3.69 lbs / 1.67 kg	14.7 lbs / 6.68 kg	36.9 lbs / 16.7 kg	73.7 lbs / 33.4 kg
70	3.43 oz / 97.2 g	5.48 oz / 156 g	13.7 oz / 389 g	4.28 lbs / 1.94 kg	17.1 lbs / 7.78 kg	42.8 lbs / 19.4 kg	85.6 lbs / 38.9 kg
80	3.92 oz / 111 g	6.28 oz / 178 g	15.7 oz / 445 g	4.91 lbs / 2.22 kg	19.6 lbs / 8.90 kg	49.1 lbs / 22.2 kg	98.1 lbs / 44.5 kg
90	4.40 oz / 125 g	7.04 oz / 200 g	1.10 lbs / 501 g	5.50 lbs / 2.50 kg	22.0 lbs / 10.0 kg	55.0 lbs / 25.0 kg	110 lbs / 50.1 kg
100	4.88 oz / 139 g	7.81 oz / 222 g	1.22 lbs / 556 g	6.10 lbs / 2.78 kg	24.4 lbs / 11.1 kg	61.0 lbs / 27.8 kg	122 lbs / 55.6 kg

Courtesy Taylor Technologies, Sparks, Md.
*Treatment amounts are based on 100% calcium chloride dihydrate.

Table 11-12.   Amount of cya required to achieve the desired stabilizer level

Desired increase (PPM)	Pool volume (gallons)					
	1000	5000	10,000	20,000	50,000	100,000
	Amount (lb)					
10	0.083	0.42	0.83	1.7	4.2	8.3
20	0.17	0.84	1.6	3.4	8.4	16.6
30	0.25	1.3	2.5	5.1	12.6	24.9
40	0.33	1.7	3.3	6.8	16.8	33.2
50	0.42	2.1	4.2	8.5	21.0	41.5

Courtesy BioLab, Decatur, Ga.

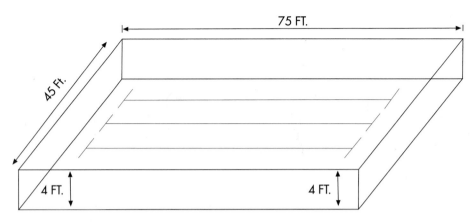

Fig. 11-1. Example 1.

Rectangular
Pool Volume
Length X Width X Average
depth X 7.5 Gallons = Pool gallons

Circular
Pool volume
Diameter X Diameter X Average
depth X 5.9 Gallons = Pool gallons
or
π X Radius^2 X Depth X 7.5 Gallons =
Pool gallons
$\pi = 3.14$

Oval
Pool Volume
Maximum length X Maximum
width X Average depth X 5.9 Gallons = Pool gallons

NOTE: Average depth is calculated by taking the depth of the deep end, adding it to the depth of the shallow end, and dividing by two in a pool with a constant slope. 7.5 represents the gallons in 1 cubic foot of water.

When the pool volume must be calculated for irregular shaped pools with a variety of depths, the pool should be divided into separate geometric sections and calculated individually, and then the results of each section should be totaled.

The first three of the following are for constant depth pools, whereas the last three examples pertain to pools with variable depths.

EXAMPLE 1

A rectangular pool is 75 feet long, 45 feet wide, and has a constant depth of 4 feet. How many gallons does this pool contain (Fig. 11-1)?

Length X Width X Depth X 7.5 gallons	=	Pool capacity in gallons
75 ft X 45 ft X 4 ft X 7.5 gallons	=	101,250 gallons

EXAMPLE 2

A circular swimming pool is 20 feet across (diameter) and has a constant depth of 3.5 feet. How many gallons does this pool hold (Fig. 11-2)?

Diameter X Diameter X Depth X 5.9 gallons	=	Pool capacity in gallons
20 ft X 20 ft X 3.5 ft X 5.9 gallons	=	8260 gallons

EXAMPLE 3

An oval pool is 25 feet at its maximum length and 15 feet at its maximum width. The pool has a constant depth of 4.5 feet. What is the pool capacity of this pool (Fig. 11-3)?

Maximum length X Maximum width X Average depth X 5.9 gallons	=	Pool volume
25 ft X 15 ft X 4.5 ft X 5.9 gallons	=	9956 gallons

EXAMPLE 4

A rectangular pool has a shallow section and a deep section. The pool is 75 feet long (25 yards) and 42 feet wide. The shallow section is 35 feet long and extends from the shallow end of the swimming pool to the beginning of the deep section. The deep section begins where the shallow section ends at a depth of 4 feet and ends at a depth of 8 feet. In calculating the pool capacity, this pool should be divided into two sections. For the purposes of this problem the shallow section will be volume 1 and the deep section will be volume 2. After both volumes are computed, the two are added together for the entire pool capacity. The diagram in Figure 11-4 will aid in the calculations.

Volume 1 = shallow section

Length X Width X Depth X 7.5 gallons	=	Volume
35 ft X 42 ft X 4 ft X		

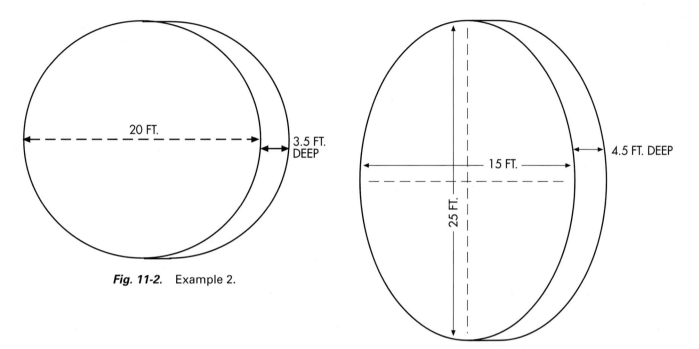

Fig. 11-2. Example 2.

Fig. 11-3. Example 3.

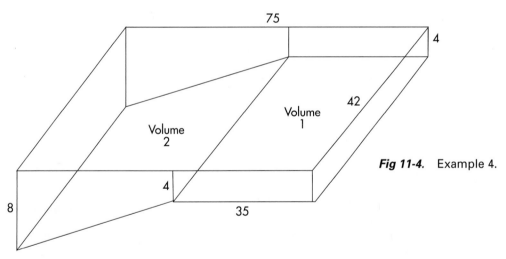

Fig 11-4. Example 4.

7.5 gallons	=	44,100 gallons

Volume 2 = deep section

Length X Width X
Average depth X   = Volume
7.5 gallons

40 ft X 42 ft X
4 ft + 8 ft X 7.5 gallons   = Volume
2

40 ft X 42 ft X 6 ft X
7.5 gallons   = 75,600 gallons

Volume 1 (shallow section)..............44,100 gallons

Volume 2 (deep section)...................+ 75,600 gallons

Answer   119,700 gallons

pool volume

EXAMPLE 5

A pool is 75 feet long and 45 feet wide with three different sections within the one pool. The shallow section is 45 feet long by 45 feet wide and runs from 3.5 feet deep to 5 feet deep. The middle or sloped section of the pool runs from 5 feet deep to 14 feet deep where the diving section begins. This section is 15 feet long and 45 feet wide. The diving section of the pool is 14 feet deep and is 15 feet long and 45 feet wide. What is the

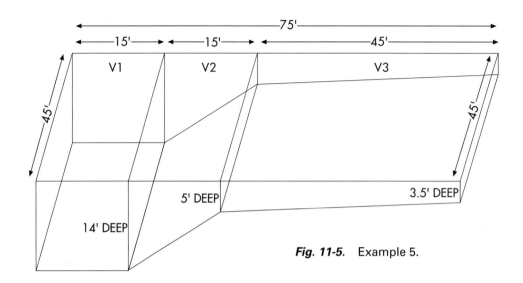

Fig. 11-5. Example 5.

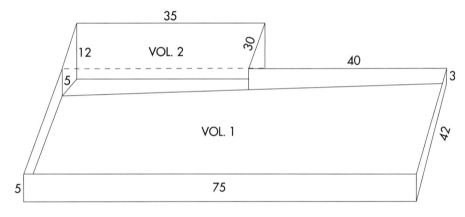

Fig. 11-6. Example 6.

volume of this pool in gallons? For ease of calculations, this pool will be divided into three sections, diving section (volume 1), middle section (volume 2), and shallow section (volume 3) (Fig. 11-5).

Volume 1 = diving section

$$\frac{\text{Length X Width X Depth X 7.5}}{} = \text{Volume 1 (diving section)}$$

15 ft X 45 ft X 14 ft X 7.5 = 70,875 gallons

Volume 2 = middle section

$$\frac{\text{Length X Width X Average depth X 7.5 gallons}}{} = \text{Volume 2 (middle)}$$

15 ft X 45 ft X

$$\frac{14 \text{ ft} + 5 \text{ ft}}{2} \text{ X 7.5 gallons} =$$

15 ft X 45 ft X
9.5 ft X 7.5 gallons = 48,093 gallons

Volume 3 shallow section

$$\frac{\text{Length X Width X Average depth X 7.5 gallons}}{} = \text{Volume 2 (shallow)}$$

45 ft X 45 ft X

$$\frac{5 \text{ ft} + 3.5 \text{ ft X 7.5 gallons} =}{2 \text{ ft.}}$$

45 ft X 45 ft X
4.25 ft X 7.5 gallons = 64,546 gallons

Volume 1 = 70,875 gallons

Volume 2 = 48,093 gallons

Volume 3 = + 64,546 gallons

Answer = 183,584 gallons

EXAMPLE 6

An irregular-shaped pool has a main, racing pool section and a deeper diving section attached but off to one side. The main pool is 75 feet long and 42 feet wide and ranges in depth from 3 feet at the shallow end to 5 feet at the deep end. This section can be called volume 1. The diving section is 30 feet long and 35 feet wide. The water depth in this section runs from 5 feet to 12 feet. This section can be called volume 2. What is the capacity of this pool in gallons (Fig. 11-6).

Volume 1

$$\frac{\text{Length X Width X Average}}{\text{depth X 7.5 gallons}} = \text{Pool volume}$$

$$\frac{75 \text{ ft X } 42 \text{ ft X}}{3 \text{ ft} + 5 \text{ ft X 7.5 gallons} =}{2}$$

75 ft X 42 ft X 4 ft X 7.5 gallons = 94,500 gallons

Volume 2

$$\frac{\text{Length X Width X Average}}{\text{depth X 7.5 gallons} =}$$

$$\frac{30 \text{ ft X } 35 \text{ ft X}}{5 \text{ ft} + 12 \text{ ft X 7.5 gallons} =}{2}$$

30 ft X 35 ft X 8.5 ft X 7.5 gallons = 66,937 gallons

Volume 1 = 94,500 gallons

Volume 2 = + 66,937 gallons

Answer 161,437 gallons

Summary

Swimming pool chemical manufacturers often provide chemical dosage charts with their products. Pool owners and operators should ask for these charts. When in doubt about how to adjust water chemistry, the chemical distributor should be contacted. When using chemical dosage charts, chemical adjustments become quite easy. Calculating the pool volume is the only chore left for the pool operator, and if this chapter has not been fully understood, a local pool store or dealer should be consulted.

References

1. Kowalsky L (editor): Pool/spa operators handbook, San Antonio, Tex, 1991, National Swimming Pool Foundation.
2. Williams KG: The aquatic facility operator's manual, Hoffman Estates, Ill, 1991, National Recreation and Park Association, National Aquatic Section.

Bibliography

BioGuard Lab: *The pool book*, Decatur, Ga, 1981.
Johnson, R: *Swimming Pool Operations Manual*, Harrisburg, Penn, 1991, Pennsylvania Department of Community Affairs.
Kowalsky L (editor): *Pool/spa operators handbook*, San Antonio, Tex, 1991, Swimming Pool Foundation.
Mitchel K: *The proper management of pool and spa water*, BioLab, Inc., Decatur, Ga, 1988, BioLab.
Pool and Spa News, Los Angeles.
Service Industry News, Torrance, Calif.
Taylor C: *Everything you always wanted to know about pool care*, Chino Calif, 1989, Service Industry Publications.
Taylor Technologies: *Pool and spa water chemistry, testing and treatment guide with tables*, Sparks, Md.
Washington State Public Health Association: *Swimming pool operations*, Seattle, 1988 The Association.
Water quality and treatment: ed 3, 1971, The American Water Works Association.
Williams KG: *The aquatic facility operator's manual*, Hoffman Estates, Ill, 1991, National Recreation and Park Association, National Aquatic Section.

Review Questions

1. If the combined available chlorine level in a pool is 0.5 ppm, how many ppms must be added to the pool in FAC to reach breakpoint?

2. One pound of gas chlorine added to a 120,000 gallon pool will raise the FAC by how many ppm?

3. When FAC chlorine levels are excessively high, what chemical can be added to the pool to lower those levels?

4. How many pounds of Sodium Bicarbonate must be added to a 100,000 gallon pool to increase the TA by 50 ppm?

5. Describe the exact procedure for lowering TA.

6. What is the formula for determining the volume of an oval-shaped pool?

7. When is sodium thiosulfate added to a pool and what is the recommended dosage?

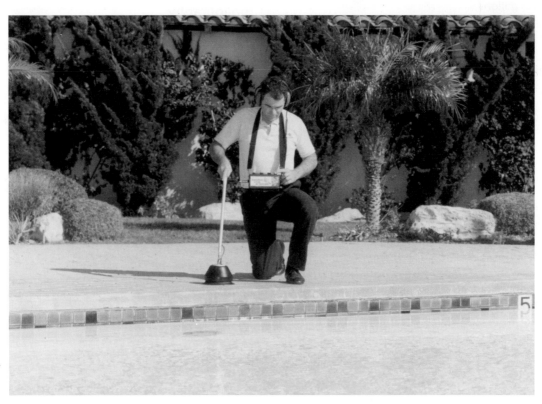

12

POOL PROBLEMS

Key Concepts

- *Algacide*
- *Algistat*
- *"Quats"*
- *Polyquats*
- *Chloramines*
- *Cloudy Water*
- *Iron Content*
- *Copper Content*
- *Unbalance Water*
- *Chlorine Neutralizer*

To provide the reader with a practical trouble-shooting guide for correcting common swimming pool problems, this chapter is organized differently from the others. For every pool problem presented, the following areas are discussed: cause, symptom, treatment, and prevention. By presenting material in this manner, a more comprehensive understanding of pool problems can be achieved. In this fashion, readers can become more familiar with how and why pool problems arise and how to cure them. Not every pool problem is discussed in this chapter; only those that occur often and are serious in nature. The pool problems most often puzzling pool operators discussed in this chapter are the following:

- Algae
- Chlorine odor
- Discolored water
- Sand/DE in pool
- Excessive chlorine
- Foam
- Eyeburn/skin irritation
- Cloudy water
- Corrosion

- Scale
- Water loss

Algae
Cause

Although there are hundreds of different types of algae, only those species that affect pools are discussed here. Algae grows in both indoor and outdoor pools, but outdoor pools provide an ideal environment for algae growth. The emphasis therefore is placed on algae in outdoor pools, although indoor pools may also develop algae problems.

Algae are the simplest forms of the plant kingdom, and these microscopic, single-celled plants thrive in all bodies of water. Algae has a great tendency to grow in and around swimming pools and can be found even in the best maintained aquatic facilities.

Algae growth is promoted by heat, humidity, sunlight, heavy swimmer loads, rain, and above all, insufficient disinfectant level. Dissolved minerals and scale formation also provide pool surfaces that aid algae growth and proliferation.[1] Some pool operators claim that high CYA levels promote algae growth, but others refute this claim.

Algae itself in the pool is not harmful to swimmers. It is unsightly and gives the *appearance* of a poorly maintained pool. But algae growth can create other severe pool problems. Algae on pool decks and bottoms can be extremely slippery and may lead to falling accidents. If untreated, algae can also turn pool water green, reducing visibility. In addition to these problems, algae growth will attract the disinfectant's killing power, rendering the disinfectant less effective in killing bacteria and other organic wastes. Untreated algae can also harbor bacteria growth.

Whenever the disinfectant level in a pool drops and/or the pH level increases, algae may begin to flourish. In outdoor pools this is particularly true, but even more so when these conditions combine with high temperatures, swimmer loads, and following thunderstorms.

Symptoms

Algae growth is quite easy to detect. Pool bottoms, walls, and decks become slippery at the initial stages of algae growth. Algae plants come in different types and the following colors are most often experienced at pools:

Green algae

Green algae is a free-floating algae that can turn the most well-kept pool "pea soup" green in a matter of hours.

Green algae most often begins to grow in pools that are disinfected periodically rather than continuously. It is more likely to begin after summer storms. Once green algae begins to grow in a swimming pool, it is extremely difficult to kill.

Blue/green algae

Often called black algae, this type of algae appears to be black and typically attaches itself in cracks and on rough surfaces in pools with inadequate disinfectant levels. Blue/green algae often appears as black spots on pool bottoms and walls and in expansion joints in pool decks. If left untreated, this type of algae is not only unsightly and slippery but can also harbor bacteria like amoebas and hookworm.[1]

SIDEBAR 12-1

THE USUAL

SUSPECTS

The basic rules for the prevention and remediation of algae problems apply no matter what type of algae you encounter: A good sanitizer residual coupled with good circulation affective filtration and thorough cleaning routines generally does the trick.

But the various strains of algae commonly found in pools do possess specific characteristics that call for specialized treatment regimens. Here's a brief rundown of the possibilities.

• *Green algae*, a fast-growing strain, will spread like wildfire in pools where the chlorine or bromine residuals are consistently low or absent. Although brushing is always a good idea in pool maintenance, green algae is free-floating and will quickly reattach after brushing.

A chemical assist is called for here, with polyquats being perhaps the most effective killer—and also being helpful in that they help to flocculate the organics left behind by dead algae, not only reducing halogen demand but also aiding in filtration. (Copper and silver algaecides are much less affective here.)

• *Black algae*, also known as blue-green algae, is widely considered the hardiest algae strain found in pools and spas. A surface-clinging form, it is found mostly in inadequately maintained plaster pools where it finds strong foothold in the porous plaster surface.

Its stubbornness extends mostly from a gelatinous coating that protects the algae from chemical attack. The goal before chemical treatment is stripping this

coating away with aggressive brushing—even using a wire brush in plaster pools. That done, polyquats and silver-based algaecides have proven effective. (Copper-based algaecides are much less effective here.)

• *Mustard algae*, also known as yellow algae, is another hardy strain that is very hard to kill once it finds its Way into a pool or spa. Mustard algae exhibits stubborn resistance to regular chlorination or treatment by other halogens.

Copper and polyquat algaecides followed up by rigorous brushing and vacuuming have proven effective with this strain. (Silver algaecides are generally less effective here.)

From *Pool & Spa News*, February 8, 1993.

Blue/green algae has a protective gelatinous sheath that protects it from disinfectants. In the case of blue/green and any other surface clinging algae, brushing is required before superchlorination.

Mustard algae

Mustard algae, which most often grows on pool walls that are shaded, is easily brushed off surfaces yet difficult to kill.[2] Although mustard algae may not present problems of the same magnitude as green and blue/green algae, this form of algae appears to be quite resistant to normal disinfectants and the addition of algacides. Some swimming pool algae are also pink in color (Sidebar 12-1).

Treatment

More than any other pool problem, when it comes to algae growth, the best treatment is prevention.

Regular brushing and vacuuming along with proper chemical levels will prevent most algae growth. Once algae appears in a swimming pool, it must be treated with powerful chemicals to rid it completely (Table 12-1). Before discussing specific treatments, however, it is important to understand the difference between an algicide and an algistat. An algicide is used to kill algae once it begins to grow in a pool, whereas an algistat prevents and inhibits algae growth. Disinfectants like chlorine and bromine are excellent algistats. Once algae is detectable, the addition of a algicide may be required.

Algicides

Once algae is present, an algacide is often added to the pool to remove it. Many algicides are *quaternary ammonia compounds*, which are simply referred to as *quats*. Although this type of algicide works well in

Table 12-1. 30 ppm shock table for algae removal

Available chlorine (%)	Volume of water						
	250 gals / 946 L	400 gals / 1,514 L	1,000 gals / 3,785 L	5,000 gals / 18,927 L	20,000 gals / 75,708 L	50,000 gals / 189,271 L	100,000 gals / 378,541 L
5	2.36 cups / 558 mL*	1.89 qts* / 893 mL*	2.36 qts* / 2.23 L*	2.95 gals / 11.20 L*	11.8 gals / 11.70 L*	29.5 gals* / 112 L*	59.0 gals* / 223 L*
10	1.18 cups* / 279 mL*	.94 pts / 447 mL*	1.18 qts* / 1.12 L*	1.48 gals* / 5.58 L*	5.90 gals* / 22.30 L*	14.8 gals* / 55.80 L*	29.5 gals / 112 L*
12	.98 cups* / 234 mL*	.78 pts / 372 mL*	.98 qts / 932 mL*	1.23 gals* / 4.65 L*	4.92 gals* / 18.60 L*	12.3 gals* / 46.50 L*	24.6 gals* / 93.10 L*
35	2.86 oz / 81.1 g	1.58 oz / 130 g	11.4 oz / 324 g	3.57 lbs / 1.62 kg	14.3 lbs / 6.50 kg	35.7 lbs / 16.20 kg	71.5 lbs / 32.40 kg
60	1.67 oz / 47.3 g	2.67 oz / 76.0 g	6.67 oz / 190 g	2.08 lbs / 950 g	8.34 lbs / 3.79 kg	20.8 lbs / 9.4 70 kg	41.7 lbs / 19.00 kg
65	1.54 oz / 43.7 g	2.46 oz / 69.9 g	6.16 oz / 175 g	1.92 lbs / 875 g	7.70 lbs / 3.49 L	19.2 lbs / 8.74 kg	38.5 lbs / 17.50 kg
90	1.11 oz / 31.6 g	1.80 oz / 50.5 g	4.45 oz / 126 g	1.39 lbs / 635 g	5.56 lbs / 2.52 kg	13.9 lbs / 6.35 kg	27.8 lbs / 12.60 kg
100	1.00 oz / 28.4 g	1.60 oz / 45.5 g	4.00 oz / 114 g	1.25 lbs / 569 g	5.00 lbs / 2.28 kg	12.5 lbs / 5.70 kg	25.0 lbs / 11.40 kg

Courtesy Taylor Technologies, Sparks, Md.
* For correct chlorine product to add refer to How to use the Treatment Tables.

killing algae and also possesses some germicidal properties, quats are notorious for causing foam in pools, although this foaming may be due to overdosing. When algicidal quats are used to fight algae growth, they should be used weekly and the manufacturers guidelines must be followed carefully. Algicides that have a tendency to foam should not be used in hot tubs or spas. Both quats and polyquats may cause a very slight increase in chlorine demand.

Polyquat has both algicidal and algistatic properties and has been used to control algae in pools, hot tubs, and spas. The major advantage of polyquat is that it does not foam. This compound also flocculates organic material, thus assisting filtration. Proper levels of polyquat must be maintained continually in the pool for it to function properly. Most experts recommend adding polyquats weekly.

Copper- and silver-based algicides have both been used with some success. Both metals do have a tendency to precipitate out of the water, however, and may cause pool stains (Sidebar 12-2).

The following steps should be taken when treating algae:

1. Brush all pool surfaces and skimmers aggressively with a brush compatible with the pool shell. Using an inappropriate brush may mar the pool finish. Brushing cannot be overemphasized for both treatment and prevention of algae growth. For best results the pool recirculation pump should be turned off while brushing so that living algae is not drawn back to the filter.
2. Treat affected areas by placing a granular disinfectant like calcium hypochlorite or trichlor directly on visible algae growths. This is not recommended for liner pools because bleaching or spotting may result.
3. Superchlorinate up to 30 ppm. Superchlorination instructions like predissolving and diluting shocking agents must be followed so that pool finishes are protected.
4. Add an algicide. Quats or polyquats should be added 24 hours after superchlorination.
5. Clean filters Filters and filter elements must also be treated because stubborn forms of algae may continue to grow there while other forms are being killed in the pool.
6. Repeat steps 1 to 5 as needed.

Prevention

Like any other pool problem, prevention is the key, but it is particularly important to prevent algae. Once algae gets a foothold in a swimming pool, it is extremely difficult to kill completely. The following tips are key factors in preventing algae growth.

1. Keeps disinfectant levels up. Increase levels as conditions (sunlight, high swimmer loads, rain) that promote algae growth arise. Algae usually begins in the absence of disinfectants.
2. Brush, brush, brush. All pool finishes must be brushed frequently. Skimmer baskets, gutters, water lines, and filters must also be scrubbed. Care must be taken to use strong bristle brushes that will not scratch the pool/spa finish. The manufacturer should be consulted in this case. Concrete pools usually require stainless steel brushes, whereas vinyl-lined pools require a soft nylon brush. Brushes must be cleaned and disinfected after each use.
3. Clean and backwash filters regularly. Filters must be cleaned and backwashed according to the manufacturer's recommendations. Filter elements, media, and septa must also be checked and treated for algae.
4. Add an algicide during prime algae growth periods. In addition to the above precautions, nonfoaming algicides should be added when conditions are prime for algae growth. If a pool exhibits persistent algae problems, a polyquat algicide is probably a good idea. The use of all algicides must follow the suggested guidelines provided on the label.
5. Respond quickly and aggressively to the first sign of algae growth (Sidebar 12-3).

Chlorine Odor
Cause

As mentioned previously, obnoxious "chlorine" odors are perhaps the most persistent problem in heavily used pools. The odors that pool patrons object to is caused by too little, not too much chlorine, however. Chloramines or combined available chlorine are the culprit in this case. When free available chlorine combines with ammonia and other nitrogen compounds, chloramines (CAC) are formed. Perspiration, urine, saliva, body oils, and lotions are just a few compounds chlorine readily combines with to form chloramines.

Symptoms

The symptoms of chloramine development are easy to detect; pungent, obnoxious chlorine odors perme-

SIDEBAR 12-2

LINING UP

REINFORCEMENTS

The chlorine/algaecide strategy works for many pools, but what about those in which chlorine isn't the primary sanitizer?

Ionizers are a good bet here, because the copper and silver ions they release are lethal to most forms of algae. A tip from Don Girvan, vice president and general manager of John Girvan Co., a specialty-chemical manufacturer in Jacksonville, Fla.: combine ionizer use with an algae inhibitor to reduce the stress placed on the ionizer.

Bill Peck, owner of William Peck Pool Service, Poway, Calif., agrees that ionizers are effective in controlling algae, but he thinks that chlorine alone is enough. "I think the money is far better spent on a chlorine generator if you're going to spend that kind of money," Peck concludes.

What about ozonators? Girvan cites their effectiveness as oxidizers in eliminating food supplies for algae and bacteria and controlling the levels of organic compounds introduced by algae. He also credits their killing power when algae itself passes through the ozone chamber.

The problem with ozone alone, however, is the fact that pool circulation systems usually aren't perfect: In some areas, water doesn't circulate well enough to ensure adequate algaecidal contact, and there is no ozone residual left behind when the system is off, leaving algae free to regain its footholds.

"In fact, ozone has actually been associated with an increase in algae problems rather than a decrease," notes John Puetz, vice president for research at Great Lakes Biochemical, a manufacturer based in Milwaukee, Wis. The best strategy here, say the experts, is to use ozone in conjunction with either bromine or chlorine residuals.

From Pool & Spa News, February 8, 1993.

SIDEBAR 12-3

TO THE RESCUE

Preventing and killing algae is no small task. Once established, algae often grow wildly, seemingly undaunted by chlorine or any other sanitizer.

Not to fear: The pool and spa industry has responded with a number of specific products designed to eradicate even the most stubborn algae strains, including those listed below.

• Quaternary ammonium compounds (or quats) are versatile algaecides. Manufactures recommend maintaining a healthy concentration in algae-sensitive pools. That can be tough at times, because some research has shown that these compounds are subject to filtration—meaning regular applications are necessary.

• Polyquats are prime algae preventives for pools and spas. Again, because they tend to be subject to filtration, the trick is maintaining adequate levels of the product in the pool. As a big plus, polyquats act as a floccing agent for organic compounds and therefor work very will in conjunction with chlorine or bromine compounds.

• Copper-based algaecides are effective in ridding pools and spas of mustard algae in particular, but care must be used in their application because of their ability to stain pool surfaces. To counter that effect, many manufacturers recommend using a chelating agent to prevent the precipitation of copper carbonate and copper oxide onto pool and spa walls. Others recommend running vessels at a lower pH to minimize precipitation—and maximize killing power.

• Silver-based algaecides are well known for their ability to kill stubborn black algae. Like copper algaecides, however, straining is a concern, particularly in chlorinated pools.

From Pool & Spa News, February 8, 1993.

ate the facility. These symptoms are more noticeable in indoor than outdoor pools. Eyeburn and redness of the eyes may also accompany the chloramine odor. The water may also take on a dull or even cloudy appearance. It must be noted that even excessively high levels of FAC do not smell. Experienced pool operators agree, when they "smell" chlorine, they know it is time to superchlorinate.

Treatment

The treatment of chloramines is quick and simple. Once a CAC reading is determined by proper use of a test kit, the pool water is "shocked" to a FAC level that is 10 times grater than the amount of CAC. For example, if a CAC level of 0.4 ppm is found, the FAC level must be increased 4.0 ppm. Sodium hypochlorite, calcium hypochlorite, and lithium hypochlorite work well for shocking. If the pool needs to be reopened to the public immediately after shocking, a nonchlorine oxidizer like monopersulfate should be used. Whatever form of shocking is used, the target FAC level must be reached as quickly as possible. It must be emphasized that undershooting the target FAC will actually worsen the CAC problem. In indoor pools, windows and doors should be opened to allow the chloramines to be "off-gassed." See Chapter 11 for specific instructions regarding shocking.

Prevention

The best way to avoid a buildup of chloramines is to maintain disinfectants at breakpoint. Breakpoint chlorination is a maintained heightened level of disinfection whereby chloramines are unable to form. As swimmer loads increase, breakpoint levels will also have to be adjusted upward. Showering before swimming in a pool does much to prevent chloramine development. If swimmers understood this concept, they would probably shower with regularity before entering the pool. Unfortunately, many swimmers do not shower because they believe they are clean. Clean swimmers still carry body oils, lotions, perspiration, and other compounds into the water that produce CAC. Showering is a good preventive measure.

Routine shocking is also a recommended practice to prevent chloramine production, particularly just before anticipated heavy swimmer loads like swimming meets or hot humid days. In addition to shocking, disinfectant levels should never be allowed to drop to unacceptable levels.

Eye and Skin Irritation

Cause

Swimmer discomfort is often caused by high CAC levels and can be avoided by following the procedures mentioned above. If chloramines are not present in the pool water, however, and discomfort is still a problem, the pH of the water may be too high or too low. Eye and skin irritation can be caused by a pH that is above 7.8 or below 7.2.

Symptoms

CAC levels above .3 PPM can produce eyeburn. Red eyes and itching skin experienced by swimmers can also be attributed to pH levels that are excessively high or low. The CAC level should be checked first however. When the pH level becomes too high the water will actually feel slippery.

Treatment

If swimmer discomfort is actually caused by improper pH levels, the pH must be adjusted to between 7.2 and 7.6. If the pH must be lowered, either muriatic acid or sodium bisulfate (dry acid) should be used. If the pH must be raised, soda ash is commonly added to the pool. If chloramines are present, shocking is required. Refer to Chapter 11 for specifics.

Prevention

Prevention in this case is simple. Constant and vigilant monitoring of pool water will help to keep the pH within its ideal range.

Cloudy (Milky) Water
Cause

There are numerous causes for cloudy water in swimming pools. Because there are several causes, clearing up a pool can be frustrating and challenging. The cause must be specifically identified before any corrective action can be taken. It is important to note that the cloudy water discussed here is not discolored water, but rather a milky, white water that has no coloration at all. Discolored (red, blue, or green) water will be discussed separately.

Perhaps the leading cause of cloudy water is a lack of disinfectant in the water or some other chemical imbalance. Using a good test kit, the pool owner/operator should analyze chlorine, pH, total alkalinity, calcium hardness, and TDS, and a saturation index should be calculated. Often, cloudy water is produced in the absence of a disinfectant.

Another leading cause of cloudy water is inadequate or nonexistent filtration. If for any reason the pool water is not being filtered, it will turn cloudy quickly. When filtration is the cause of cloudy water a host of additional problems may exist: the recirculating pump may not be running, the filter may need backwashing or cleaning, the hair and lint strainer may be clogged, or some other obstruction may exist in the circulation and filtration system. In sand filtration systems, unbalanced water might calcify the sand media making it impossible to filter water. Oils, hair, and lint can create mud balls that can also hinder filtration. If a DE system is in use, a ripped or torn septa might be allowing the media to pass back into the pool. Cartridge filters must be cleaned and repaired often because they can become worn or clogged quickly.

Also, in a highly saturated pool, air entering the system through a faulty hair and lint strainer cover or some other location can turn a pool milky quite fast. The air turning the pool cloudy may not be detected as air and may easily fool the pool operator.

This discussion assumes that the swimming pool treatment plant is filtering at proper flow rates and turnover rates, and that the filtration system is properly sized. Insufficient turnovers and inadequate filter size will not produce good water clarity. The filtering charts provided in Chapter 5 should be referred to when determining the proper flow rate, turnovers, and filter size. If turnover rates are too slow, a new pump will probably be needed. If the filter surface area is too small, installation of an additional filter(s) may be necessary.

High swimmer load, CAC, and TDS levels may also cause cloudiness.

Symptoms

A pool that turns cloudy often does so slowly. As the water progressively turns from dull to cloudy, the pool operator must quickly and systematically check the above mentioned areas of concern.

Treatment

When cloudy water first appears, the water chemistry should be checked immediately. If any chemical parameters are not within ideal ranges, adjustments should be made promptly. In the case of inadequate filtration, the flow rate meter should be checked first. Often when cloudy water appears, little or no water is moving through the filters. If there is no flow rate, the pump and hair and lint strainer should be checked. If inadequate flow rate is present, the filters may need to be backwashed. If air is in the system, it usually comes from a faulty gasket on the hair and lint strainer or a crack in a plexiglass housing or some other apparatus on the circulation system. The suction side of the pump must be checked for air leaks and should include valves and chemical injectors but especially the hair and lint strainer and all lids. These items would have to be repaired or replaced. If a DE filter is in use, all elements and septa must be checked for tears or gaps where DE can be returned to the pool. When found they need to be replaced.

If high CAC levels are causing the turbidity, shocking is required. If high TDS levels are causing cloudiness, replacing some or all of the water is in order. If particles are simply too small for the filter to trap and remove, then the addition of clarifiers and flocculants may be used to clump these fine particles together, thus improving filtration.

Prevention

To prevent pool water from becoming cloudy, pool chemistry must be continually monitored and kept within ideal ranges. Filters must run effectively and be backwashed and cleaned regularly. When high swimmer loads and/or CAC levels appear, shocking should commence. When high TDS levels occur, some or all the water should be replaced.

Discolored Water and Staining
Cause

When pool water becomes discolored or stains on the pool shell begin to appear, the actual color exhibited can often predict the pool problem being experienced. Discoloration problems in swimming pools can be the result of high mineral content in the source water used to fill the pool or corrosive water in the pool, which erodes iron, copper, and other metals. Some copper- or silver-based algacides can also produce staining or spotting of the pool shell.

Symptoms

Green, blue/green water

If not caused by algae, green or blue/green water normally indicates copper. Highly aggressive, unbalanced water can corrode copper pipes and heater elements, thus turning the water green or blue/green.

Source water may sometimes have a high copper content. High halogen levels will also cause this discoloration.

Red or brown water

Water that is colored red or brown usually indicates iron in the water. High iron content is often found in source water, or unbalanced water may be dissolving iron pipes.

Blue or black water

Likewise, blue or black discolored water is caused by a high manganese content or by highly aggressive water.

Treatment

When discoloration and staining first appear it would be beneficial to contact a local swimming pool supplier or pool chemical dealer to see if he or she is familiar with the problem. Perhaps these experts are familiar with the source of the discoloration and can offer a quick cure to the problem. The water should be balanced immediately to ensure pool equipment is not being dissolved. Depending on the metal causing discoloration, either sequestering or chelating agents are used to combat the problem. Although these agents are slightly different, they are often used interchangeably in the swimming pool industry. Sequestering agents are most often used and hold the offending metals in solution so that they are not visible. If sequestering agents are used regularly, however, a chelating agent may eventually be required. Chelating agents bring these metals out of solution so that they can be filtered or vacuumed from the pool. Numerous pools are plagued with high iron contents and as a result must use a chelating agent regularly. Stains and spots on the pool shell may require draining for acid washing. If there is a high mineral content in the water that creates discoloration, it is extremely difficult to prevent.

Corrosion of Pool Equipment
Cause

Corrosion is a natural process, but when swimming pool water is unbalanced, very aggressive, corrosive water conditions may result. Aggressive water can corrode many pool parts but particularly those made of metal or copper like pipes, heat exchangers, ladders, light rings, and more. Additionally, if disinfectant levels are allowed to remain above the recom-

mended levels for extended periods of time, the corrosion process will be accelerated. Also, when TDS levels become excessive, electrical conductivity increases, thereby promoting corrosion.

Symptoms

The malfunctioning of swimming pool heaters is often one of the first symptoms of corrosive water to appear. Because heat sinks and heat exchangers are usually made of copper and copper is susceptible to corrosive conditions, this is one of the first pool components to be adversely affected by aggressive water. As mentioned earlier, if pool water becomes colored, metals are often being dissolved. Pump impellers and other metal fixtures in contact with pool water may be eaten away. In addition, copper, iron or manganese may begin to stain the pool walls and floors.

Treatment

Corrosive water can be corrected by simply balancing the water with the aid of the saturation index. Increasing pH, total alkalinity and calcium hardness may be in order, depending on the results of the saturation index. Second, disinfectant levels may have to be lowered if they are above the upper limits of the recommended ideal range. TDS levels and water temperatures may also need to be lowered. See Chapter 11 for specific instructions on making water less corrosive.

Prevention

Fortunately, preventing corrosive water is simple. Water must be kept balanced by constant calculation of the saturation index. Disinfectant levels should be kept within ideal ranges except for superchlorination. TDS levels and temperatures should not be allowed to get too high.

Sand/DE in Pool
Cause

If sand or DE finds its way into the swimming pool, it is usually caused by filter problems. In the case of sand filters, the media will be deposited on the pool bottom near inlets. There are several causes for this. The pool pump may be oversized, pushing sand back into the pool. The laterals may be broken and need to be replaced. The filter bed may have mud balls and channeling in it and may need to be cleaned and raked or replaced. Finally, there may simply be too much sand in the filter.

DE filters will often allow the media to enter the pool through holes or openings in the filter screens or return manifolds. Sometimes, human error is responsible for this problem. If return valves to the pool are mistakenly left open during the backwash cycle, DE can be pushed back into the pool through inlets in white clouds.

Symptoms

Malfunctioning sand filters will deposit sand granules on the pool bottom near pool inlets. DE filters not operating properly will turn the pool water milky white.

Treatment

Treatment calls for checking the source of the problem, the filter and correcting it. Sand filters may need new sand, new laterals, or possibly a downsized pump. DE filters may require repairing or replacing the filter septa or manifold. Close attention to backwashing procedures may also correct this problem if filter screens and manifolds are in good repair.

Prevention

Regularly scheduled maintenance to the filter, filter elements, and filter media will prevent the media from entering the pool. Unfortunately, this area is often neglected at many pools.

Excessive Scale Formation
Cause

Excessive scale formation, like many other pool problems, is caused by unbalanced water. Scale is produced when the pH, total alkalinity, and calcium hardness levels become to high. This type of unbalanced water is basic and scale forming. Slight scale formation has positive effects because It can actually become a protective coating for heater elements, valves, impellers, and fittings. But when scale formation becomes extreme, it can roughen pool and spa finishes, cause filter calcification, and reduce circulation. Excessive scale can also clog pipes, tubes, injectors and chemical feeders. In regions that have extremely hard water, even the most rigorous water balancing programs may not prevent scale build-up.

Symptoms

Typically, excessive scale formation may slow and even stop swimming pool circulation and filtration.

Roughened pool and spa finishes, filter clarification, damaged heater elements, slowed circulation and clogged swimming pool parts are just a few of the side-effects caused by excessive scale formation. Scale can be observed as a hard, white precipitate.

Treatment

Treating for scale requires the pool owner/operator to return the pool water to balance by lowering pH, total alkalinity, or calcium hardness, depending on which values are high. See Chapter 11, for specific directions on reducing scaling properties in water. Basic water usually requires muriatic or dry acid for balancing. Using a sequestering agent (sequestrant) may also be required to inhibit scale formation. Sequestrants may be required in geographical regions with extremely high calcium hardness levels. In rare cases involving exceedingly high levels of calcium hardness, the pool water may need to be drained and refilled with fresh water low in calcium hardness.

Prevention

Preventing scale formation requires balanced water. Using the saturation index regularly will help in this regard. If scale is a constant problem, a sequestering agent may have to be added regularly.

Excessive Chlorine
Cause

Shocking, faulty chlorination equipment or human error may cause chlorine levels to become excessively high. Above 10 ppms, chlorine can begin to cause discomfort to swimmers. Above 25 ppms or so, chlorine will start to bleach bathing suits.

Symptoms

Actually, high chlorine levels are difficult to detect without a test kit and can be tricky as well. As mentioned previously, when chlorine levels are very high, test reagents may be bleached out indicating no chlorine is present. High chlorine levels do not permit chloramine production, and as a result, *no "chlorine"* odor is present. High chlorine levels may cause eye and skin irritation however, particularly when pH levels are low.

Treatment

Sodium sulfite, sodium bisulfite, or sodium thiosulfate can all be added to quickly reduce high chlorine levels. Adding too much chlorine neutralizer however, will make it difficult to return chlorine levels within acceptable ranges. Large amounts of a neutralizing agent may also significantly lower pH so a watchful eye must be kept on this value as well. See Chapter 11 and a local swimming pool company for questions concerning high chlorine levels.

Prevention

A vigilant water testing program will ensure that chlorine levels will be kept within ideal ranges. Test reagents must be kept fresh so that faulty readings do not confuse the pool owner/operator. All chemical controllers and feeders must receive regular preventive maintenance.

Foam
Cause

Foaming water occurs more often in spas and hot tubs than in swimming pools. Although foam on the surface looks unsightly, it is not much of a problem unless it spills over onto decking and creates a slip hazard or obscures a view of the bottom. Foaming pool/spa water has several causes. Soft water sudses and foams easily so low calcium hardness may promote this problem. Some algicides, particularly the quats as opposed to polyquats, cause foaming. In spas with high TDS stemming from lotions, creams and shampoos, foaming may also be encouraged. Finally, pranksters have been known to add detergents to pools and spas.

Symptoms

Foam on a pool or spa surface is readily detectable. In severe cases, a foaming spa resembles a bubble bath.

Treatment

Although the fast-fix method of combating foam is to add a defoamer, it is often better to attack the cause of the problem. Calcium hardness may have to be raised, TDS lowered and a polyquat algicide used instead of a quat. If foaming persists, then a defoamer may be warranted.

Prevention

Residential spas and hot tubs should not be filled with treated water from a water softener. If soft water must be used to fill a hot tub, spa or pool, the calcium

hardness must be increased immediately. Showering before soaking or swimming might also reduce foaming, particularly in hot tubs and spas. Nonfoaming algacides should be used.

Excessive Water Loss
Cause

Water loss that is excessive would be more than 1 inch in a 24 hour period. For every 1000 square feet of surface area, an inch of pool water represents 620 gallons. This type of water loss is probably due to a leak rather than evaporation or splash-out. Leakage in the pool shell can occur around inlets, outlets, and copings, but most large leaks are often detected in the main drain box. Broken or corroded pipes may also cause major water loss. Vinyl lined pools are easily punctured by sharp objects. Vandalism can easily damage vinyl liners. Water loss occurs naturally at swimming pools through evaporation and splash-out. Pool rules and pool covers can help prevent natural water loss.

Symptoms

Excessive water loss is usually detected by the addition of large amounts of make-up water to keep the pool full. When large amounts of make-up water needs to be added to the pool, particularly after slow periods, a leak should be suspected.

Leaks in the pool shell are best detected by using a SCUBA diver with a syringe or squirt gun filled with dye or food coloring. By injecting this coloring in pool water near suspected leaks, the movement of the dye can be followed to the leak. Vinyl liner pools only need to be inspected for cuts and punctures in the shell. Wet spots may also be noticed outside the pool shell on adjacent ground. Professionals may be required to detect hard to find leaks (Fig. 12-1).

Treatment

Fixing a leak in a swimming pool is often a difficult task. If the leak is on the pool bottom, naturally the pool must be drained. Vinyl lined pools are easily repaired when full and waterproof patch kits are available in most swimming pool stores. SCUBA diving makes this chore much easier. If the leak is in the filter room or other pool plumbing, pipes and fixtures may need to be replaced. Whatever the cause, the leak may require either patching or replacement by a professional.

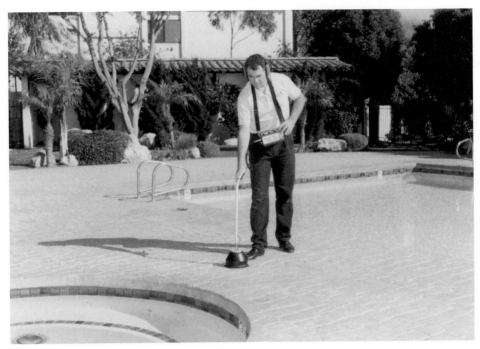

Fig. 12-1. Professionals may be required to detect hard-to-find leaks. (Courtesy National Leaks Detection, Palos Verdes Estates, Calif.)

Prevention

Whenever a pool or spa is emptied, the shell should be checked for cracks or gaps and repaired as necessary. Properly balanced water will prevent corrosion of pool pipes and parts. Do not allow sharp objects in a vinyl-lined pool and protect against vandalism.

Summary

This chapter dealt with pool problems that occur most frequently in swimming pools throughout the country. Because source water differs dramatically from region to region, when a pool problem suddenly effects a given pool, local experts should be consulted early during the trouble-shooting process (Table 12-2).

References

1. Mitchel K: *The proper management of pool and spa water,* Decature, Ga, 1988, BioLab.

Bibliography

BioGuard Lab: *The pool book*, 1981, Decatur, Ga.

Johnson R: *Swimming pool operations manual*, Harrisburg, Penn, 1991, Pennsylvania Department of Community Affairs.

Kowalsky L (editor): *Pool/spa operators handbook*, San Antonio, Tex, 1991, National Swimming Pool Foundation.

Mitchel, K, *The proper management of pool and spa water*, Decatur, Ga, 1988, BioLab.

Pool and Spa News, Los Angeles.

Pope, JR Jr: *Public swimming pool management.* I and II. Alexandria, Va, 1991, National Recreation and Park Association.

Service Industry News, Torrance, Calif.

Taylor C: *Everything you always wanted to know about pool care*, Chino, Calif, 1989, Service Industry Publications.

Taylor Technologies: *Pool and spa water chemistry, testing and treatment guide with tables*, Sparks, Md.

Water quality and treatment: ed 3, 1971, The American Water Works Association.

Williams K G: *The aquatic facility operator's manual*, Hoffman Estates, Ill, 1991, National Recreation and Park Association, National Aquatic Section.

Table 12-2.   Pool Problem Summary

Pool problem	Symptom	Cause	Treatment
Cloudy, milky water	Cloudy, milky	No disinfectant; poor filtration, unbalanced water; DE in water, air in system	Add chlorine; clean filter; balanced; check filter; repair leaks
Malodorous, irritating water	Red eyes; itching skin	Chloramines; improper pH	shock; adjust pH to 7.2-7.8
Green water	Clear green	Copper	balance pool; use clarifier
	Cloudy green	Algae	shock, brush; algicide
Red or brown water	Red/brown	Iron, rust	balance pool; use clarifier
Blue or black	Blue or black	Manganese	balance pool; use clarifier
Pump problems	Noisy; hot	Turn-off power	call for service
Sand in pool	On pool bottom near inlets	Cracked laterals; oversized pump	call pool company
Excessive water loss	Water level keeps dropping	Leak in main drain or pool plumbing; hole in vinyl liner	call pool service company; patch hole
Excessive foaming	Foam and suds	Unbalanced water; detergent	balance pool; add defoamer; dump spa
Corrosion of metal parts	Metal staining; wearing out pool parts	Unbalanced water; low pH, low TA	Balance water
Scaling	Clogging of filter and pipes; scale on pool walls	Unbalanced water; high pH, high TA, high calcium hard	Balance water
Excessive chlorine	Free chlorine above 8 ppm/ mgl; bleaching	Shocking; overdosing	Add sodium thiosulfate
Scum ring at water line	"Bathtub" ring around pool/spa	Body oils, dirt, lotions	Use specified tile or vinyl cleaner

Review Questions

1. Describe the difference between an algicide and a algistrat.

2. How many species of algae can cause pool problems?

3. What is a disadvantage of using quats?

4. Once algae becomes noticeable in a swimming pool, is it relatively easy to eliminate?

5. List 3 possible causes of cloudy, milky water.

6. Match the following symptoms with the appropriate cause of the discolored pool water: blue/green; red or brown; blue or black; with manganese, copper, or iron.

7. What causes rough pool finishes, clogged pipes, and filter calcifation?

8. Where are most large water leaks in pools located?

SECTION IV
SPECIALTY POOLS

This section concentrates on pools and topics that are slightly different from the standard residential or public pool. Chapter 13 discusses hot tubs and spas, which is probably the fastest growing area in the swimming pool industry. Of particular interest in this chapter is "hot water chemistry." The reader will find that as water temperature increases, so do the challenges for the hot water pool owner or operator. Typically, hot tubs and spas require higher levels of disinfectant and much more attention to water balance. TDS is also a problem in this environment. Many different safety concerns are also outlined in this chapter.

Chapter 14, Water-Parks and Theme Parks, is written by an expert in this area, P.J. Heath. P.J. is a highly regarded author and speaker who specializes in all phases of water-park operations. This chapter presents a wealth of information that will assist the reader in establishing a risk management program for water-parks. Water-parks entertain many more patrons than standard pools and thus require closer supervision. These parks also offer tremendous variety in their attractions. Rides, special park procedures, and guarding techniques are discussed in detail.

Chapter 15 concentrates on winterizing procedures for seasonal pools. Both residential and public pools are considered in this discussion. The underlying theme of this chapter is that winterizing is important and must be taken seriously. More damage can occur to a swimming pool and its equipment during the off-season than during the hottest summer months. It is also emphasized that organization is the key to good winterizing.

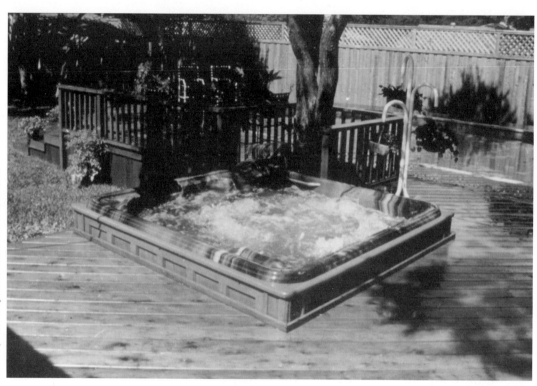

13

HOT TUBS AND SPAS

Hot tubs and spas are considered separately in this text because they present unique problems apart from swimming pools. In fact, some spa specialists strongly believe that spas are *not* swimming pools and therefore should not be treated as such. Although spas and hot tubs are the fastest growing facilities in the swimming industry and they offer many hours of relaxation, recreation, and therapy, unique challenges are associated with their use.

Hot water soaking has been a popular form of relaxation and therapy for centuries. The Romans, Japanese, and many other cultures have enjoyed the benefits of hot water immersions. Soaking in a hot tub or spa relaxes tired muscles, promotes circulation, and helps relieve mental stress.

According to the Arthritis Foundation, about 37 million Americans, or one in seven, have some form of arthritis.[1] Although there are many different kinds of arthritis, most forms are characterized by inflammation. A hot tub or spa can provide the warmth, hydrotherapy, and buoyancy needed to relax and exercise the affected joints and muscles of the body in the convenience of one's own home. The warm water allows muscles to relax, which in turn makes exercising and daily tasks easier to perform. Arthritics

should consult their personal physicians before purchasing or exercising in a spa. If treatment is the primary reason for purchasing a hot tub or spa, all or part of the purchase *may* qualify as a medical expense and tax deduction. To receive this deduction, the owner should consult a doctor, lawyer, and accountant.

Today as many as 4 million hot tubs and spas are in the United States, and nearly 3 million can be found in private residences. More than one third of all privately owned hot tubs and spas are located in California[2] (Fig. 13-1). Soaking in a hot tub or spa produces benefits that many swimming pools cannot. These benefits can be physical, psychological, or both. Physical benefits include reducing muscle soreness as well as aches and pains. And of course, the reduction of modern day stress and tension and the promotion of overall relaxation are achieved through the combination of hot water and hydrojet action of the water in a hot tub or spa. As a result, hot tubs and spas have become vital components for health clubs, hotels, hospitals, rehabilitation clinics, housing developments, and private residences.

Water temperatures in hot tubs and spas should range from 98° to 104° F. These high water temperatures, coupled with relatively high soaker loads and organic debris, make spa maintenance troublesome in some cases. The warmth and moisture offer an ideal breeding ground for bacteria, algae, and fungi. Four people in a 500-gallon spa is equal to 160 people in a 20,000 gallon pool. Heavy soaker loads plus the heat and moisture promote problems that must be controlled through proper chemical disinfection.

Definitions

Hot tub, spa, whirlpool, Jacuzzi, and *therapy pool* are all terms that have been used interchangeably throughout the years. Although steam rooms and

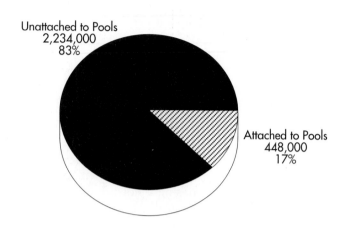

Rank	Region	Total Spa/Hot Tubs Owned	Percent of Total
6	North Atlantic	179,000	7%
10	Mid Atlantic	78,000	3%
2	South Central	425,000	16%
9	Southwest	116,000	4%
4	West Central	197,000	7%
8	East Central	127,000	5%
3	Florida	232,000	9%
5	Northwest	181,000	7%
11	New England	60,000	2%
7	Southeast	129,000	5%
1	California	958,000	35%
	Total	2,682,000	100%

Fig. 13-1. **A,** Spa and hot tub ownership. **B,** Spa and hot tub ownership by region. (From NSPI: *Pool and spa market study for the year 1991*, Alexandria, Va, The Institute.)

saunas are closely related to the hot water pools just mentioned, they are not considered in this discussion because they do not offer body immersion in water. This discussion is limited to hot tubs and spas that have chemically treated water. Jacuzzi is a brand name of hydrotherapy jets and related pool equipment, whereas whirlpools and therapy pools are often associated with athletic training rooms and rehabilitation hospitals. Hot tubs and spas use several pumps for different functions. Separate pumps are required for filtration, water jets, and air jets.

Hot tubs

California probably made hot tubs popular in this country because of the availability of redwoods and the wine industry making these barrels plentiful. For the purposes of this book, hot tubs refer to wooden barrels or tubs that have hot water and hydrotherapy jets. In addition to redwood, hot tubs can also be made of mahogany, teak, cedar, and other woods. Hot tubs are found in residences rather than commercial establishments (Fig. 13-2).

New wooden hot tubs, when first filled, may turn the water brown. Rust- or coffee-colored water is caused by nontoxic tannic acid leeching out of the wood. The water should be replaced frequently during the first 4 to 6 weeks, but eventually the discol-

oration of the water decreases with time. High water temperatures, high chlorine levels, and low pH levels increase the leeching process. A similar concern of wooden hot tubs is the bleaching of the wood that occurs as the lignin or natural cellulose glue present in woods reacts with sanitizers. When first filled with water, hot tubs may leak until the wood swells and becomes watertight.

The wooden hot tub should be emptied periodically to remove stubborn stains. Commercial cleaners and very fine sandpaper should be used but never acid. Wooden hot tubs should not, however, be drained and left empty for long periods of time. When this occurs, the hot tub may shrink and cause leaks. The grain of the wood in hot tubs may also provide more breeding grounds for bacteria to flourish. Hot tubs made of wood appear to be more suitable for residential rather than public use.

Spas

A more recent version of the wooden hot tub is a fiberglass, acrylic, or stainless steel prefabricated shell that is available in a variety of shapes, sizes, colors, and seating arrangements. Spas can be installed in-ground or above-ground, inside or outside (Sidebars 13-1 to 13-3). Above-ground spas are less expensive and movable, which is a big advantage

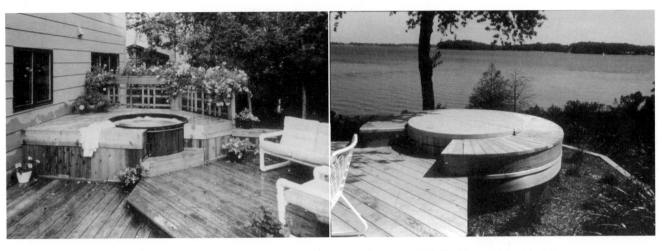

Fig. 13-2. **A,** Wooden hot tub and decking. (Courtesy NSPI, Alexandria, Va.) **B,** Wooden hot tub with cover.

SIDEBAR 13-1
SPA
INSTALLATION—
SITE CHECK LIST

☐ Check local building and safety codes and obtain permits before starting installation.

☐ Make sure the chosen installation site is not too close to trees or foliage where falling leaves or pine needles may fall into the spa or roots may cause excavation problems.

☐ Check for adequate run-off drainage. Don't block designed run-off areas. Don't install a spa in such an area.

☐ Make sure spa and equipment sites are accessible and properly ventilated.

☐ Determine direction of the prevailing wind. If not protected from wind, operating expenses for heating will go up.

☐ Determine whether difference in elevation between spa and equipment is too great (see Chapter 5).

☐ Check for overhead wires (see NEC Code and Chapter 17).

☐ Check for underground cables and septic tanks.

☐ Check for easy access from house to spa.

☐ Check any gates that provide entry. They must be self-latching and self-closing.

☐ Check for proper fencing, if required.

☐ Check depth of fill dirt that may lie over a base. Check the type of base (rock or boulders).

☐ Check possible obstacles to piping, including plumbing and utility lines, concrete, sprinkler lines, and walks.

☐ Check for privacy from surrounding areas.

☐ Check that required permits are in order or make appropriate additions.

☐ Make sure there is access to electrical service and available power.

☐ Check that there is access to the gas lines and meter, if required.

From NSPI: *Basic pool and spa technology*, ed 2, Alexandria, Va, 1992, The Institute.

SIDEBAR 13-2

STARTING OVER

Before agreeing to transport a well-loved hot tub to a new location, would-be rebuilders and their customers should certainly consider whether replacing the tub is the wiser move, say the experts.

You must get your customers to think about the expense and labor involved in the move; for your part, you need to assess the age and condition of the tub.

A rule of thumb from Steven Gasperson, general field manager for Salinas, Calif.-based Blackthorne, "If a tub is more than 10 years old, moving it probably isn't worth the effort." And always, always, *always*, he cautions, be sure to look at the tub yourself before making any promises.

From *Pool & Spa News*, Oct 5, 1992, Los Angeles.

SIDEBAR 13-3

WHILE YOU'RE

AT IT

There can be much more to moving a tub than simply relocating it whole or pulling it apart for later reassembly. Your goal, after all, is to make the tub as "good as new" to satisfy your customers.

As you work with the wooden tank, here are some possibilities you should consider:

• *Pumping the croze*: This tub repair entails pumping silicon into the joint between the bottom of a stave and the tub's floor—but is required *only* when the tub is actually leaking.

• *Stave replacement*: If a stave is cracked or otherwise out of sorts, the challenge is getting a good match. The best bet here, obviously, is to go back to the tub's manufacturer. If you can't find a stave of the same brand and the right size, you'll need to resort to underwater epoxies and other such products to repair the bad stave.

• *Hoop cleaning/replacement*: The hoops on older hot tubs are subject to rust damage; some may even need replacing if the nuts and threads are affected. Often, however, it's possible to free up rusted parts with WD-40 or similar product.

• *Jet/fitting/plumbing replacement*: Replacing these items is generally a good idea to help ensure that the tub is in prime condition well after the move—or to update old-fashioned systems and to make the tub more efficient. If your customer chooses not to replace the jets altogether, be sure to put a hood bead of silicon where the jets crimp together around the stave to ensure they are properly resealed.

From *Pool & Spa News*, Oct 5, 1992, Los Angeles.

(Figs. 13-3 to 13-5). Larger spas are often in-ground models made of gunite or concrete, and many of these are tiled. The fiberglass and acrylic spas should be much easier to clean than the wooden hot tubs (Fig. 13-6).

Hot water chemistry

As mentioned earlier in this text, increased water temperatures create some interesting challenges in water chemistry. Disinfection and water balance are much more difficult to maintain in hot water than in normal swimming pool water (78° to 84° F). Perhaps the two greatest challenges for hot tub and spa owners is the production of chloramines and the increase of TDS levels. Bacteria growth is also an ever-present concern.

One of the problems posed by hot water chemistry is increased bacteria proliferation. Many bacteria thrive and reproduce better in warm water. Therefore it is not surprising that as the popularity of hot tubs

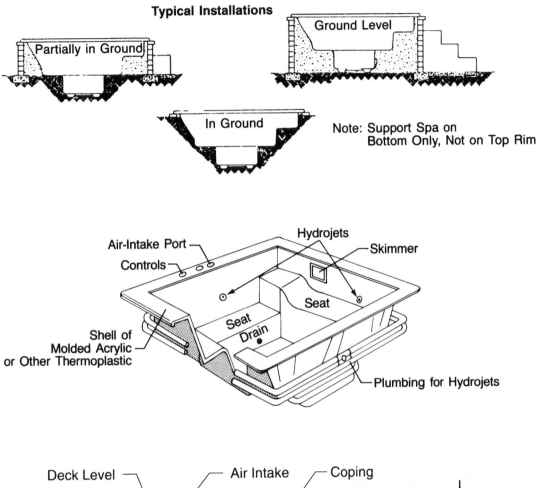

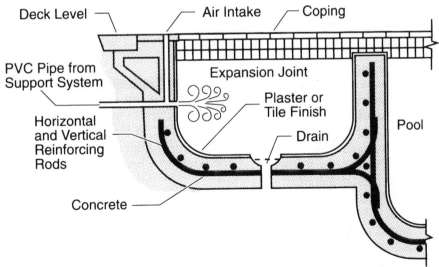

Fig. 13-3. In-ground spa structures. (From NSPI: *Basic pool and spa technology*, ed 2, Alexandria, Va, The Institute.)

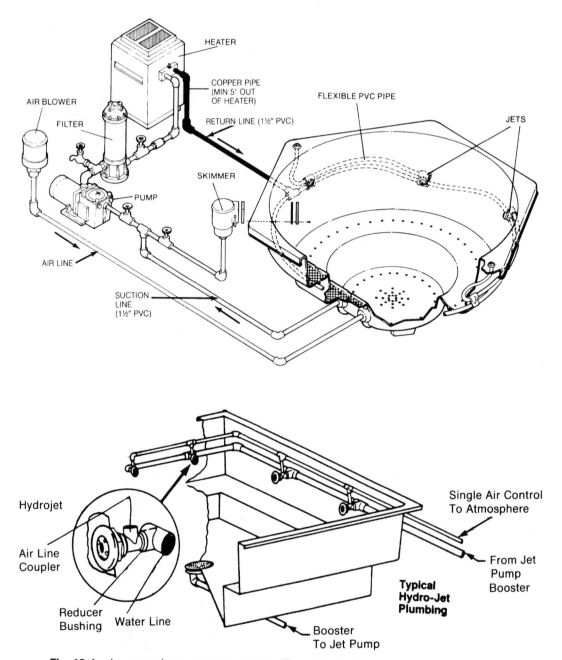

HEATER

COPPER PIPE
(MIN 5' OUT
OF HEATER)

FLEXIBLE PVC PIPE

AIR BLOWER

FILTER

RETURN LINE (1½" PVC)

JETS

PUMP

SKIMMER

AIR LINE

SUCTION
LINE
(1½" PVC)

Hydrojet

Single Air Control
To Atmosphere

Air Line
Coupler

From Jet
Pump
Booster

Reducer
Bushing   Water Line

**Typical
Hydro-Jet
Plumbing**

Booster
To Jet Pump

Fig. 13-4. In-ground spa support system. (From NSPI: *Basic pool and spa technology*, ed 2, Alexandria, Va, The Institute.)

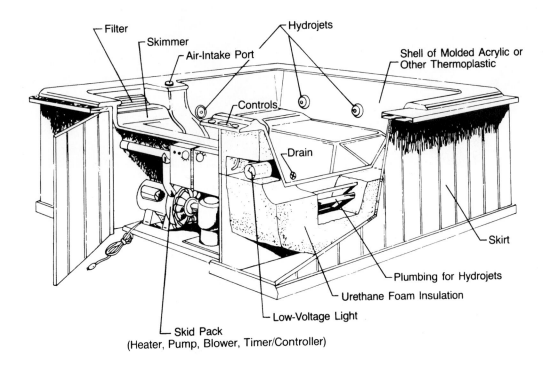

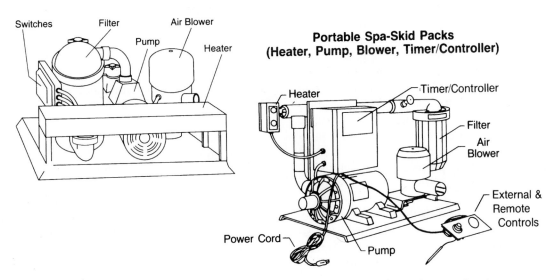

Fig. 13-5. Portable spa and spa packs. (From NSPI: *Basic pool and spa technology,* ed 2, Alexandria, Va, The Institute.)

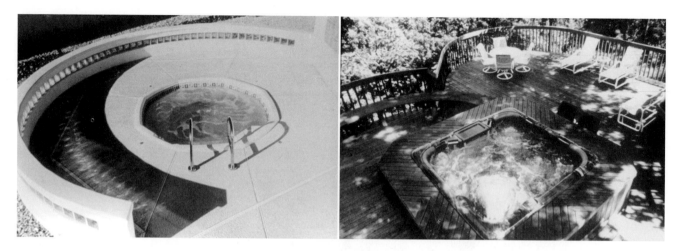

Fig. 13-6. Spas and decking. (Courtesy NSPI, Alexandria, Va.)

and spas has increased, so has the number of outbreaks of dermatitis and folliculitis resulting from exposure to *Pseudomonas aeruginosa*. Pontiac fever, or Legionnaires disease, has also been associated with hot water pools. Considering that pseudomonads thrive and may even double in number every 20 minutes in water temperatures between 100° and 105° F, hot tubs and spas make a perfect home for these rod-shaped bacteria.[3] Pseudomonads also enjoy smooth surfaces such as fiberglass, acrylic, and PVC piping that accompany hot tubs and spas. Associated with the increased bacteria proliferation in hot water pools is the fact that high water temperatures tend to dilate the pores of the body while the water jets can "jack-hammer" bacteria into the skin, making soakers more susceptible to any bacteria present. This is why soap showers are recommended before *and* after hot tub or spa use.

Compounding this problem is the fact that disinfectants are less effective at higher temperatures. Because of reduced killing power at higher temperatures, more chemicals must be added to a hot tub or spa to keep it clean, clear, and bacteria free.

Soakers in hot tubs and spas perspire much more than in pools, and therefore more chloramines are produced. Additional chemicals are required to burn out the chloramines, and as more chemicals are added TDS levels also rise. In addition, as temperatures increase, calcium carbonate becomes less solu-

ble and precipitates out of solution. As a result, water chemistry in hot tubs and spas must be continually monitored and adjusted. Recommended chlorine and bromine residuals are much higher than in standard pools.

Another problem associated with hot tubs and spas is the turbulence of the water created by the hydrojets. This water agitation increases evaporation of both water and chemicals. Chemical levels in these hot water pools must be checked hourly. It is especially difficult to keep sufficient amounts of disinfectant in the water in public spas with high soaker loads.

For all the reasons mentioned above, hot tubs and spas require a tremendous amount of disinfectants, which in turn result in a significant TDS production. Hot tubs and spas are also a good place to experiment with alternative sanitizers in an attempt to avoid chloramine and TDS buildup. Both ozone and potassium monopersulfate show promise in this regard. Of the halogens, bromine is preferred over chlorine because bromine tends to be more stable at higher temperatures and bromamines are effective sanitizers, whereas chloramines are not. Dichlor, the stabilized chlorine, is also becoming popular with hot tub and spa users, but because it contains CYA to protect chlorine from the damaging effects of ultraviolet (UV) rays in the sun, it should not be used indoors. Trichlor, another stabilized chlorine, should

Table 13-1. Ideal Chemical Ranges for Hot Tubs and Spas

Parameters	Minimum	Ideal	Maximum
Free available chlorine (ppm)	1	3-5	10
Combined available chlorine (ppm)	None	None	0.2
Bromine (ppm)	2	3-5	10
pH	7.2	7.0-7.6	7.8
Total alkalinity (ppm) for hypochlorites	60	80-100	180
Total alkalinity (ppm) for gas, bromine		100-120	
TDS (ppm)	300	1000-2000	3000
TDS (ppm)	150	200-400	500
Calcium hardness	10	30-50	150*

* Except when limited by local health departments, usually to 150 ppm.
From NSPI: *Basic pool and spa technology*, ed 2, Alexandria, Va 1992, The Institute.

not be used in hot tubs or spas because it is too acidic. Trichlor in hot water pools may lower the pH sufficiently to cause damage to both the equipment and the shell.

Because water chemistry changes so rapidly in hot tubs and spas, disinfectants should probably be added by reliable and accurate automatic controllers rather than added manually. Particularly for hot tubs and spas with high soaker loads, proper disinfection and oxidation may be impossible to maintain if done manually. Too often in the case of hot tubs and spas, proper chemistry cannot be maintained for long periods and the only solution is to empty the tub or spa. "Dumping" a hot tub or spa is an unavoidable ritual that should be performed weekly in public spas with higher soaker loads and bimonthly for moderately used spas and hot tubs. However, well-maintained residential hot tubs and spas with low soaker loads do not need to be dumped as frequently. Shocking hot tubs and spas should also be a regular practice. Public spas should probably be shocked daily, preferably at the end of each day.

Chemical standards

The chemical standards in Table 13-1 are recommended by the National Spa and Pool Institute for hot tub and spas.

Soaker loads for hot tubs and spas

Because hot tubs and spas can quickly become overburdened with too many people in them, resulting in excessively high soaker wastes, many states suggest using the following formula to calculate soaker loads for hot tubs and spas. Basically, the surface area of the hot tub or spa divided by 10 dictates the number of people allowed in the spa at given time. The formula for the area of a circle (most hot tubs and spas are circles) is πr^2, where $\pi = 3.14$. If a spa has a 12-foot diameter, the radius is half of the diameter or 6 feet. The soaker load of this 12-foot spa is determined by using the following formula:

$$3.14 \text{ times } 6^2 \div 10$$

or

$$3.14 \text{ times } 36 \div 10 = 11 \text{ soakers}$$

In the case of a rectangular or square spa, the area is determined by multiplying length times width, and that total is divided by 10. Soaker loads for hot tubs and spas must be monitored aggressively. If recommended soaker loads are exceeded, there is a good chance the water chemistry and balance will become even more difficult to control.

Filtration

Good filtration is also extremely important for hot tubs and spas. Although many public and private pools have 6- to 8-hour turnovers, hot tubs and spas must turn over their pool capacity every 30 minutes. In fact, in heavily used public hot tubs and spas, complete turnovers will occur every 5, 10, or 15 minutes. In addition to quick turnovers, the filtration systems must have superior ability to trap dirt and particularly body oils. Hot tubs and spas should also provide at least 5 times the filter area for the hot water pool as for an equivalent amount of swimming pool water. Sand filters often become ineffective in hot tub and spa applications because oils, grease, and a high mineral content eventually clog the sand media, which must then be replaced. Regenerative DE filters seem to work quite well in hot water environments, and cartridge filters may also do a good job if the owner or operator is willing to purchase new cartridges frequently. Because rapid buildup of body oils on filter medium and septa is a constant problem associated with hot tubs and spas, these filter elements must be cleaned and degreased more often than traditional swimming pool filters. A watchful eye must be kept on all flow gauges, and strict enforcement of the shower rule will aid in effective filtration.

Public spas should be filtered 24 hours a day, although many owners or operators do not follow this guideline to conserve energy. This is a questionable practice because these hot water pools require more time to regenerate after large soaker loads. Owners of residential hot tubs and spas may in fact turn off heaters and filters for long periods of time for energy conservation, but it is a good idea to filter for at least 2 to 4 hours before and after each use.[3,4] Once again, good water balance must be maintained in hot tubs and spas so that the filter medium and related equipment can run effectively. In addition, several filter aids and clarifiers such as enzymes and organic polymers are available for hot tubs and spas.

Heaters

Regardless of what type of heater is used for a hot tub or spa, a good quality cover, preferably a hard, tight-fitting cover, should be used. When not in use, the tub or spa needs to be covered so that heat and the energy used to produce that heat can be preserved. This cover will also protect children from climbing or falling into the hot tub or spa. Heat loss, of course, is even more of a problem for outdoor installations. Proper insulation of the shell is also recommended whenever possible.

Before a heater is purchased, several types and models should be researched. Spa specialists should be consulted for their recommendations. Several pros and cons accompany each type of heater. Fuel source and heater size in British thermal units (BTU) should be discussed fully with pool suppliers. Hot tub and spa heaters should have an automatic high temperature shut-off switch so that excessive temperatures do not become a problem.

Water balance is of paramount importance to the functioning and longevity of the heater. Unbalanced water that is aggressive corrodes heater elements. Most heater components are made of copper, which is sensitive to low pH values. When hot tubs and spas are installed in homes with a water softener, adjustments must be made to keep calcium hardness levels up; otherwise the pool heater and other components will be destroyed quickly. Conversely, highly basic water with an elevated pH forms calcium deposits in the heater, making the system inefficient and unable to produce sufficient heat. Because the heater contains the hottest water in the system and calcium carbonate is *less* soluble at higher temperatures, it is most likely that calcium buildup will occur here. Many hot tubs and spas have continual heater problems because water balance goes unchecked. Water balancing is much more important and difficult to maintain in hot water pools than in standard pools.

Safety

Elevated water temperatures found in hot tubs and spas can create physiological changes in users, which can lead to accidents. Hot tubs and spas are not intended for use by everyone and have numerous restrictions. At higher temperatures (104° F) and for extended stays (greater than 15 minutes), hot water can elevate the core temperature of the body and produce hyperthermia. Hyperthermia can be accompanied by drowsiness and elevated blood pressure.[4] Alcohol can exaggerate this condition. Researchers at Boston University found that pregnant women who used spas, hot tubs, and saunas during the first 8 weeks of pregnancy were 3.5 to 7 times more likely to deliver a baby with birth defects.[5] Therefore the following conditions should preclude individuals from using a hot tub or spa and may lead to serious injury:

1. High blood pressure
2. Children under the age of 12
3. Use of prescription medication
4. Pregnancy
5. Heart disease
6. Diabetes
7. Hypertension

SIDEBAR 13-4

TOO HOT TO HANDLE

Although spa use clearly has its benefits, there are some people for whom the physiological changes a spa causes can be too taxing.

As a result, medical and allied expers caution people with the following conditions to consult their physician before soaking:

• *High- or low-blood pressure*: A doctor needs to determine in these cases whether the patient can withstand the sudden (albeit temporary) changes in blood pressure that hot water causes.

Heart disease: Many medical experts agree that the heart cannot handle the stress presented by the rise in blood pressure that comes with soaking in hot water, although recent studies see some benefit. The best advice is to consult a doctor.

Lung disease or illness: This category includes patients with emphysema and bronchitis whose lungs would not be able to accommodate increased blood flow and heart rates.

• *HIV-positive blood*: In advanced stages, these patients are generally too weak to withstand the hot water and its effects. (It should be noted that there is no medical evidence that the AIDS virus is transmitted through spa water.

• *Multiple sclerosis*: The muscle-weakening effects of the spa saps too much strength from these patients.

• *Thermal-nerve deficiency*: This causes inability of sufferers to recognize when they are being burned or monitor their temperature.

• *Asthma or allergies*: The sudden change in temperature may be hazardous for these patients.

• *Seizures*: The effects of hot water may affect the brain in a way that could bring on seizures.

• *Diabetes*: Soaking in a spa or hot tub can affect comsumption of insulin, and the body may not be able to take the change in activity within the body.

Pregnancy: Fetuses exposed to hot water in the first month of pregnancy are more vulnerable to spina bifida and other neural-tube defects.

Acute or new injury: In most cases, an injury is going to be swollen for a couple of days; this swelling indicates that there's quite a bit of blood circulation occurring in that area, and hot water may serve to aggravate the injury.

Lost sensation: It's important that spa users be able to tell whether they're too hot, so people who have a loss of feeling should consult with their doctor before soaking.

Patients with certain other conditions should also consult practitioners before using a spa, incuding those with vascular disease, kidney disease, open wounds or pressure sores, skin infetions or contagious rashes, malignant or active tuberculosis, acute fever, or impaired balance. In addition, obesity and incontinence can be factors precluding spa use.

It should also be noted that discretion should be used in deciding whether infants and very young children should soak at all, because their bodies are not yet sufficiently developed to regulate their own temperature.

And, of course, users need to be warned not to use the spa after taking prescription drugs that affect the body's heart rate, blood pressure, or its ability to regulate temperature.

Finally, those who are using alcohol (or recovering the morning after) should stay away from spas. Alcohol and certain drugs have several of the same effects on the body as hot water, thus amplifying the effects of both; at the same time, those substances impair the body's temperature-regulating mechanisms.

Modified from *Pool & Spa News*, Feb 8, 1993, Los Angeles.

8. Epilepsy
9. Use of alcohol or recreational drugs
10. Body infections or open sores

Whenever any doubts remain concerning the above or any other concerns, a physician should be consulted (Sidebar 13-4).

Many other rules and regulations should be followed to ensure the safety of hot tub and spa users:

1. A 15-minute time limit
2. A maximum temperature of 104° F
3. No use of tub or spa if bottom cannot be seen clearly
4. A soap shower *before* and *after* entry
5. No diving, handstands, or underwater swimming
6. No use alone
7. Only slow, stretching exercises allowed
8. No lotions of any type permitted
9. No use of electrical appliances in or around hot tubs and spas. (Radios, hair dryers, and other appliances have caused extreme electrical shocks.)

Drain covers

Another area of concern with hot tubs and spas is drains and drain coverings (Fig. 13-7). Orifices not properly covered have been known to keep victims submerged long enough to drown them. The suction in this case can be extremely strong, and an emergency cutoff for the pump should be readily accessible to all hot tub and spa users. There should be at least two suction orifices for each pumping system. Every drain or suction orifice must be covered with an antivortex plate to prevent entrapment or entanglement. If any drain or suction orifice is not properly covered, the hot tub or spa should be closed. Individuals with long hair must either keep it covered or up off the shoulders, and hair should not be allowed underwater. Entanglement and entrapment accidents have occurred in hot tubs and spas, but misuse and alcohol have usually been linked to these occurrences.

Foaming

A number of factors contribute to foaming of the water in hot tubs in spas. High TDS is a major contributor to foaming and sudsing. Low calcium-hardness levels also contribute to this condition. In addition, soaps, body oils, and suntan lotions tend to foam very quickly. The air jets that are powered by pool pumps cause these materials to foam readily.

Not only are these suds unsightly, they also smell, create a bathtub ring, and can also create slippery, unsafe conditions. Defoamers are often used by hot tub and spa owners, but controlling TDS and calcium-hardness levels, banning oils, and requiring showers are also helpful in keeping foam to a minimum.[6]

Ventilation

Good ventilation is a must for rooms that contain hot tubs and spas. Gases must be pulled from the area during superchlorination, which is done often in these specialty pools. Also, as chloramines develop, symptoms of exposure are reduced with good ventilation. Because heat and humidity are extremely high in this environment, it would be wise to have quick air changes to protect equipment and appliances in the room.

Signage

Rules and regulations must be clearly posted around hot tubs and spas. Because there are so many precautions involving hot tub and spa use, much information needs to be presented. "No Diving" signs must also be posted both vertically (on walls) and horizontally (on floors). "No Diving" signs on the deck should be within approximately 18 inches of the spa's edge. Water depths should also be clearly marked. In addition to all the signage required, someone should check the spa regularly to be certain that rules are being followed. Although lifeguards are not normally assigned to hot tubs and spas, someone on staff should check on the patrons periodically. When a new hot tub or spa is installed, consideration should be given to placing the spa in a location where it can be visually monitored from adjoining areas. Closed-circuit television coverage of hot tub and spa use may also be a good idea in some instances.[3] These precautions should apply to residential hot tubs and spas as well as public facilities.

Timers

Installation of a 15-minute timer is highly recommended to prevent prolonged immersions in hot tubs and spas that may lead to hyperthermia and other related problems. This timer switch should be designed to turn off the hydrotherapy jets every 15 minutes and should be located at least 10 feet away from the water. If someone is using a hot water pool alone (which is not recommended), the timer switch will force the soaker to leave the water at least every

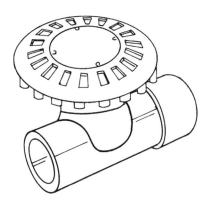

Anti-vortex drain cover to prevent whirlpool
effect caused by drain suction.

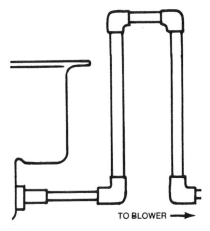

TO BLOWER ➔

Plumb a loop in air blower line near spa to
keep water out of line.

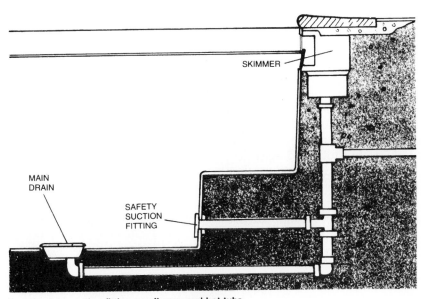

Install safety suction fitting on all spas and hot tubs.

Fig. 13-7.   In-ground spa support system. (From NSPI: *Basic pool and spa technology*, ed 2, Alexandria, Va, The Institute.)

15 minutes. The emergency shut-off switch should also be located in this area.

Accidents

It must be emphasized that the majority of accidents occurring in and around hot tubs and spas are alcohol related. Most adults injured in these specialty pools are legally drunk at the time of the accident. The combination of hot water immersion and alcohol consumption can cause drowsiness, weakness, and irregularities in the heart. Drownings are often the result of an intoxicated person slipping, tripping, or falling in this environment. In addition, accidental electrocutions take place in hot tubs and spas because patrons misuse electrical appliances such as radios, televisions, VCRs, hair dryers, and others. All electrical appliances should be kept away from this environment, and GFIs are a must. Alcohol consumption should be discouraged before and during hot tub use. Patrons should also be checked periodically.

Younger children, particularly those with long hair, have become entangled with drains and grates. As mentioned previously, children under 12 years of age should not use hot tubs or spas. If a younger person is allowed to use a hot tub or spa, the child should be carefully supervised by an adult.

Summary

Hot tubs and spas are perhaps the fastest growing appliances in the swimming industry. Some experts believe they are the most popular request for home improvements. Not only do hot tubs and spas provide many hours of recreation and relaxation, they also provide hydrotherapy for many individuals. Hot tubs and spas require special attention because of the hot water they use and because not everyone can use a hot tub safely. NSPI publishes a booklet called "What's Cool, What's Hot," which contains consumer tips for buying a spa or hot tub. They also have a comprehensive list of dealers selling these hot water pools. For further information, call NSPI at (800) 395-SOAK.

References

1. Arthritis Foundation: *Spas, pools and arthritis*, Atlanta, Georgia.

2. NSPI: *Pool and spa market study for the year 1991*, Alexandria, Va, 1992, The Institute.

3. Crow SA: *Aquatic international*, Mar/Apr 1992.

4. Kowalsky L(editor): *Pool/spa operators handbook*, San Antonio, Tex, 1991, National Swimming Pool Foundation.

5. Health update, *Better Homes and Gardens*, Feb 1993.

6. Johnson R: *YMCA pool operations manual*, Champaign, Ill, 1989, YMCA.

Bibliography

BioGuard Lab, Inc: *The pool book*, Decatur, Ga, 1981.

BioGuard Lab, Inc: *The spa book*, Decatur, Ga, 1981.

Johnson R: *YMCA pool operations manual*, Champaign, Ill, 1989, YMCA.

Kowalsky L (editor): *Pool/spa operators handbook*, San Antonio, Tex, 1991, National Swimming Pool Foundation.

Mitchel K: *The proper management of pool and spa water*, Decatur, Ga, 1988, BioLab.

NSPI: *Maintaining your spa or hot tub: how to protect your investment*, Alexandria Va, 1988, The Institute.

Osinski A: Safe and clean, *Aquatics International* Sept/Oct 1992.

Pool & Spa News, Los Angeles.

Service Industry News, Torrance, Calif.

Taylor C: *Everything you always wanted to know about pool care*, Chino, Calif, 1989, Service Industry Publications.

Taylor Technologies, Inc: *Pool and spa water chemistry: testing and treatment guide with tables*, sparks, Md.

Walsh D: Spa trouble shooting, Torrance, Calif, 1992, *Service Industry News*.

Williams KG: *The aquatic facility operator's manual*, Hoffman Estates, Ill, 1991, National Recreation and Park Association, National Aquatic Section.

Review Questions

1. What is the difference between a hot tub and a spa?
2. Do public, hot water pools require more attention to chemical levels than conventional public swimming pools?
3. What is the formula for determining the soaker load in most public spas?
4. Which spa component is particularly susceptible to unbalanced water?
5. List five safety rules that should be enforced at all hot tubs and spas.
6. What is the function of an antivortex plate?
7. What is the function of a timer switch located near a spa but away from the water's edge?
8. What should the water temperature in a spa never exceed?

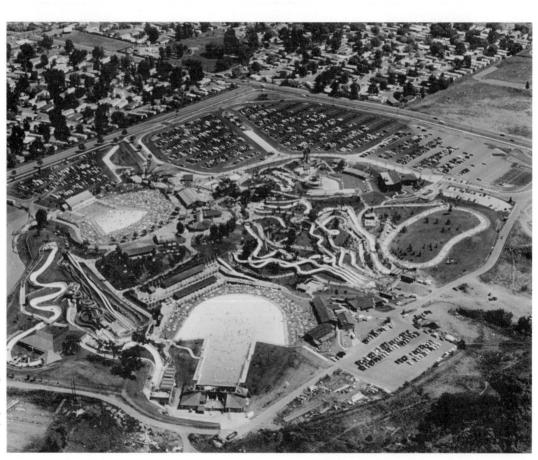

14

WATER PARKS

PJ HEATH

Water Park Statistics

Number of water parks

There are approximately 725 private sector water parks in the United States. In 1993, members of the World Water Park Association total 540. Of the 725 private sector water parks, approximately 90 are "large" water parks, based on an annual attendance of more than 100,000 guests. A total of 75 public sector parks are believed to be operating. However, many are not identified because they have only one or two small slides discharging into the city pool.

The definition of a *water park* generally hinges on the presence or absence of waterslides. This is the single most important criterion for identifying a Water Park. The top attractions or rides that make up a typical water park include waterslides, snack bar, children's rides, wave pool, slow river, activity pools, wet children areas, and a sit-down restaurant. Other attractions or rides that may be found at water parks may include a carousel, live entertainment, miniature golf, bumper boats or cars, roller coaster, ferris wheel, go-karts, animated figures, animal activities or shows, dark rides, and batting cages. Of these attractions and rides, waterslides are the most common and dark rides and batting cages are the least common.

Water park attendance

A world Water Park Association survey reports that U.S. Water Park attendance rose to a record high of 42 million in 1991. This was an increase of 31% over the previous 2 years. During 1991, no drownings were reported in an attended attraction.

Water park operating expenses

Water parks spend about 37% of their operating budgets on full-time and seasonal personnel.

Insurance is only 6% of the Water Park operating budget. The following is a ranking of operating expenses in order of highest percentage of overall operating expense:

1. Seasonal employees—20%
2. Full-time employees—17%
3. Food or beverage—12%
4. Marketing or promotion—10%
5. Maintenance or grounds—9%
6. Insurance—6%
7. Utilities—5%
8. Local services—5%
9. Other—15%

Capital expenditures at water parks

The following is the a ranking of the type of projects financed in order of most common to least common:

1. Water ride
2. Children's ride
3. Adult ride
4. New or enhanced theme
5. New entrance, facility
6. New service for guests
7. New dining facility

Personnel

Seasonal water park employees outnumber full-time employees at a ratio of approximately 2.5 to 1. This ratio is even greater for water parks that employ more than 250 seasonal employees. The water park personnel distribution by percentage is as follows:

- 31% employ 51 to 100 employees
- 29% employ 250 or more employees
- 27% employ 1 to 50 employees

- 6% employ 151 to 200 employees
- 4% employ 101 to 150 employees
- 2% employ 201 to 250 employees

The percentage of water park employees by age is as follows:

- 51% ages 17 to 19 years
- 29% ages 20 to 55 years
- 14% ages 14 to 16 years
- 4% ages 56 years and older

- 1% ages 14 years and younger

Approximately 36% of water park seasonal employees earn less than $4.00 per hour. In all water parks, 82% earn $5.00 or less per hour. The hourly wage for seasonal employees ranges from about $4.00 per hour to more than $7.00 dollars per hour.

Accident/incident rate

Before 1983, a number of industry factions attempted to compile incident statisitcs and develop design and operating parameters based on those statistics. Notably, the Consumer Product Safety Commission (CPSC) published its guidelines for recreational waterslide flumes in 1981, along with several authors' published analyses that purported to present the state of the art for accident control.

Unfortunately, the CPSC document was published just after the conventional flume slide was no longer the mainstay of water parks. This CPSC document failed to address the speed slides, free-fall rides, double and triple drops, enclosed tubular slides, body flumes, and other nonslide attractions that erupted on the scene during the nearly 4 years it took the National Spa & Pool Institute (NSPI) committee to get their finding published.

With the industry forced to grow and develop without definitive guidelines for design, construction, and operation, many rides and parks were constructed with little accurate consideration for guest safety.

At the Centers for Disease Control, injuries were being attributed to "waterslides" even though no definition of such an attraction was or is in the National Electronic Injury Surveillance System (NEISS). In the NEISS system the sliding board, backyard pool, and "Slip n' Slide" yard toy injuries were being reported as waterslide injuries. Amusement park log flume ride incidents and other rides totally unrelated to water were also included. This type of baseless information and some accurate reporting of "disastrous"

experiences in one or two parks built in the late 1970s have led several "self-proclaimed" experts to publish analytical reports that inaccurately present the state of the industry to the unknowing public. One such article, "A Cluster of Injuries at a Water Slide in Washington State," presents an analysis of a series of incidents in the late 1970s. This article states these series of incidents as being typical of the industry, when in fact there has never been another facility built with such results. Several submissions and rehashes of this article were published as new information without basis.

The problem affecting any analysis of water park safety is the lack of coordinated and verifiable incident, injury, and attendance data. Insurance carriers will not publish loss statistics, the trade association has been unable to develop a valid membership survey on the subject, owners and operators are reluctant to be candid with private surveys, independent consultants will not share their client histories, and the government has not considered this subject of sufficient importance to incorporate it into the consumer safety network. One of the difficulties in injury assessment stems from the lack of definition of reportable incidents. Tabulating every visit to the first aid room and all first aid given on the run by guards and attendants, water parks were recording treatable incidents at the rate of 5 per 1000 visitors in the early 1980s, with hospital or emergency room incidents occurring at the rate of 1 per 8000 park visits. In the early 1990s, using the same reporting basis, it appears that a reportable injury rate of 3.5 to 4.0 per 10,000 visitors and a hospital or emergency room rate of 1.5 to 1.8 per 100,000 is anticipated.

In the early 1980s, a drowning rate of 5 to 7 per season of 15 to 20 million visits was recorded. However, in the 1990 and 1991 seasons, no guest drownings were recorded in 38 to 40 million visits each year. A drowning rate of 5 to 6 drownings per 1 million visits annually is expected.

The early statistics noted above occurred during the water park industry's formative years. There was little information available to govern park design and operation. The later figures are the result of these influencing factors:

- The World Water Park Association guidelines for operating safety were published in 1985 and updated with the latest revision occurring in 1991. (NOTE: Although this publication is not definitive, it presents a compilation of industry practice as it has developed.)
- The emergence of specialty lifeguard training by

the firm of Ellis and Associates developed techniques applicable directly to the circumstances and attractions in the water park environment.

- The American Red Cross developed new techniques for lifeguarding skills.
- An awareness of risk management and its benefits by park management was a result of the insurance market shrinking in the mid 1980s. The recognition by park management of the voids in their risk management programs spawned the emergence of private risk management firms such as Glynn Barclay & Associates, Inc., which focused on the needs of the industry.

Private risk management firms have produced staff training systems that establish better control of guest activity, thereby reducing the cause of many injury-producing incidents. They have also developed management techniques and procedures that reduce exposures generated by the park facilities and hardware.

Industry evolution has eliminated many of the operators and manufacturers who would not participate in the growth of risk management in the industry.

Continued development of risk management concepts and procedures should further reduce the rate of injury experienced in the water park and general leisure industries.

High-risk locations

Running is the number one cause of accidents in water parks. Another area of trouble occurs with one guest colliding with another on a waterslide. Other potentially hazardous areas are discussed later in this chapter.

Water Park Attractions

In this section, information about water park rides and attractions are discussed in general and generic terms. (NOTE: Lifeguards should understand the manufacturer's specific operating guidelines for each attraction or ride they are operating.) Every facility should check state and local codes and regulations to ensure compliance.

A good operating routine does not mean a Water Park can avoid all hazards or risk of injury. However, such routines can reduce and maintain injuries at minimum levels. It is the responsibility of lifeguards to make considerable efforts to lessen guest injury during normal use. Lifeguards cannot predict or foresee all the different guests' personalities, behavior, or physical ability. This creates the possibility (not probability) that injury will happen as the result of inappropriate or abusive guest activity.

The following sections pertains to seven common attractions and rides. Safety considerations are presented in a "fact sheet listing" for easy and quick reference. The safety considerations are not inclusive because of the special considerations of every attraction or ride.

Children's flumes

Children's flumes are short-length flumes with an uncomplicated design that controls rider speed (to some extent) and allows each rider to clear the ride with little or no risk of injury (under normal use and supervision) (Fig. 14-1).

Safety considerations

Staff

1. Staff oversee the flume area.
2. Staff demonstrate skill at working with young children.
3. Staff are aggressive and continuously talk and physically move people away from the slide discharge area.
4. The staff's areas of responsibility for this attraction comply with the "10/20" rule.

Attraction

5. Flumes are smooth on the slide surfaces to eliminate exposure to skin abrasions.
6. The main drains incorporate covers with openings no smaller than 3/8 inch in diameter and no longer than 1 inch.
7. Depth markings are placed on the deck near the pool's edge (or on the coping of the pool) and on the interior wall of the pool except in rimflow or deck level pools where the wall is below the water level.
8. The deck and step surfaces are nonslip.
9. All ledges in the splashpool are painted in a contrasting color.
10. All gates to flumes, splashpools, and doors contain self-closing and positive self-latching mechanisims at a height above a toddler's reach (minimum of 4 feet).
11. Flumes are "locked" when not in use.
12. The deck surface can be completely drained.
13. Appropriate precautions are taken to prevent slips and falls in the approach and entry areas.

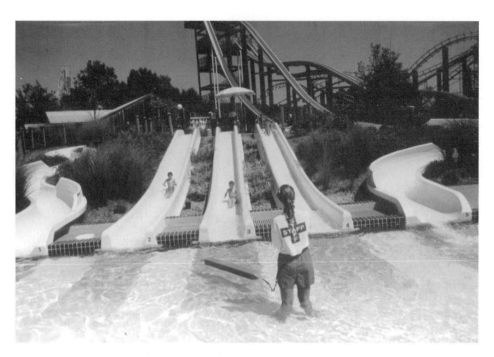

Fig. 14-1.   Children's flume slide. (Courtesy Splash Magazine.)

14. Water flow rate down the flume conforms with the manufacturer's recommendations.
15. The splashpool or water run is of adequate depth and conforms with the manufacturer's recommendations.

Guest

16. U.S. Coast Guard-approved life jackets are available to those who wish to wear one.
17. Children are not engaged in "uncontrolled play."
18. Strict rules to educate children and parents against running, horseplay, and other risks of slipping are maintained.

Children's play areas

Play areas vary in design and attraction content (Fig. 14-2). Items that may exist in play areas include "climb-on" apparatus, small straight slides, water fountains, wall falls, rope swings, water guns, small tunnel chutes, small obstacle mazes, themed characters, and landscaping.

Safety considerations

Staff

1. Staff oversee the play area. Staff are attentive to activity and potential accidents.

2. Staff are positioned to continuously monitor the play area. Staff are located in effective vantage points that allow the entire play area to be monitored.
3. Staff demonstrate skill at working with young children. Staff demonstrate friendly, firm behavior that is effective in communicating with children; children listen and obey a large majority of staff instructions.
4. Staff conduct daily cleaning and checks for broken glass and other litter.
5. Staff do not permit too many children on the same piece of equipment at the sametime.
6. The staff's areas of responsibility for this attraction comply with the "10/20" rule.

Attraction

7. Concrete pool bottom surfaces are slip resistant by providing adequate barefoot friction to prevent falls but not cause injury to feet.
8. Surfaces intended for guest activity are slip resistant and moderate in slope and elevation changes.
9. Pool drains are equipped with multiple antivortexing drain or suction inlets to pumps.
10. Steps and ledges are painted a contrasting color.

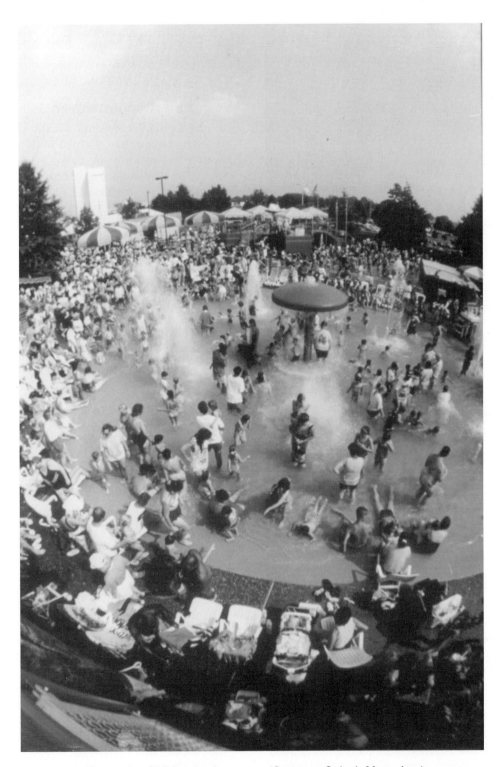

Fig. 14-2.   Children's play areas. (Courtesy Splash Magazine.)

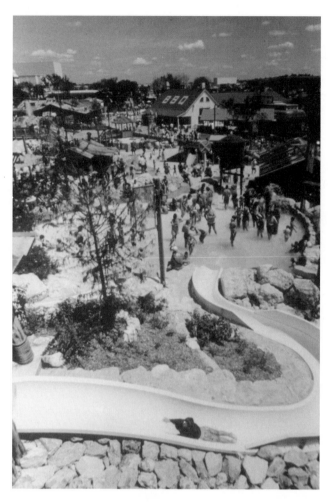

Fig. 14-3. Inground standard flume slide. (Courtesy Splash Magazine.)

11. There are no exposed ends of tubing that should be covered by plugs or caps.
12. There are no accessible sharp edges or points on the equipment.
13. There are no broken or missing rails, steps, rungs, or seats on any of the equipment.
Guests
14. Strict rules to educate children and parents against running, horseplay, and other risks of slipping are maintained. Rules are stated clearly and briefly, prevent or deter hazardous or risky behavior, and are consistently enforced.

15. Children are not engaged in "uncontrolled play."
16. Children are not permitted to use damaged equipment.
17. U.S. Coast Guard–approved life jackets are available to those who wish to wear one.

Standard ride flumes

Standard ride flumes are usually serpentine (winding) structures that feature a slide path with an appropriate mixture of straight and drop sections (Fig. 14-3). These rides generally expel a slider at an exit speed of approximately 30 feet per second or less (about 20 miles per hour) and are characterized by short drop sections and winding paths rather than spiral, whip, or straight slide paths.

Safety considerations

1. The chief risk in standard ride flumes and splashpools is the possibility of guest collisions. Other potential risks to guests include the following:
   Slips and falls in approach and entry areas
   Impact with flume sidewalls
   Impact with splashpool water surface or floor
   Abrasions to skin from side walls and slide bottom
   Ejection from flumes in turns
   Falls and collisions within the waterslide run
2. Lifeguards are the key to minimizing guest risk and injury. Therefore lifeguards must be alert and aware of the waterslide activity.
3. Guests travel at different speeds because of differences in body weight, friction from swimming apparel, and rider position or posture.
4. When guests slide on mats with low water flow, the loss of mats may slow their progress, requiring the next guests to delay their starts. The lifeguard or attendant needs to be constantly aware of slider progress.
5. On "no mat" slides, lifeguards need to be aware that materials such as denim slide much slower than synthetic materials.
6. Restrictions on guest dress should be clearly posted.
7. On slides designed for multiple sliders or use with sleds for multiple sliders, lifeguards should follow manufacturer's guidelines.
8. Collisions primarily occur in the splashpool area.
9. Sliders have a tendency to watch for their

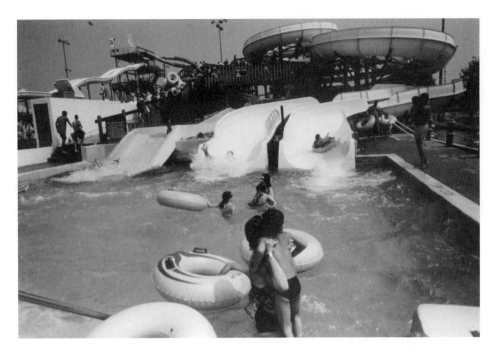

Fig. 14-4. Intertube slide. (Courtesy Splash Magazine.)

friends coming down behind them or they become confused and disoriented on entry into the splash pool. Lifeguards must be aggressive and continually talk and physically move people away from the slide discharge area.

10. Another hazard at the splashpool exit is the improper storage of mats. Mats on walk paths present serious fall hazards to spectators and sliders.
11. No sliding in the standing position is allowed.
12. No backward sliding is allowed on any standard waterslide or chute.
13. Only specifically designed slides should allow headfirst sliding. However, headfirst sliding may be possible on slides that have landing flaps or decelerating runout sections as a braking mechanism or in conjunction with a splashpool.
14. Headfirst sliding on "no mat" slides requires special slider instrucitons.

Innertube ride—chute and pool rides

This type of ride is primarily serpentine and features a slide path that allows innertube access through a combination of turns with an appropriate mixture of straight and drop sections and intermittent splashpools (Fig. 14-4).

Safety considerations

1. The chief risk on innertube chute and pool rides is the collision hazard at the bottom or splashpool area of each chute.
2. Guest exposure to concrete sidewalls can produce skin abrasions.
3. Improper or uncontrolled guest access to the slide chute presents a risk of collision or injury. Lifeguards should patrol and monitor chute access.
4. Intermediate pools should be of sufficient depth to permit rollovers without injury to the rider.
5. Generally the tube style does not present a safety hazard.
6. Water flow rate down the chute should conform to the manufacturer's recommendations.
7. Concerning water flow rate, the following may occur:
   Extremely low water flow or barely wet surfaces (0 to 150 gallons per minute [gpm]) result in high rider speeds.
   Increase the water flow (up to 600 gpm) decreases the rider speed.

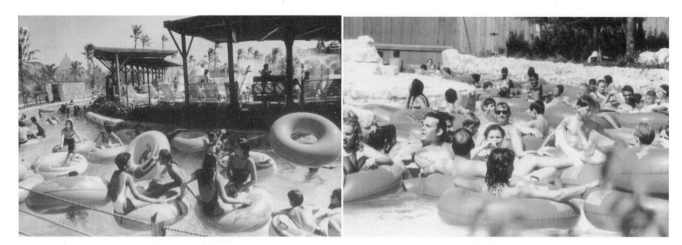

Fig. 14-5. Intertube ride—slow river. (Courtesy Splash Magazine.)

Further water flow increases (up to 1500 gpm) decrease rider speed.

At a water flow rate greater than 1500 gpm, the rider speed tends to equal the speed of the water.

High flow rates tend to decrease the differences in acceleration and exit speed among various guests.

8. Lifeguards should be aware of the design of their facility's innertube chute, since some designs result in whirlpools and back eddies.

Innertube ride—rapids rides

Rapids rides are identified by an innertube slide path that is continuous or nearly continuous. The path may be designed in a random serpentine, curved, or "stream" shape. This ride can include devices that cause "choppy water" and obvious bumps in the slide path.

Safety considerations

1. The splashpool approach and design should give the rider a balanced entry, producing a landing pattern that allows minimal risk for rider turnovers and in-pool collisions.
2. A facility should have a procedure that allows guests to release their tube and exit the pool without diverting attention to tube recovery.

Innertube ride—slow rivers

Slow rivers are a very popular attraction in a water park. They are usually a flat circuitous stream moved by booster pumps providing a riverlike flow rate (under 5 miles per hour) in which riders are transported on various flotation devices or by body floating or walking (Fig. 14-5).

Safety considerations

1. The entry and exit locations in a slow river require consideration of the potential for rider impact with rails, stairwells, and ramp ways.
2. Tunnels, bridges, waterfalls, and other features should have adequate clearance to ensure that riders can avoid a collision.
3. Rivers flowing faster than 5 miles per hour need special provisions for guest entry and exit to provide convenience and to ensure safety.

Wave pools

Wave pools (Fig. 14-6) are classified into two general categories:

1. Wave action (WA) pools have a motion that is oscillating (seesaw motion) or standing (no rolling waves). These pools produce waves by cyclic pulsing; therefore wave action pools cause little cross flow. As a rule, waves are generated in cycles of approximately 3 seconds and produce a crest to valley depth of up to 4 feet or greater. This type of wave pool usually operates several minutes "on" followed by a period of calm or greatly reduced water action. Wave patterns will vary among facilities depending on experience and manufacturer's recommendations. In some facilities, AW pools have special

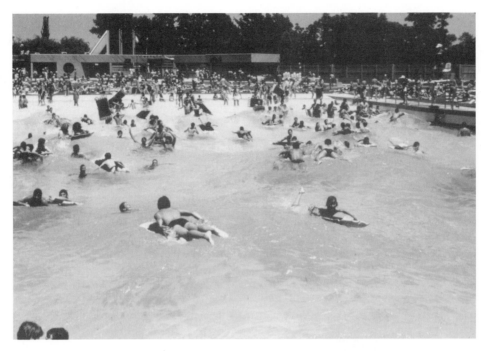

Fig. 14-6. Wave pool. (Courtesy Splash Magazine.)

equipment to generate waves in patterns and heights to allow body board and boogie board riding, rafting, and exhibition surfboarding.

2. Solitary transitional (ST) wave pools create waves that make a moving wall of water that runs the total length of the wave pool. Providing the ST wave pool has the equipment and design, waves up to 6 feet high or greater can be generated for a few seconds to several minutes. In ST wave pools the waves are controlled by the design of the pool bottom. Characteristically, ST wave pools develop flow (wave) patterns below the average water level of the pool. This information is outlined in the manufacturer's operating procedure.

Safety considerations

1. Generally, the same local codes and health department requirements for water quality, signage, depth markers, and other parameters apply to wave pools as well as standard pools.
2. Slip resistant surfaces should be on all walkways.
3. Slips and falls are most likely to occur in shallow areas (0 to 24 inches) of the wave pool.
4. Underwater draughts and falls can occur in

wave pools that have significant undertows and back flow.
5. ST pools have strong back flows or cross flows of water after passage of the main wave.
6. Pool grab rails and ladders should be inspected daily for tightness.
7. Signs should be visible from the pool and deck stating that only strong swimmers should proceed beyond a designated point.
8. Signage should be posted noting that small children must be under continuous adult supervision while in the wave pool.
9. The use of mini-surf, surf, and boogie boards may be permitted only when the manufacturer has designed the wave pool for these activities. The manufacturer's guidelines for the operating procedures, emergency procedures, crowd control, and rules for use during these activities should be followed.
10. Masks, fins, and snorkels should not be permitted in wave pools during wave action periods.
11. Lifeguards should be alert to tired guests and novice or weak swimmers.
12. Lifeguards should have overlapping areas of responsibility to scan.
13. When a lifeguard determines a swimmer is

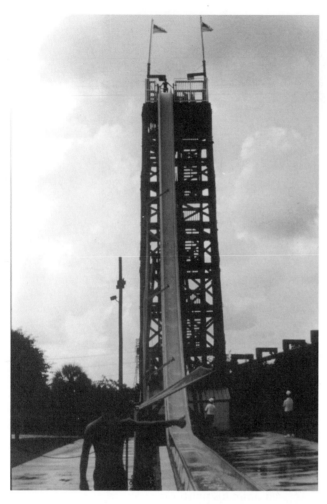

Fig. 14-7.   Speed slide. (Courtesy Splash Magazine.)

being placed in danger, voice or whistle commands should direct the swimmer to shallower water.

14. A signal or warning should be sounded or seen before resuming wave action. Lifeguards should be aware of guests running from the deck to "hit the waves" when the signal is given.

15. It is important that lifeguards be rotated from station to station and to other assignments to break boredom and increase alertness.

16. Signs should warn guests that waves can be overpowering and that collision and falls are possible.

17. ST pools are tiring. Lifeguards should scan the

pool after the wave action has stopped to pick out those guests that should exit or move to shallower water to rest.

18. Collisions generally occur during the wave cap; in shallow water, scraping the bottom is possible. Lifeguards should respond immediately to any signs of guest distress.

Speed slides

Speed slides are identified by chutes or roller tracks that may be straight, serpentine, helical, or whiplike and that have long or steep drops (Fig. 14-7). These slides exit sliders into a splashpool or run out at speeds of approximately 20 miles per hour or greater. Depending on slide design, guests may be positioned on the slide in a number of ways. Guests may be seated in a chain of four or be lying feet–first or headfirst on sleds and mats according to the manufacturer's recommendations. Many speed slide designs permit sliding without mats or sleds.

It is important for every speed slide to have an exit system that safely decelerates (slows down) the guest, who may be traveling at a speed of 40 miles per hour. In addition, the guest's body position (attitude) must be correct during the entry into the splashpool. A speed slide may use one of the following exit systems: run-out (trough lane), direct to splashpool, landing flap to splashpool, or combination run-out and pool. The combination run-out and splashpool is a longer, somewhat level continuation of the slide trough containing water. The slider's speed is reduced by pushing against this water with the body, creating a braking action.

Safety considerations

1. Only one slider enters at a time.
2. Lifeguards need to consider the rider's height, weight, and age against the slide design and operational limits.
3. Absolutely no headfirst sliding is allowed except where approved by the manufacturer's and/or park safety supervisor's instructions.
4. Sliding feet-first on the back is usually the position.
5. Depending on the speed of the slide, legs may need to be crossed at the ankles and arms crossed over the chest.
6. Lifeguards should not dispatch the next slider until the first slider is out of the runout and moved from the flume exit center line.
7. Any slider who appears to be under the influ-

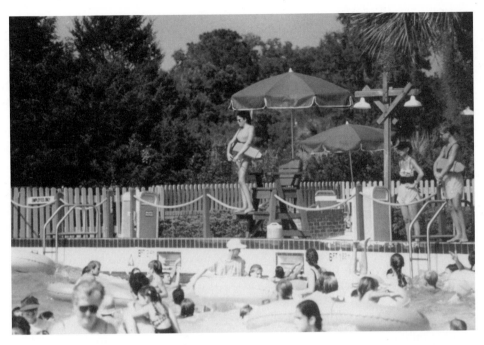

Fig. 14-8. Lifeguard on duty at wave pool. (Courtesy Splash Magazine.)

ence of drugs or alcohol should not be permitted to use the speed slide. (This rule should apply to all activity-oriented attractions in the facility.)

8. Good instructional signage informing the guest what to expect and how to slide and exit safely on the speed slide is extremely important.

9. Guests who may not be suited for speed slide use include but are not limited to the following:
   a. Guests who are frail due to age
   b. Pregnant guests
   c. Young children without supervision
   c. Guests who are very obese (overweight)
   d. Physically challenged guests or guests wearing a prosthesis
   e. Guests who have demonstrated previous horseplay
   f. Guests with a history of heart condition, back problems, or fear of heights

Lifeguarding at a Water Park

Lifeguarding is the development and application of the skills and techniques necessary to control and prevent aquatic accidents (Fig. 14-8). It is very demanding, monotonous at times, and tiring. Lifeguarding is not as glamorous as portrayed on television and in motion pictures. However, lifeguarding is challenging and can be personally rewarding.

The major responsibility of the lifeguard is to prevent accidents and to respond in the event of an emergency. No people are in a better position to prevent accidents in a water park than alert lifeguards sitting and standing in position watching their areas of responsibility. Lifeguards act as human "radar," constantly scouting their areas of responsibility for any potential problems.

Over the past decade a demand for new standards of training for lifeguards has developed with the emergence of water parks. In the past any student who completed a "lifesaving course" was considered a qualified candidate to hold a lifeguard position. It is the contention of several authorities in the aquatic industry that lifeguards should be skilled far beyond the competence of an advanced lifesaver. When a drowning or serious injury occurs, the performance of the lifeguard becomes the issue, and in a court of law the training and certification of the lifeguard is closely examined. Therefore trained professional lifeguards are a necessity and not a luxury, regardless of the type or size of the water park.

Although there are some similarities between traditional swimming pools and water parks, there are also significant differences. According to Ellis and Associates, many water parks encounter more patrons in one summer season than many traditional pools see in several years. In addition, it appears that although water park rides are exciting and challenging, many visitors are not skilled or prepared to handle the waves, currents, "white water," and hydraulics that many water parks provide. In addition, some water parks are profit driven rather than service driven, so management of the park is also different. Management and lifeguards cannot run a water park safely and efficiently armed with only traditional pool rules and skills.

There are several differences between lifeguarding at a water park and the public swimming pool. Some of the differences include the following:

Water parks	Public swimming pools
1. Draw new guests everyday	1. Draw same guests from local community
2. Have a greater number of lifeguard staff	2. Have only a few rescues per season
3. Draw a larger number of guests	3. Are funded by local government or are nonprofit
4. Have large expense attractions	4. Offer aquatic education programs
5. Are operated for profit	5. Attract swimmers of all types and for different reasons
6. Have frequent water rescues daily	
7. Have greater news media coverage	
8. Attract the recreational swimmer	

The Job of the lifeguard

Lifeguards at water parks may be called on to fill many different roles while on duty. They may find themselves in the roles of host, friend to a lost child, provider of first aid treatment, disciplinarian, referee of human behavior, complaint manager, or a professional who is "cool-headed" in an emergency. Lifeguards must be authority figures who are respected for their knowledge and skills (Fig. 14-9).

The romantic or glamorous status of the lifeguard is only imagined in the minds of uninformed employers, swimmers, and inexperienced lifeguards. The truth is that a lifeguard's job is full of serious responsibilities. Although a lifeguard's responsibilities and duties are differ among facilities, the primary responsibilities remain the same and include the following:

1. The prevention of accidents through assuming responsibility for the guests in the facility
2. The immediate response to an emergency requiring the technical skill and knowledge of a trained lifeguard and the administration of appropriate emergency care

The basic premise of lifeguarding is that preventing accidents is more desirable than performing successful rescues. Therefore lifeguards should keep guests from getting into dangerous situations.

Knowledge of and adherence to the following principles is an indication that the lifeguard accepts responsibility for the safety of the guest:

1. Danger areas of water park attractions should be continuously and closely supervised. Lifeguards should anticipate problems by watching guests closely. In a water park, high-risk areas include but are not limited to the following:
   a. *Physical hazards*—for example, shallow water, underwater steps, deep water, slippery surfaces, cloudy water, algae, and objects floating in the water
   b. *Chemical hazards*—for example, chlorine gas, acid, and cleaning chemicals
   c. *Environmental hazards*—for example, lighting in and around a water attraction and glare on water surface from sunlight or artificial light
   d. *Behavioral hazards*—for example, running, pushing people, throwing people, riding a slide in the wrong position, horseplay, and swimming in or around a splashpool
2. Rules should be enforced tactfully and consistently. (Rule enforcement is covered in detail later.)
3. Lifeguards should be heard and seen by facility guests. The use of a whistle and uniform are universally recommended for lifeguards. A bright colored uniform will help guests spot the lifeguard quickly. Being seen also includes remaining in the assigned location that is visible to all guests. Lifeguards should realize that a quick response is expected when the situation

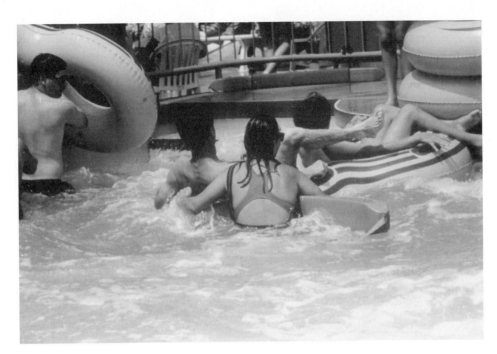

Fig. 14-9. Lifeguard assissting tube riders. (Courtesy Splash Magazine.)

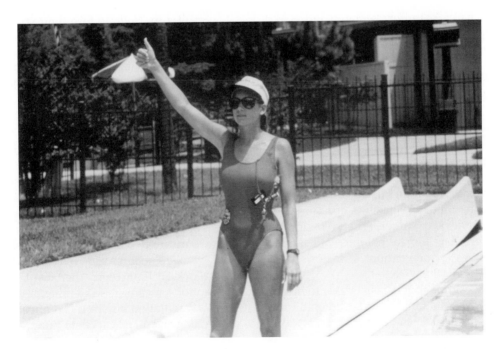

Fig. 14-10. Lifeguard with eye and head protection from sun. (Courtesy Splash Magazine.)

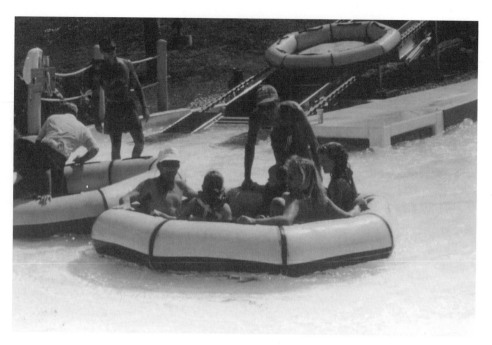

Fig. 14-11. Lifeguard assisting riders out of tube. (Courtesy Splash Magazine.)

warrants. Therefore uniforms that include laced shoes or pullover sweatshirts could hamper a rescue effort.

Personal health hazards of lifeguarding

Lifeguards face several health hazards while performing their duties (Fig. 14-10). All lifeguards should know what hazards exist and how to protect themselves from harm. As a rule the lifeguard's supervisor does not have the time to constantly remind the lifeguards to protect themselves. It is the responsibility of individual lifeguards to take care of themselves. All the following hazards are caused by the environment and/or weather. (The following are "universal" suggestions and are not intended as individual prescriptions for prevention. A doctor should be consulted for medical advice.)

1. *Skin hazard*—Although it is fashionable to have a rich, dark, deep suntan, roasting the epidermis to get that "fashionable look" has a cost. The cost may result in the skin cancer known as *melanoma*. Scientists have correlated other hazards to sunlight that include a suppression of the immune system (a possible contributor to other forms of cancer) and damage to skin cells that causes the cells to lose their soft, pliable properties. The prudent lifeguard avoids the concentrated ultraviolet (UV) radiation of the sun that occurs between 11:00 AM and 2:00 to 3:00 PM.

The closer a person gets to the equator, the more intense the sun's UV rays. The risk of skin cancer doubles about every 300 miles a person travels toward the equator, so the "sun time" and sunscreen strength should be adjusted accordingly. The intensity of the rays also increases with altitude, so necessary precautions should be taken when applicable. Lifeguards should wear protective clothing, stay under a sun umbrella if possible, or wear sunscreen. There are two basic types of sunscreens. Physical blockers such as zinc oxide or titanium dioxide block all light rays. Chemical blockers found in lotions, creams, and ointments selectively absorb UV radiation before it can affect the skin. When using chemical blockers, lifeguards should pay attention to the sun protection factor (SPF). The SPF is a number on a scale of 2 or higher that tells how long a person can extend exposure time in the sun by using a particular sunscreen. A product with SPF 8 will increase the time it takes for a person to turn red by a factor of 8. Following are tips for selecting a chemical blocker sunscreen:

Light-skinned persons should use a sunscreen with an SPF of at least 6 and possibly as high as 15 or higher.

A sunscreen with two or more UV-absorbing ingredients should be selected.

A long-lasting formula that penetrates or clings to the skin and is not rinsed off easily should be selected. A water-in-oil lotion is a good example. (Lifeguards should not apply coat after coat, which may prevent perspiration and increase the risk of heatstroke.)

Some people who are allergic to certain diuretics, sulfa drugs, or hair sprays may develop rashes as a reaction to PABA. If a reaction occurs, a doctor should be consulted regarding the use of a PABA-free sunscreen.

Lifeguards should apply a sunscreen 30 minutes to 2 hours before sun exposure to give the sunscreen time to penetrate the outer layer of skin. Another skin hazard that a lifeguard should be aware of is the development of skin irritation from wearing a wet swimsuit for an extended period. Lifeguards should remove wet suits when possible and use talcum or baby powder with cornstarch to dry out moist body areas.

2. *Eye hazard*—Good sunglasses can provide safe, comfortable vision, especially while a person is around water. The main purposes of sunglasses are to reduce the amount of vision light and provide protection from glare and UV rays.

Sunglasses should block out 75% to 90% of visible light. Some sunglasses carry a tag stating their "transmission factor" (the amount of light passing through). Unless specially treated, few sunglasses provide protection from UV rays. The UV rays can damage the eye's retina; however, sunglasses with a special clear coating can block a large percentage of the UV rays from reaching the eye. Lifeguards should wear UV-protected sunglasses because of the amount of time spent in the sun and the constant watch over the water surface.

Dark lenses that do not have a UV coating can harm the eye. They will cause the pupil to dilate, exposing the retina to more UV rays than usual. A burning or gritty feeling in the eye after exposure to bright sunlight may be a sign of eye sunburn, which requires prompt treatment from an ophthalmologist.

3. *Dehydration hazard*—To avoid dehydration, lifeguards should drink plenty of water over an extended time and stay in the shade to avoid profuse sweating and excessive loss of body fluid. In short, they should protect their bodies as much as possible.

Guest Relations

Positive guest relations can only be achieved by having water park employees who are courteous and tactful to the guests in the park (Fig. 14-11). The importance of positive guest relations is twofold. First, the guest has bought the right to have an enjoyable time. This right includes exceptional treatment from the staff. Second, the best defense against a potential lawsuit is positive guest relations. A well-treated and respected guest will respond positively to most situations, whereas a guest who is treated poorly or neglected is more likely to get "mad" and file a lawsuit.

All water park employees should encourage guests to voice their opinions about the facility and its operation. This is not an easy task because guests generally do not like to complain and employees do not like to hear it. In a survey conducted by the World Water Parks Association, only about 4% of the guests voiced a compliant; the other 96% voted with their money by not coming back to the facility. A total of 8 out of 10 unsatisfied guests tell their friends about "unhappy experience" at the facility. Employees should give the guests the opportunity to tell them about an "unhappy experience" so that the employee can help make it happy.

You Should Remember

Your best defense against a lawsuit is positive guest relations. Give guests the opportunity to tell you about an "unhappy experience" so that you can help make it happy.

The following should be implemented by the staff to facilitate positive guest relations:

- *Media*—The water park should have a plan of

action to follow when the media is making an inquiry about an incident or accident. The plan should designate a facility spokesperson to handle any questions asked by the media. All other staff should direct the media to the spokesperson and refrain from any comments. Staff should *never* say, "I have no comment." This statement can be construed as implied fault with an attempt to cover it up. The media is the water park's only link to "future guests," and the impression given could affect guest attendance and ultimately the employee's job.

- *Guest complaints*—All complaints should be received in an appreciative manner and necessary action should be initiated as soon as possible. The guest can provide the staff with valuable insight and constructive criticism that may help prevent a potential accident or disaster. Regardless of how valuable or constructive a guest's comment may seem , the guest has bought the right to voice dissatisfaction with a product or service. The staff is obligated to listen with interest and concern.
- *Lost and found*—The facility should have a policy and location for lost and found items and persons. If an item is found by or turned in to an employee, it is that employee's responsibili-

ty to see that the proper owner has an opportunity to claim the item. The old rule of "finder's keepers" does not apply. A guest has paid not only for use of the facility but for honest, customer-oriented service that respects guest property. In addition, the facility should have a plan of action for lost or missing persons. Lost children must be taken under the guardianship of the staff until the parent or responsible adult is found.

- *Park information*—The staff is responsible for knowing all water park information or the person who can answer a guest's question. It is frustrating to the guest to be led on a "wild goose chase" to find the answer to a simple question. Employees should know the correct answer or know who will have the correct answer.
- *Correcting guests*—Employees cannot treat all guests the same. The approach and delivery of a corrective statement differs from child to adult and from child to child. In general, use positive commands that show concern and respect for the guest. Employees must remember that they are not only in the business of preventing accidents and saving lives but also promoting goodwill between the guests and the water park.

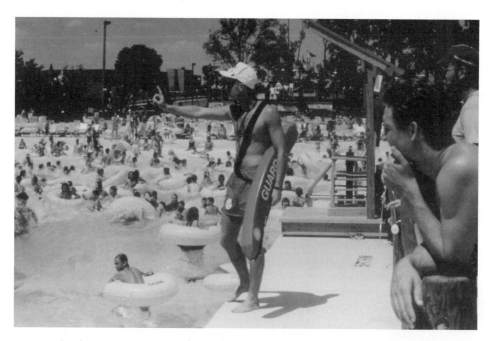

Fig. 14-12. Lifeguard enforcing the rules. (Courtesy Splash Magazine.)

Enforcement of the Rules

The first point that employees must understand is that they are symbols of authority and, as such, must demonstrate respect for authority by personally adhering to all park rules and policies (Fig. 14-12). It is difficult to expect guests to comply with rules designed for their safety if employees are not obedient to the same rules. When enforcing the rules, employees should consider several points:

- *Consistency*—To be consistent means to enforce the same rule in the same way every time. Uniform rule enforcement means that if two different guests are violating a rule, both should be stopped. Rules should be fair for everyone.
- *Delivery/demeanor*—Employees should try to explain to the guest the reasons for rules when enforcing them. An employee is correcting guests, not punishing them. The delivery of the correction is crucial. For example, look at the following two statements and decide which statement is most effective:
  1. "Mister, you can't bring that bottle in here."
  2. "Excuse me, sir, for your safety, bottles are not allowed in the pool. Broken glass in the pool is almost impossible to find and clean up. You may get a paper cup at the concession stand."
  Use a little diplomacy when explaining the rules. *Diplomacy* can be defined as "telling guests to do something in such a way that they actually look forward to following the instruction." The second statement is by far the better of the two. It states the rule, explains why, and offers a solution while using diplomacy. In contrast, the first statement is condescending and abrupt. The old saying "you can catch more flies with honey than vinegar" has some merit and application here.
- *Education of guests*—Because most accidents occur when employees are not present, employees must interject safety education at every opportunity. It is important that the employee explain why certain actions are dangerous and why other actions are desirable.
- *Adults versus young children*—In general, adults and children differ in their motivations and experiences. Children are accustomed to being told what to do. Adults are more self-directed. Children are not likely to be interested in the reasons for a rule, whereas adults want to know immediately what the reason is for the rule. The reason a child is running through the park will usually be different from the reason the adult is running across the park. Thus the employee should adapt corrections to the age level of the guest.
- *The "out-of-control" guest*—An effective way to deal with an out-of-control guest is for the employee to remain in control. The emotions of rage, hostility, and anger usually need "fuel" to keep them alive. An out-of-control employee will serve as that fuel, whereas an employee who remains calm and calls for assistance will not encourage the rage and anger to continue. Another type of out-of-control guest is the one who ignores and/or defies the rules and authority of the employee. The same principles, as stated above, should be used by the employee.

> ## *You Should Remember*
>
> *Don't expect guests to comply with rules designed for their safety if you do not obey the same rules. Enforce the same rules in the same way every time. Remember that you are correcting guests, not punishing them.*

Guest/Safety Perceptions

Every guest in a facility begins to form a mental impression about the park and the staff on duty. These mental impressions or perceptions can be positive or negative depending on the appearance and condition of the park and staff. The environment should look safe as well as be safe.

There should be signs, safety equipment, and other equipment (for example, trash cans) available for guests and employees. The park should look clean and neat, with everything in its assigned place. Every staff member is responsible for the appearance and condition of the park. If something is out of place or out of order, see that it gets the proper attention needed to correct it.

Employees are a very important part of the facility "team" and contribute to the total environment. If employees look and act like professionals, the park looks like a well-run park. Employees are "on-stage," and the guests watch what employees do and do not do. Therefore employees must not only be professionals but look like professionals at all times.

Some employees may be talented enough to effectively watch an attraction or ride and carry on a conversation with two of their friends. However, the perception in the mind of the guest is that the employee is not paying attention. Why should employees care what the guest's perception is, as long as they are doing their job? The reason is that every guest is a potential witness in a court of law.

If the guest carries a negative impression of the employee on the witness stand, this will weaken the employee's defense. Perceptions are received at "face value" and not judged as right or wrong. The fact that the employee was talking to friends is the fact that will remain in the guest's mind and the jury's mind, regardless of whether the employee was also performing other duties. A prosecuting attorney will focus on the fact that the employee was supposed to be giving the attraction or ride *total* attention to do the job correctly.

You Should Remember

Perceptions can be positive or negative, depending on the appearance and condition of the park and staff. Therefore you must not only be a professional but look like a professional. And the environment should look safe as well as be safe.

Water Parks Employee Operations
Chain of command

A chain of command is the ranking of employees in the order of superiority or command within the organization. The ranking structure is usually mapped out in a diagram. The basic concept behind the chain of command is that someone is in charge and thus is ultimately responsible for the facility operation. All employees should know the chain of command so that they understand who has the responsibility and

authority to make decisions at the various levels of the command. It is extremely important that the chain of command is used effectively to ensure the smoothest facility operations possible.

Rotation system

Although ride operations are not physically demanding, the sun, heat, humidity, and crowd noise produce stress-induced fatigue and subsequent drowsiness. Employees should remain at a station for no more than 20 to 30 minutes. A change of location can boost the alertness and attentiveness of employees. Rotations can be organized to include a combination of time at attraction 1, followed by walking duty through the park, time at attraction 2, a "little patrol" or miscellaneous assignment, and then completion of the rotation cycle with a break period.

Uniforms

Facility employees need to be clean and neat in appearance for guest relations purposes, and all employees should be outfitted in a uniform. The uniform may consist of specified pants, shirt, jacket, whistle, hat with a visor, and sunglasses. The hat, pants, and jacket are necessary for quick identification by both employees and guests. It is often difficult to detect employees from guests on peak attendance days without employees wearing a visible uniform.

You Should Remember

1. The chain of command tells you who is in charge and responsible for the facility operation.

2. A change of location can boost the alertness and attentiveness of the employee.

3. All employees should be outfitted in a uniform.

Rescue equipment

Rescue equipment for Water parks may be specified in the local and state codes. The park should adhere to these codes as a minimum acceptable standard. Each employee should be aware of the location and use of the rescue equipment.

Equipment that may be used or needed includes megaphones or bullhorns, whistles, warning signs, emergency lighting, backboard, stretcher, first aid kit, blankets, rescue tubes, ring buoys, and resuscitator or resuscitation mask.

Communications

It is important that each employee learn the signals and communication system used at the park. The communication must be simple, clear, and easily understood to be effective in an emergency. In many facilities a "10-code" system (for example, "10-4" means "OK" or "I read you"; "10-20" means "state your location") is established and used to communicate during operations. All employees should know the communication system used in their park.

Telephone

A telephone should be available for use in an emergency. If possible, one phone should be designated only for official business and emergencies. It is recommended that a verbal code be established to aid in quick communication of common information. If such a code is used in a park, it should be explained in the emergency action plan.

The telephone numbers for emergency services should be posted near the phone and should be easily readable. If a pay phone is designated as the emergency phone, $0.25 (a quarter) should be available near the phone. (In some areas of the country, it is not necessary to have a coin to call emergency services.)

Electronic devices

Technology continues to advance and allows communication systems to improve in the delivery, speed, and accuracy of information. Some of the electronic devices used are walkie-talkies, lights (stop and go), electronic gates, buzzers, and public address systems. If modern technology is not available, flags can be used. For example, flags can be used to dispatch guests down the slide when the landing is clear of sliders.

> ## You Should Remember
>
> *It is important that you learn the signals and communication system used at your park. The communication must be easily understood to be effective in an emergency.*

General ride operating procedures

Large water park facilities, commonly known as *theme parks*, may have carnival amusement rides at the facility. The following procedure applies to this type of ride.

When operating any ride or attraction, the employee's primary concern should be guest safety. A vast majority of park rides are automatic. Therefore the attendant's job is to make sure that guests are able to make the transitions from ride entrance to ride unit and from ride unit to ride exit in absolute safety. To ensure this safety, the ride attendant must remain alert and be prepared for any unexpected problems that may occur at any time during operation. Due to automation and modern technology, some rides are easy to operate, and there is the temptation for attendants to neglect their duties and responsibilities. However, each employee is personally responsible for the safety and welfare of the guests and must constantly be conscious of those duties.

> ## You Should Remember
>
> *Your job is to make sure that guests are able to make the transitions from ride entrance to ride unit and from ride unit to ride exit in absolute safety. You are personally responsible for the safety and welfare of the guests and must always be aware of your duties.*

Opening procedures

The following opening procedure or equivalent procedure should be completed by each ride operator before allowing guests to use the ride:

1. Check in with your supervisor or at the main office to obtain any new information or working material needed for your shift's operation.
2. Do a visual inspection of your ride to ensure that no one is working on it, and make sure all moving units have a clear path to operate.
3. Start the ride 2 or 3 times and listen for strange noises that may be mechanical problems. Test brakes and make sure all gauges register properly.
4. Inspect all safety straps and bars to ensure that they are in proper operating order.

5. Complete necessary checklist or documentation to verify completion of opening procedures.
6. Notify supervisor of ride status and open ride to guests at the appropriate time.

Loading and unloading procedures

Because guests are only in the park for a relatively short period of time, it is extremely important that ride attendants attain the highest capacity that is safely possible for their ride. Profit is just as important as safety, but profit should *never* "overrule" safety procedures. The following is a general guideline for loading and unloading procedures:

1. After you collect the ticket from the guest, direct him or her to the ride unit.
2. Be sure to provide assistance to those guests who may need help. Always instruct guests to keep their hands and legs inside the ride unit.
3. Do not allow guests to eat or drink on or during the ride.
4. Review the rules with the guests to ensure a safe ride.
5. Load guests in numbers closest to the maximum comfortable load per ride unit. If there is not a line, it may be best to allow guests to ride separately to distribute or balance weight, depending on the attraction or ride.
6. Check all safety belts or straps to ensure they are properly fastend around each guest.
7. Dispatch unit or start ride when all waiting guests are clear and all riding guests are secure and ready.
8. After the ride has completed its normal "trip time," help guests out and direct them to the eixt(s).
9. Last, show positive guest relations by wishing guests "a great day" or "a good time" while visiting the park.

You Should Remember

When loading a ride with guests, profit is just as important as safety, but profit should never overrule safety procedures.

Closing procedures

The following closing procedure or equivalent procedure should be completed by each ride operator before leaving the facility:

1. After the guests are clear of the ride, clean all ride units and pick up litter around the ride.
2. Bring the ride to the "night storage" position.
3. Turn off all appropriate power switches and lights.
4. Cover any ride units if necessary.
5. Take all working materials to the main office and report any maintenance that needs to be done before the next operating day.
6. Check with the supervisor about any new information and check out for that day.

You Should Remember

The opening and closing procedures for rides may vary. Therefore you should know the procedures for the rides in your area of responsibility.

General Water Park Lifeguard Operating Procedures

Operating procedures are designed to give an overall view of the lifeguard position at your facility. The procedures and training, combined with your common sense and good judgement, will aid you in being successful as a lifeguard. The following are examples of opening , operating, and closing procedures for lifeguards. The procedures may vary among water parks. Therefore the following is just an *example* and not a recommendation for any specific water park. The water park management team must develop procedures that suit your facility.

Opening procedures

Each day, lifeguards have opening procedures. The number of lifeguards may vary because of attendance levels at various times of the season. However, each of the following opening procedures is completed before the gates are opened to guests regardless of the number of lifeguards on duty.

1. Lifeguards check in and advise supervisor that they are present and starting work.

2. Lifeguards check the communications system to determine proper operations. Any problems are reported to the supervisor.
3. All furniture is arranged in an orderly manner and cleaned as needed.
4. The pools are vacuumed or brushed.
5. All sidewalks, stairs, and pool decks are swept.
6. All tables, trash cans, and urns are cleaned and put in position.
7. Guard-stand safety equipment is cleaned and checked for proper function. All equipment is positioned for rescue use. (Your facility's opening procedures explain exactly where the equipment is to be located and positioned for rescue use.)
8. All items such as brooms and pans are stored out of sight of guests. Each broom should be returned to its original storage location.
9. All lifeguards are in their duty station in proper uniform when the gates open at 11:00 AM.

Operating procedures

Operating procedures should be explained for each attraction that requires a lifeguard. This example is for a wave pool:

1. Lifeguards are responsible for the safety of each guest in their area of responsibility.
2. Constantly be alert for weak swimmers. The deeper water is only for strong swimmers during the wave action.
3. Guests are not allowed to hold onto ladders during the wave action or any other time.
4. Watch for nonswimming guests on rafts. Remember that rafts are not personal flotation devices designed to keep a swimmer afloat.
5. Watch for guests entering the wave pool with floating devices. Only Coast Guard–approved life vests are allowed. Ring buoys, inflated rubber boats, and water wings are not allowed in the wave pool. Tell guests where they may use the items safely.
6. No masks, fins, or snorkels are allowed in the wave pool. Tell the guests that masks are permitted at the shallow end of the activity pool if the mask is made of tempered glass or has a platic face plate.
7. No pushing or horseplay is allowed in the pool or on the deck area.
8. No one may jump or dive into the pool. Guests may enter the pool only through the shallow end.

9. No running is allowed in the pool or surrounding deck area.
10. Keep guests off the buoy lines.
11. All lifeguards stand at their assigned positions during the wave action.
12. Available lifeguards on duty cover the assigned positions or stand while the duty lifeguard makes the rescue and returns.
13. Lifeguards are required to wear rescue tubes while in the watch position.

Closing procedures

The manager on duty notifies the lifeguard or attendant to close the attraction or pool. Once the lifeguard has been instructed to close, the following procedure is begun:

1. Clear guests from the pool by use of the whistle and by announcing that the pool is closed and all guests should exit.
2. Lifeguards clean the bathroom nearest their attraction.
3. Furniture is stacked and put in night storage.
4. Pool decks and sidewalks must be swept.
5. Rental tubes left out by guests are returned to the tube rental stand and counted.
6. Trash cans and cigarette urns are emptied.
7. Assigned personnel clean the parking lot of trash and debris.
8. Lifeguards squeegee all decks of excess water.
9. Lifeguards are responsible for collecting life jackets around their areas of responsiblity.
10. Your supervisor inspects your area and clears you so you can clock out. Remember to sign your time card. No signature means no pay.

You Should Remember

*Operating procedures are designed to give an overall view of the employee position at your facility. The **operating procedures** and **training**, combined with your **common sense** and **good judgment**, will assist you in being a successful employee.*

Thunder and Lightning Storms

At least 100 Americans are killed by lightning each year, which is more deaths than caused by tornadoes, hurricanes, or floods. However, to keep things in perspective, the chances of dying in a drowning accident are 50 times (5000%) greater. When lightning strikes a person, the person generally goes into cardiac arrest and/or respiratory failure. The prudent employee can understand that lightning is too fast, too powerful, and too unpredictable to risk the chance of allowing guests to use the facilities during a thunderstorm.

Action procedures during thunderstorms

Definitive information as to when guests may return to activities once a storm has ended does not exist from any auhoritative agency or organization. Therefore the employee needs to refer to the supervisor's judgment and the park's policies. The judgment of the supervisor and the park policy should consider several points in determining when to clear the facility and when to resume activity.

Evacuating the park guests from the facility

All guests should evacuate the surrounding area at the first sound of thunder. The criterion for this action is not based on the sighting of lightning but rather on the sound of thunder, since thunder occurs as a result of lightning. The park's emergency action plan for evacuation should be implemented by the employee who hears the first sound of thunder. This may mean that a supervisor is advised of the situation and begins the evacuation procedure. Because lightning is attracted to the tallest object in the area, guests and staff should not congregate under umbrellas, trees, or any tall objects. All persons in the facility should go indoors or take cover in their automobiles.

Return to normal operations

The National Weather Service does not consider a thunderstorm "over" until there has been no sound of thunder for at least 15 minutes. However, an additional factor to consider is whether the sky is dark and threatening. Unless there are obvious signs of clearing, a thunderstorm should not be considered "over." It may be necessary for supervisor or employee to consider an additional 5- to 15-minute safety margin before allowing the guests to return to park activities.

Park policy

All facilities should state their activity rules and regulations in writing for guests to see before using any attraction. It seems prudent to state that the facility will be cleared at the first sound of thunder and that guests will not be allowed to reenter the ride or attraction area until 15 to 30 minutes after the last sound of thunder.

The Americans with Disabilities Act

This section briefly discusses the general ramifications of the Americans with Disabilities Act (ADA) as it relates to water parks. It is not intended to be comprehensive or complete regarding ADA information or compliance. You will need to do some additional homework. Two resources you may want to use follow:

1. For more specific information about ADA requirements affecting employment, contact the Equal Employment Opportunity Commission, 1801 L Street NW, Washington, DC 20507 (202) 663-4900.
2. For more specific information about ADA requirements affecting Public Services and Public Accommodations contact the Office on the Americans with Disabilities Act, Civil Rights Division, U.S. Department of Justice, P.O. Box 66118, Washington, DC 20035-6118 (202) 514-0301

What is the act?

The ADA gives civil rights protection to approximately 43 million individuals with disabilities that are like those rights provided to individuals on the basis of race, gender, national origin, and religion. It guarantees equal opportunity for individuals with disabilities in employment, public accommodations, transportation, state and local government services, and telecommunications.

Who are persons with a disability?

Persons with disabilities are those with a physical or mental impairment that substantially limits one or more major life activities. These are activities that an average person can perform with little or no difficulty. Examples are walking, speaking, breathing, seeing, hearing, learning, caring for oneself, working, and performing manual tasks. Other activities such as sitting, standing, lifting, and reading are also major life activities. The ADA also includes persons with acquired immunodeficiency syndrome (AIDS), epilepsy, paralysis, and learning disabilities such as dyslexia. The ADA protects relatives and others who associate with persons with disabilities from discrimination. However, temporary impairments such as broken limbs, sprains, concussions, appendicitis, common colds, and influenza are generally not disabilities covered by the ADA.

How does the ADA affect Water parks?

The water park industry is most likely affected by Titles I and III of the ADA, which cover employment and public accommodations. **Title I** was conceived to enable approximately 14 million persons with disabilities of working age to compete in the workplace on the basis of the same performance standards expected of a person without a disability. An employer must make "reasonable accommodations" for an otherwise qualified person's known mental or physical limitation unless doing so would pose an "undue hardship" on the water park.

Reasonable accommodation is any modification or adjustment to a job or the work environment that will enable a qualified applicant or employee with a disability to participate in the application process or to perform essential job functions. Reasonable accommodation also includes adjustments to ensure that a qualified individual with a disability has the same rights and privileges in employment as nondisabled employees.

A Water Parks may be required to modify facilities to enable a person to perform essential job functions and to have equal opportunity to participate in other employment-related activities. For example, if an employee lounge is located in a place inaccessible to a person using a wheelchair, the lounge may be modified or relocated or comparable facilities may be provided in a location the would enable the person to take a break with co-workers.

Another example of reasonable accommodation is to reassign nonessential functions to other employees. When a person applying for park manager has the required education, supervisory experience and the ability to coordinate a host of programs and happens to be blind, the inability to see water park patrons shall not be the obstacle to assuming the position. Assuming other park staff could assume the

nonessential task of visual supervision, that requirement could be reassigned. However, this example would not hold true for a lifeguard because the ability to visually sweep an assigned area of the water and quickly identify potential hazards is an essential function of a lifeguard.

Title III of the ADA applies to public accommodations and commercial facilities owned or operated by private entities whose operations affect commerce and certain examinations and courses. Some examples include water parks, hotels, restaurants, golf courses, grocery stores, retail stores, doctors' offices, bowling alleys, exhibition halls, transportation facilities, and vehicles. The intent of Title III is to include Americans with disabilities into the mainstream of society in the most integrated setting possible. The ADA states, "No individual shall be discriminated against on the basis of disability in the full and equal enjoyment of the goods, services, facilities, privileges, advantages, and accommodations of any place of the public accommodations."

The term *public accommodations* means a private entity that owns, leases or leases to, or operates a place of public accommodation. Both public accommodations and commercial facilites are subject to the alteration and construction standards of the ADA accessibility guidelines. In addition, public accommodations must engage in "readily achievable barrier removal."

The ADA dictates the removal of architectual and communication barriers that are structural in exiting facilities and where such removal is "readily achievable," in other words, any modification that is not expensive or difficult to complete. The ADA lists a host of different type of modest measures possibly taken to remove barriers that are likely to be readily achievable. The obligation to engage in readily achievable barrier removal is an ongoing process. As time passes, barrier removal that initially was not readily achievable may later be required because of new circumstances.

How do you train water park staff to deal with persons with disabilities?

Careful training can modify behavior and develop new attitudes in recognizing the abilities of persons with disabilities. The most effective training should include some element of experimental learning according to Angie Chesnut, author of Breaking Down Barriers: A Complete Guide to Business

Relationships with People with Disabilities. For example, a requirement of training may be for the staff to be confined to a wheelchair or become a person with sight impairment. The staff would remain in this condition throughout the day and would be required to function in the normal environment of the facility or show. The disabled staff would experience barriers in pathways such as furniture, steps, curbs, and power cords. Through this experimental learning, opportunities may arise for the staff to "feel" the challenges and frustrations experienced by disabilities or physical impairments and therefore have a greater understanding of persons with disabilities.

It is not too late to begin a formal in-service training program with your staff. In-service training topics or activities related to persons with disabilities may include the following:

1. Discuss the proper etiquette when dealing with a disabled person.
2. Consider ADA Title III—What does it mean to this facility?
3. Understand impairments and disabilities such as Alzheimer's disease, amputees, aphasia, arthritis, cerebral palsy, cerebral-vascular accident, epilepsy, mental illness, mental retardation, multiple sclerosis, and muscular dystrophy.
4. Discuss special situations at your facility. For example, certain amusement rides or attractions may not be "reasonably safe" for persons of selected disabilities.
5. Write or review a standard operating procedure guide for handling persons with disabilities.
6. Evaluate your ability to accommodate persons with disabilities.
7. Ask a local community expert to speak about selected topics regarding persons with disabilities, for example, a physical or occupational therapist.
8. Have a person with a disability speak about a selected topic at your in-service training.

A critical area for training is helping employees understand company policies regarding hosting guests with disabilities. For example, safety considerations may prevent certain guests from using a ride. Obviously, employees must know how to handle a situation or contact a supervisor if questions arise. This type of training is ongoing as new attractions are opened. For example, if a ramp to allow wheelchairs is added to a gift shop, employees of the shop need to learn about how to assist guests in wheelchairs.

Bloodborne Pathogens and Water Park Personnel

The Occupational Safety and Health Administration (OSHA) has issued regulations to protect people from the hazards of bloodborne pathogens such as human immunodeficiency virus (HIV) and hepatitis. This regulation was primarily intended for emergency evacuation teams, hospital employees, and others who deal with the injured; the regulations also appear to apply to any employee who is likely to come into contact with human blood. For example, the legislation may apply to a park's first-aid personnel, lifeguards, and others who might be called to assist patrons or other employees injured at the facility.

The regulations require a number of things such as protective gear, information and training, record keeping, and the administration of preventive injections to appropriate personnel. The regulations are found in 29 Code of Federal Regulations (CFR) 1910.1030. If you have employees who are likely to encounter human blood because of their job duties, you should check with your attorney or the OSHA office to determine exactly what the regulations require.

What are water parks to do?

There are four steps the standard requires employers to take regarding the prevention of any possible transmission of bloodborne pathogens:

1. Identify water park staff who are at risk of exposure to bloodborne diseases. For example, first-aid personnel, emergency medical technicians, registered nurses, and possibly lifeguards.
2. Activate an infection-control plan to reduce exposure to blood. For example, supply first-aid personnel with resuscitation masks, protective eyewear, and latex gloves.
3. Offer hepatitis B vaccinations to any staff member who is occupationally exposed to blood and other body fluids on a regular basis. A "regular basis" may be as regular as once a month.
4. Request staff who have occupational exposure to attend a mandatory training program about bloodborne diseases and precautions against them. Mandatory training is primarily important because so many people are ignorant about how HIV and AIDS are transmitted and how they can be prevented.

It is important that documentation be maintained.

Water parks should have or begin maintaining the following documents: annual training of staff, employee request to receive the hepatitis B vaccination, hepatitis B vaccination refusal form, the blood-borne pathogen exposure medical follow-up form, and program audit forms such as engineering controls needed, protective equipment, work practices, housekeeping and laundry, biohazard labeling, medical waste, and program audit summary. If you wish to research this subject further contact the U.S. Public Health Service, the Center for Disease Control, or your local or state OSHA agency for additional guidelines.

Reducing Liability at Water Parks

The following is a list of questions you should consider when reviewing your Water Parks's overall operation. You may want to add to this brief list to include unique or special areas at your Water Parks.

Operations: Personnel and ride areas

1. What are the preemployment testing procedures the park uses in selecting its staff?
2. What are the preemployment training procedures the park uses to train its employees before their first day on the job?
3. What are the ongoing training procedures and meetings the park uses throughout the season? Is the documentation of these trainings current and well stated?
4. Do you have copies of all management and employee documents that are a part of the training process? This will include but not be limited to employee handbooks, newsletters, standards of performance, job descriptions, operating procedures, bulletins, and training manuals.
5. Does a staff member spend time observing the park's employees in action?
   a. How do they enforce rules?
   b. Are they consistent?
   c. Are the employees alert?
   d. Do they conduct themselves in a professional manner?
   e. Do they present a positive image of the park?
   f. Do they know how to handle the typical emergency situations?
6. Does your park have a first-aid room and an injury treatment system? Where is the nearest ambulance service? Hospital? Does the park have a backboard? Is the staff well trained in the use of the backboard? Does the park have a communication system for emergencies?
7. Is the park's management team well trained? Can they handle the employees? What is management's training and background? Can management handle emergencies?
8. What formal training is required by the park for its various employees? Is all the training approved through a national certifying agency? Do all employees have cardiopulmonary resuscitation (CPR) and first-aid training?
9. Are maintenance workers provided with funding to attend operator and equipment maintenance workshops? If not, what measures are taken to train these people?
10. Is there a standard form and system for reporting accidents in your park?
11. Are emergency and accident management procedures written and rehearsed to ensure a prompt, organized response to an accident?
12. Have emergency and accident management procedures been reviewed by your attorney, local paramedics, and/or hospital officials?
13. Are emergency and accident management drills conducted at least twice a month, one of those times during peak facility use?
14. Is current safety literature available to you and your staff?
15. Are all accidents carefully investigated and reviewed with the proper authorities and corrective action taken?
16. Are safety checks of facilities and equipment made by staff members weekly, with the report or check sheet filed in the appropriate office?
17. Are you familiar with all local, county, state, and professional safety and health standards that may affect the operation of the facility?
18. Does your staff carefully inspect equipment each day before use to ensure its safe use? Is a report filed?
19. Does your park clearly mark potentially hazardous conditions or areas with proper signage?
20. Is the current ride or attraction permit on file, if applicable in your state?
21. Is the electrical inspection up to date?
22. Are pool operations reports maintained and submitted to the health department when required?

23. Is a bacteriological analysis conducted weekly on any pools?
24. Are chlorine and pH tests conducted as required?
25. Is the water turnover rate maintained at an acceptable rate that meets local health standards?
26. Are SCBA masks available and in working condition?
27. Is water clarity maintained as required by law (usually measured by a 6-inch black disk being visible on the bottom from anywhere on the deck around the deep end)?
28. Is the water level maintained above gutter or skimmer level?
29. Is a test kit available with fresh chemicals?
30. Are depth markings the proper size and at the correct locations (usually 4-inch numbers written in red or black and located wherever depth changes 1 foot or every 25 feet)?
31. Is there a detailed maintenance and repair record kept by management?
32. Are you aware of what activities are considered to be high risk?
33. Is a positive morale held by employees? What is done to maintain a positive morale?
34. Does the staff have a room or area that is a comfortable atmosphere where guards may relax when off duty?
35. Are the filter and mechanical equipment rooms secured and kept in a clean and accessible condition? Is there adequate lighting for clear visibility of each equipment component and gauge for maintenance purposes?
36. Are the components of the pool bathhouse (clothes storage space, dressing areas, shower room, drying room, toilets, and lobby) in clean operating condition?
37. Are employees routinely evaluated and praised for the duties they perform?

Physical environment

1. Are walkways safe and well maintained?
2. Is there adequate instructional signing throughout the park? Is the signage clear in its intended meaning? Is it informative, professionally produced, and well maintained?
3. Are the buildings and other areas to which the guests have access free of hazards? Are the buildings and structures well maintained? Do they enhance the overall appearance of the park?

4. What is the condition of ramps and stairs? Are they slippery, do they have adequate handrails, and can small children slip through the rails?
5. Are the rides and attractions safe and in good working order? Are the rides and attractions causing injuries? If so, why? How can this be prevented?
6. Does the overall physical appearance of the park reflect a caring management attitude and attention to detail? Does the park appear to be professionally operated?
7. Where are chemicals and equipment stored? Is the storage area off limits to unauthorized personnel?
8. Is the snack bar or food service area clean and properly maintained according to local health department regulations?
9. Does the park have sufficient lighting for night operations (overhead and underwater lighting)?
10. Do your warning signs accomplish the following three basic objectives?
    a. To tell people about a threat to their well-being posed by dangerous conditions or products
    b. As a safety measure to change people's behavior so that they act safely
    c. To remind people of 1 and 2
11. Are signs posted to warn guests of the physical, chemical, environmental, and behavioral hazards?

Bibliography

Bureau of Business Practice: *1992 safety manager's guide,* 1992, Simon & Schuster.

Chesnut A: *Breaking Down Barriers: a complete guide to business relationships with people with disabilities,* Hackett, Ark, 1992, Trio Research Services.

Clayton RD, Thomas DG: *Professional aquatic management,* ed 2, 1989, Human Kinetics Books.

Gabrielsen MA (editor): *Swimming pools: a guide to their planning, design, and operation,* ed 4, 1987, Human Kinetics Publishers.

International Association Of Amusement Parks and Attractions: *Funworld,* 1991 Amusement Industry Abstract, Feb 1992, The Association.

International Association of Amusement Parks and Attractions: *Funworld,* Peter Herschend, Jul 1992, The Association.

James W: *Con-Serv and Associates* (in press).

Johnson RL: *YMCA pool operations manual,* 1989, Human Kinetics Publishers.

Paulozzi LJ, McKnight B, Marks SD: A cluster of injuries at a water slide in Washington State, *Am J Pub Health* 76:284, 1986.

Peterson JA: *Risk management for park, recreation and leisure services*, 1987, Management Learning Laboratories.

Pope JR, Jr: *Public swimming pool management II*, 1989, National Recreation and Park Association Printing Office.

Smith DS, Smith SJ: *Water wise*, 1987, Smith Aquatic Safety Service.

University of California: Buying guide: sunscreens, *Berkeley Wellness Letter* 1:3, 1985.

University of California: Buying sunglasses: the eight Key questions, *Berkeley Wellness Letter* 4:3, 1988.

US Department of Transportation: *Emergency action guide for selected hazardous materials*, ed 8, 1987, The Department.

World Water park Association: *WWA considerations for operating safety*, 1989, The Association.

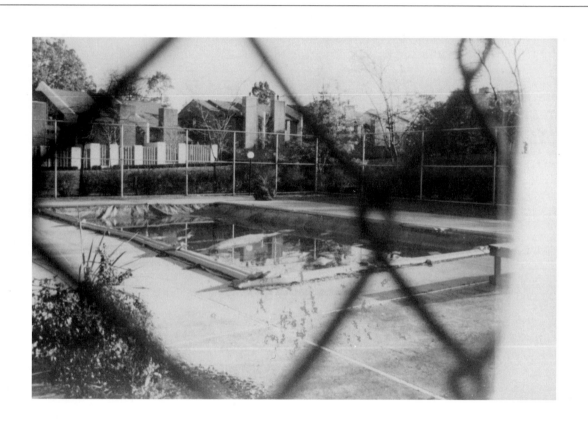

15

WINTERIZING

KEY CONCEPTS

• *Emptying the Pool*

• *Propylene Glycol*

• *Decks*

• *Equipment*

• *Security*

• *Circulation Equipment*

• *Filtration Equipment*

• *Winter Covers*

• *Utilities*

Most pools in the United States are outdoor pools. A significant number of these pools are located in cooler portions of the country and, as a result, must be winterized to protect them and their parts, particularly the plumbing, from freezing water. Moisture destroys much of the pool equipment, particularly when the pool is not in use. If equipment cannot be protected from moisture, it should be removed to a dry environment during the off-season. *Winterizing* pools means different things to different people, but the meaning of this term depends on where the pool is located. The colder the climate, the more involved winterizing is. It should be emphasized that many pool service companies can provide excellent winterizing services for $150 to $450 depending on the size of the pool (Fig. 15-1).

Winterizing is basically a prevention program. When a seasonal pool is winterized, the most important areas of concern are the following[2]:

1. Preventing damage to the pool shell caused by hydrostatic pressure
2. Preventing rust and other deterioration
3. Preventing vandalism

4. Preventing spring start-up problems by an organized and systematic closing procedure

Whether to empty the pool or keep it full during the winter months is a popular topic of discussion with many pool experts. For a variety of reasons, many individuals favor a "full" pool. Regardless of how winterizing is approached, if done correctly and completely, it will be easier to open the pool the following summer. In addition, more damage can be done to a pool in the offseason than during the peak summer months. This chapter begins by illustrating the disadvantages of emptying pools in freezing climates. The discussion of winterizing then progresses from the pool shell to the decks and finally to the surrounding buildings.

Emptying the Pool

Although some individuals empty the pool to be certain to prevent damage caused by the expansion of freezing water in pipes, this practice is not recommended, particularly in colder climates. Perhaps the most serious result of emptying the pool is "floating" a concrete pool, which can occur if the surrounding water table is high and the hydrostatic pressure relief valves are either clogged or insufficient in number. The hydrostatic relief valves can be normally be found in the main drain boxes and allow surrounding ground water to enter the pool harmlessly rather than damaging the pool shell (Fig. 15-2).

In this case, when the water with all its weight is removed from the pool, the shell of the pool becomes relatively light compared with the weight of the surrounding ground water. As a result the pool "pops" right out of the ground, damaging both the shell and piping. This can occur whenever the level of the water in the ground is higher than the water level in the pool. This is a serious concern in colder climates.

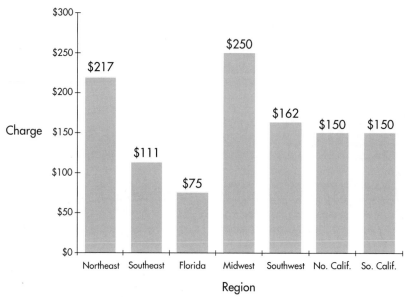

Fig. 15-1. Average charge to winterize a residential pool. (From *Service Industry News*, Torrance, Calif.)

Emptying a vinyl liner pool can also create problems. Shrinkage and wrinkling can occur to the liner in a vinyl-lined pool.

Another problem associated with an empty pool is that even if small amounts of water are left between tile joints, cracks in concrete, and coping, tremendous damage can result because of the "freeze-thaw" cycle.

An empty pool can also be hazardous to both humans and pets. Particularly in the early spring, children can be attracted to the rainwater that collects in the empty pools. During the fall, skateboarders and in-line skaters are tempted by the still dry, large, flat surfaces. The diving area becomes particularly attractive for advanced tricks. Of course, keeping these individuals out of the pool shell after the water has been drained becomes difficult.

An advantage of emptying a pool before winter is that pool personnel can inspect the condition of the pool shell. Cracks, joints, and blemishes can be both inspected and repaired easily in an empty pool. Many question whether this advantage outweighs the risks associated with emptying the pool, however.

Winterizing a "Full" Pool

Many aquatic experts agree that keeping the pool full or nearly full is the best way to winterize a pool with some precautions. Not only is it safer for the plumbing, but a full pool is actually safer to people and pets as well.

Although costly, some pools are winterized by simply covering them with a security cover. This is done more often in climates that do not experience harsh winters. The pool is kept completely full and water is circulated and heated slightly only when the temperatures reach the single digits. The movement of the water for the most part prevents it from freezing, and the heater can be turned on when the temperatures become extreme. Even if water does freeze in the pool, most of the expansion takes place upward rather than sideways, so damage does not take place. Placing logs or tires in a winterized pool that is full is no longer recommended. Very little chlorine is needed because sunlight and swimmers do not use it up. Although utilities (water and electric) must be paid during the winter months, some argue that when a pool is winterized in this fashion, there are few summer start-up costs.

When most pools are winterized, the water level is lowered about 16 inches or to just below the inlets. Although the recommended water level varies with each type of pool, at least a foot of water should always cover the shallow end floor. The type of cover used may determine what water level is most appropriate. There are two reasons for slightly lowering the water level in the pool. First, sufficient water in the

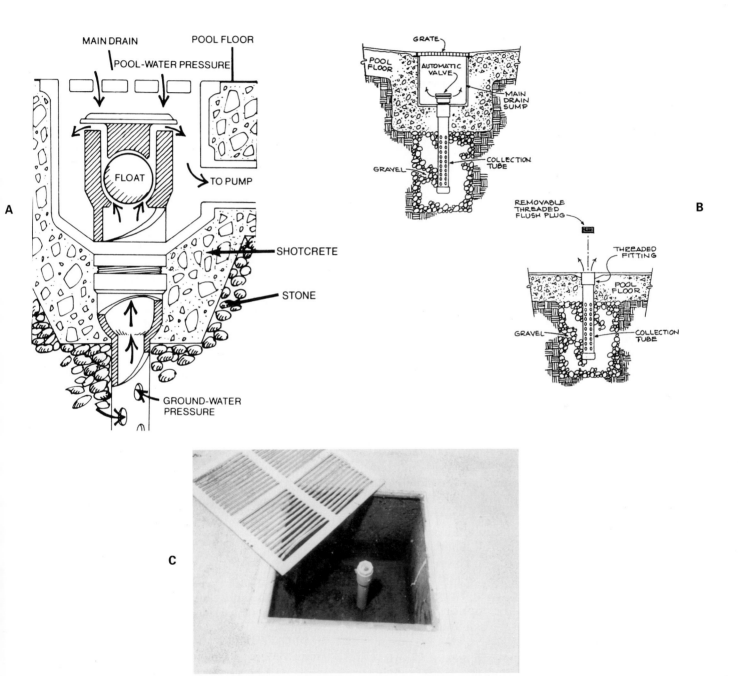

Fig. 15-2. **A,** Main drain with hydrostatic relief valve. **B,** Other hydrostatic pressure relief valves. **C,** Underwater photograph of hydrostatic pressure relief valve. (**A** from NSPI: *Basic pool and spa technology*, ed 2, Alexandria,Va, The Institute; **B** from Pool and Spa News, June 15, 1992.)

pool remains to protect the pool shell from floating and prevents the pools sides and bottom from "frost heaving." Second, it allows the skimmers and other supply lines to be drained so that they can also be protected from freezing.

The water level in a winterized pool should never be allowed to reach the tile edge that surrounds some pools because if freezing occurs, ice can either crack the tile or damage the coping.

Because the pool should be vacuumed thoroughly and the filters cleaned before winterizing, both vacuuming and backwashing should be performed to "waste" so that these maintenance functions and the lowering of the water level are completed simultaneously.

Once the pool level is lowered to the desired level, one of two precautions should be taken to protect these lines. Antifreeze should be added to the skimmers and other lines that cannot be kept dry during the winter. But care must be taken to use a recreational antifreeze such as **propylene glycol**, which is a biodegradable, recreational antifreeze. Automotive antifreeze should never be used in a swimming pool application. Automotive antifreeze is toxic, whereas recreational antifreeze is nontoxic. Antifreeze is usually preferred in extremely cold climates because even small amounts of water left in lines can freeze and cause significant damage.[3]

Some pool technicians prefer to blow all lines dry with small compressors or reversing industrial vacuums rather than using antifreeze. Care must be taken to rid the lines of all water when lines are blown and to make sure that valves and fittings are airtight so that water does not find its way back into the lines. Special plugs are inserted in the outlets to ensure that these lines remain dry. Although all skimmers should be plugged, it is difficult to keep rain or melted snow from reentering skimmer boxes, so antifreeze still may be required in skimmers even though the lines have been blown dry. Another option is to place expansion bags or bottles in the skimmer to protect them.

Blowing lines dry has become an area of expertise in the pool industry. Pool technicians isolate equipment and lines throughout the circulation system and then systematically drain them and blow them dry. Although some technicians cap or plug all lines and close all valves, some experts prefer to leave valves returning to the filter room equipment open to allow invading water room to move in case it does freeze. This process usually begins in the filter room where

the filter, heater, and pump are drained with drain plugs remaining open. The lines are usually blown dry from the filter room back to the pool and this includes the main drain line.[4]

When a vinyl-liner pool is winterized, the risk of "floating" is not as great as with a concrete or fiberglass pool, but vinyl-liner pools should still remain nearly full during the winter. If vinyl-lined pools are emptied completely, the liner can shrink, wrinkle, or crack. Another precaution must be taken when "shocking" the pool for winter. Postseason shocking with sanitizer is recommended to prevent algae growth, but if the sanitizer level becomes too high in a vinyl pool, the liner can be bleached or damaged. Some experts recommend keeping shocking levels below 6 to 8 ppm, whereas others urge the use of lithium hypochlorite, which is not as harsh on liners as some of the other sanitizers.

The water should be balanced for the winter in the same fashion it is done in the summer. The only other precaution that should be taken is the addition of an algicide. Although there is not much light or warm water in a winterized pool, the water will remain stagnant for long periods, so algae growth can become a problem in the fall and spring if an algicide is not added (box).

Chemicals Commonly Used for Winterizing

Winterizing chemicals fall into four major categories:

- *Sanitizers*—Calcium hypochlorite (cal hypo), lithium hypochlorite (lithium hypo), sodium dichlor, sodium hypochlorite (liquid chlorine), gas chlorine, nonchlorine microbicide (Baquacil), and bromine (activated by addition of a high level of oxidizer such as chlorine, ozone, or potassium peroxymonosulfate)
- *Algicides*—Copper, silver, quats, polymers, herbicides, chlorine enhancers, and algae inhibitors
- *Stain and scale preventers*—Sequestering agents, chelating agents, and pH adjusters
- *Maintenance chemicals*—Antifreeze, tilecleaner, cover cleaner and protectant, polish, clarifier, filter cleaner, and enzymes

Courtesy Service Industry News, Torrance, Calif.

Pool Decks and Equipment

After the pool shell has been winterized, attention must be turned to the pool deck and its equipment. Once the deck has been completely cleaned, of utmost concern is protecting the pool deck from the damage inflicted by freezing water. All construction joints, expansion joints, and any other areas where two solid materials meet should be carefully protected with quality caulking or other long-lasting sealants. If water enters these joints or other cracks and then freezes, the pool deck will deteriorate rapidly.

While the pool deck is being protected, all deck equipment should also be cared for. Ladders, diving boards, lifeguard chairs, pool furniture, and safety equipment should be removed from the pool deck and stored indoors if at all possible. Any nuts, bolts, and washers used to secure these items in place should also be stored but only after heavy lubrication to prevent rust and corrosion.

When ladders and handrails are removed, the anchors, cups, and bolts should be placed in a bag and tied to the ladder or handrail so that they are not misplaced. The same is true for lifeguard stands. Diving board bolts must be greased and stored with the board.

Water fountains should have the supply water turned off and should be drained, removed, and stored in a warm, dry place.

Circulation and Filtration Equipment

To prevent rusting and overall deterioration of circulation and filtration equipment, special care must be taken to protect it during the winter. Basically, all equipment should be drained of water, cleaned, lubricated, and removed to a warm, dry place. Any parts that show signs of rust should be scraped and painted with a rust retardant. Each of the following items must be carefully protected:

The pump

The power to the pump should be turned off and the terminal box should be weatherproofed. All water must be drained from the pump. If the pump is left outside and water remains inside the pump, the freezing water could cause it to crack. Whenever possible, the pump should actually be removed to a warm, dry place. If the pump cannot be removed, it should be cleaned, lubricated, and then covered. When pumps and motors are covered for winter, they should not be completely sealed because condensation that forms will not be allowed to escape, thus damaging the pump. The lid and basket for the hair and lint strainer should also be removed. The strainer basket is an ideal place to keep freeze plugs and other pool parts. A light coating of grease should be applied to the hair strainer lid and pot. The off-season is a good time to have the pump sent out for inspection, overhauling, or repairs.

The filters

All filters should be backwashed and cleaned before the winterizing process begins. The pressure relief valves should be opened on pressure systems and drain plugs removed so that all water is removed. Sand beds should be inspected and cleaned as needed, and in the case of D.E. filters, the filter elements should be removed, inspected, cleaned, and repaired. They should also be covered to protect them from rodents and debris.

Pipes and plumbing

All water must be turned off. All drain plugs should be removed, lubricated, and stored in a safe place. Standing water cannot be allowed to remain in the pipes. Experts should be consulted if questions arise concerning winterizing pipes and plumbing. All valves should be opened and kept open during the winter unless the system is below the normal operating water level of the pool. Opening the valve allows all the water to drain from them, particularly if a pool-side plug is dislodged.

Chlorinators and chemical feeders

These items must be drained of water and cleaned for the winter. Parts such as injectors, diaphragms, and check valves must be cleaned carefully and lubricated. Whenever possible, chlorinators and feeders should be moved to a warm, dry place. Chlorinators should be kept dry during the winter to prevent corrosion. The off-season is perhaps the best time to overhaul or repair this equipment.

Pressure gauges and flow meters

Both these items should be unscrewed, removed of water, dried, lubricated, and stored in a safe place. All small parts should be bagged and marked. Many pool operators tie these bags to the hair and lint strainer or some other larger associated apparatus.

Chemicals

All chemicals must be dealt with during the colder months. If at all possible, chemicals should be returned to the supplier. Dry chemicals must be tightly sealed and kept dry and off the ground. Liquid chemicals and reagents must not be allowed to freeze. It is important to know the shelf life of each of the remaining chemicals as the end of the season approaches. For example, sodium hypochlorite has a short shelf life, and storing over the winter will only result in wasting the chemical. Sodium hypochlorite must be ordered conservatively at the end of the season. If any liquid chlorine is still remaining when the pool closes, it should be used in the pool for super-chlorination or other pool sanitation chores. Empty gas cylinders should be returned to the chemical supplier. Test kits and reagents should be moved to a warm, dry, safe environment, but it may be wise to discard reagents at the end of the season and to purchase fresh reagents at the beginning of the next season. Algicides should be kept on hand during the off-season in case warm periods are experienced while the pool is closed.

Other Equipment

Pool Heater

The power source to the heater must be turned off. The water must be drained and the heating elements should be cleaned according to the manufacturer's recommendations.

Pool Lights

Pool lights must be protected from freezing water. Power to the lights must be turned off at the circuit box. Wet niche lights should be removed from a full pool that is being winterized. Once out of the water, lights should be inspected for damage and leakage, repaired, and then lubricated. The gaskets require special attention. Whenever possible, lights should be boxed or wrapped and kept in a warm, dry place. If lights are left on the pool deck, care must be taken to prevent vandalism. Another approach to dealing with underwater lights is to weigh them down after removing them from their niche and to sink them to the pool bottom after weighting them with a brick. Extra care must be taken to avoid cracking the lens when lowering them to the bottom of the pool.

Safety Equipment

All safety equipment must be moved indoors and kept dry. Self-contained breathing apparatus (SCBA) systems need to be stored indoors, protected from the weather and vandalism. First-aid kits should be inventoried and stocked with replacement items *before* the winter. If this is done, one less task will be required in the spring. Ring buoys, reaching poles, rescue tubes, and other equipment should be covered, stored indoors, and kept together. All ropes and lines should be neatly coiled and stored to save hours of work untangling them in the spring.

Maintenance Equipment

All cleaning and maintenance equipment should be stored together and organized. Tool boxes should be cleaned out and replacement tools purchased in the fall. All brushes, poles, vacuums, hoses, and other cleaning tools should be inspected, repaired, and replaced as needed. Again, it must be emphasized that the off-season is the time when these time-consuming tasks must be completed, not during the pre-season.

Equipment needs should be evaluated as the pool is being winterized while these needs are still fresh in the minds of the pool operators. In many respects, running a seasonal swimming pool is like farming. A successful summer season often depends on how much effort is exercised in the off-season.

Locker Rooms

Locker rooms deserve special attention, particularly because of the risk to frozen pipes leading to showers, sinks, and toilets. All lines should be drained and blown dry to prevent freezing. Mirrors should be covered with cardboard to prevent breakage, particularly if pool equipment is to be stored in the bathhouse during the offseason. The locker rooms should be protected against rodents as well as vandals; doors and windows must be locked securely. After the locker rooms have been thoroughly winterized, the water must be turned off for the winter.

Pool Covers

There are a variety of covers available for the winterization of swimming pools. The two most commonly used covers are **winter covers** and **safety covers**. Winter covers are large, solid, vinyl fabric covers

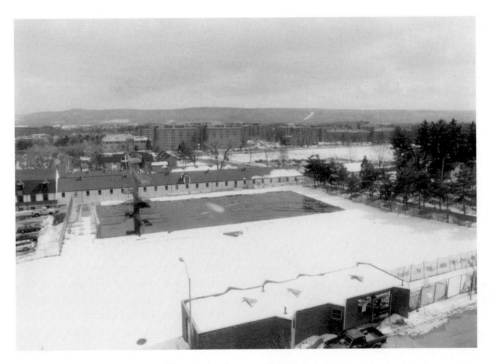

Fig. 15-3. Large winter cover.

that are held down with sand or water bags (Fig. 15-3). The purpose of the winter cover is solely to keep debris such as leaves and dirt from entering the pool. They are often held down with water or sand bags, but the trend is moving toward a strap or cable locking system that anchors these covers to the pool deck because the weighted bags often break. One disadvantage of the solid cover is that large amounts of water can collect on the surface, making it difficult to remove during the spring. One advantage of the solid vinyl winter cover is that it is relatively inexpensive.

Safety covers are strong, polypropylene mesh covers that can support people and pets that might mistakenly wander out onto the cover. They are anchored to the pool deck with a cable system and can withstand a great amount of weight (Fig. 15-4). They allow rain and melted snow to pass through the cover, but they keep all solid objects out of the pool. Safety mesh covers are used for winterizing but also provide a large margin of security.

Some **automatic pool covers** are solid pool covers that secure the pool at night during the season but can also be used to winterize the pool.

Superchlorination or heavy algicide use may damage some pool covers. If water chemistry is going to change drastically when a pool is covered, the manu-facturer's recommendations must be followed closely. In addition, regardless of what type of cover is used, the perimeter must be fastened down sufficiently to prevent the wind from getting under the cover and displacing it.

Perimeter Security

The perimeter of the pool must be securely fenced in before the pool is closed for the winter. The fence should be at least 8 feet tall, but many pools are using taller fences. All holes, gaps, and other points of unauthorized entry must be sealed. Locks should be checked to ensure that they are in good working order. The police should be notified when the pool is closed, and their advice should be sought for protecting the property against trespassers.

In addition to the fencing, lighting is very important. Mercury vapor or other bright lights should be installed. A security system should be considered if fencing is inadequate. Any electronic or battery-operated appliances should also be removed from the pool premises and secured in a warm, dry, safe environment. This includes walkie-talkies, bullhorns, radios, TVs, VCRs, computers, and cash registers.

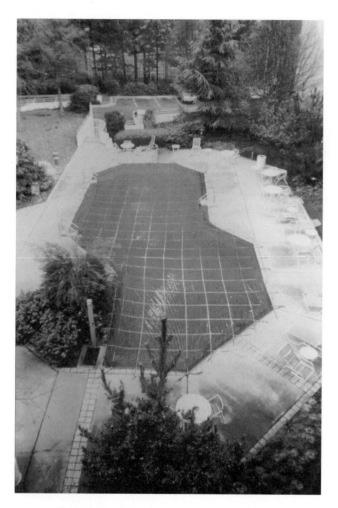

Fig. 15-4. Security cover used in winter.

Utilities

The last step in the winterizing process is the cancellation of utilities, including water, gas, and electric. Although water should be turned off, some swimming facilities have electricity maintained in the filter room and bathhouses so that they can be checked during the off-season. Also, if the electricity is left on, heat bulbs can be controlled with a timer to help control moisture. This is particularly true in the filter room.

Summary

Too often, when swimming facilities (small or large) close for the winter, the owners or operators do not take sufficient time to winterize properly. All pools should be closed for the off-season slowly, deliberately, and completely to protect against cold, moisture, insects, rodents, and vandalism. Lack of use, particularly in a moist, cold environment, often destroys pool equipment prematurely. Opening a pool for the summer is also a comprehensive task. But the harder one works in closing a pool for the winter, the easier it will be to open for summer. The summary found in the National Swimming Pool Foundation CPO manual is helpful for both closing and opening a seasonal pool (Table 15-1).

References

1. Dickman D: Winterizing, *Service Industry News*, Torrance, Calif, Oct 23, 1992, p 6.
2. Dickman D: Winterizing, *Service Industry News*, Torrance, Calif, Oct 23, 1992, p 4.
3. Walsh M: *Aquatics International* Jul / Aug 1992, pp17-21.
4. Herman E: *Pool and Spa News*, Los Angeles, Oct 7, 1991.

Bibliography

Aquatics International, Communications Channels, Atlanta.
Gabrielson AM: *Swimming pools: a guide to their planning, design, and operation*, ed 4, Champaign, Ill, 1987, Human Kinetics.
Johnson R: *YMCA pool operations manual*, Champaign, Ill, 1989, YMCA.
Kowalsky L (editor): *Pool/spa operators handbook*, San Antonio, Tex, 1991, National Swimming Pool Foundation.
Pool and Spa News, Los Angeles.
Pope JR, Jr: *Public swimming pool management*. I and II. Alexandria, Va, 1991, National Recreation and Park Association.
Service Industry News, Torrance, Calif.
Williams KG: *The aquatic facility operator's manual*, Hoffman Estates, Ill, 1991, National Recreation and Park Association, National Aquatic Section.

Table 15-1. Winterizing and Spring Opening Checklist

General Area	Winterizing	Opening
Office supplies and equipment	Store in boxes, prevent moisture, cover	Inventory
Janitorial supplies	Liquids in nonfreeze storage	Inventory
First-aid supplies and equipment	Store in boxes, prevent moisture, cover	Inventory
Ventilation equipment	Lubricate, spray rubber and fabrics with silicone	Check operation
Public address systems, stereo, radio	Remove, store in secure, dry area, and cover	Check operation
Electrical control panels	Shut off all electrical breakers, spray switches with silicone, lock panel door, tape switches for underwater lights in off position	Inventory
Keys	Remove and store in security	Inventory
Main water supply	Turn off all source and use only as needed	Check meter, check pipes systematically for breaks
Openings, rooms, etc.	Rodent control	
Electrical appliances	Store securely	
Pool Area		
Diving boards	Remove, dry, store flat, and cover	Replace bolts and nuts and lubricate
Pool furniture	Repair, store under cover	Clean, inventory
Safety equipment	Store	Inventory
Locker and Shower Rooms		
Showers	Drain and blow lines	Pressure test for leaks
Lockers	Cover	Clean and upgrade
Toilet and sink fixtures	Drain, blow lines	Replace seals
Mirrors	Cover with cardboard, spray metal fittings	Uncover and clean
Chlorinator Room		
Chlorinator	Disconnect, drain, store dry, nonfreeze	Have serviced
Water lines	Drain and blow lines	Connect
Tools	Store, spray with silicone	Inventory
Chlorine tanks	Return to supplier	Order 1-month supply before opening
Wall heaters, fans	Mask and cover, spray switch with silicone	Uncover
Gas mask	Store dry, spray rubber with silicone	Replace, check for function
Test kit	Store dry and nonfreeze	Order new reagents
Filter Room		
Pool water heater	Shut off energy supply at main source, spray switches with silicone and cover, drain	Return to operation

Modified from Pool Spa Operators Handbook, National Swimming Pool Foundation.
FAC, Free-available chlorine.

continued

Table 15-1. Winterizing and Spring Opening Checklist (Cont'd)

General Area	Winterizing	Opening
Filters, sand	Backwash, rake sand	
Filters, DE	Back wash, wash filter cover (septa)	Rake and replace sand
		Refinish tank interior, order second set of filter covers; repair old covers; operational checks for backwashing
Gauges and flowmeters	Cover with plastic bag	
Chemical feeder	Disconnect, drain, clean, lubricate moving parts, cover	Recalibrate, service
		Connect and clean lines, return to operation
Valves	Close and back off two to three turns, check for leaks	
Hair strainer	Clean	Check packing, lubricate stem
		Replace gasket, have a second strainer
Pumps	Check for leaks	
Motors	Lubricate, spray with silicone, cover but allow air circulation	
		Have serviced professionally
Chemical, liquid	Discard hypochlorite, use up inventory	
Chemicals, dry	Cover containers tightly, store off floor, keep dry, maintain inventory to hand-feed pool	Reorder
		Reorder
Outside Fixtures		
Drinking fountain	Remove and store	
Furniture	Store indoors	Replace
		Replace
Swimming Pool		
Pool level	Automatic leveler checked, circulate from drains to filter	
Underwater lights	Turn off at breaker	Balance 50% overflow, 50% drain
Pool cover	In place and tied down	Inspect and repair
		Remove and inspect cover
Chemistry	Hand feed chemicals direct to pool; maintain FAC below 1.0 ppm, pH at 7.2-7.4, check weekly; observe trend of saturation index	Back-up to code standards
Circulation	Place on time clock 4 hour/24 hours, continuous if freezing is possible	
Pool shell	Leave full	24-hour standard

Review Questions

1. In colder climates, is the preferred method of winterizing a pool when it is empty or full?
2. To protect an empty pool from excessive ground water protection, which valve must be functioning properly?
3. What specific type of antifreeze is recommended for winterizing a pool's plumbing?
4. What precautions should be taken when winterizing a vinyl-lined pool?
5. What is the difference between a safety cover and a winter cover?
6. What precautions should be taken when winterizing a pool that has underwater lights?

SECTION V
SAFETY, SUPERVISION, AND RISK MANAGEMENT

Although the chapters in this section appear to be quite different, the major theme is preventing accidents and lawsuits. Chapters 16 and 17 discuss two particularly troublesome areas in aquatics, diving and lifeguarding. Chapter 16 specifically deals with diving. The thrust of this chapter is not to encourage pool owners and operators to remove their diving boards from their facilities but rather to show them how to make diving safer. If pool personnel could prevent all adults from entering headfirst into less than 9 feet of water, headfirst entries would no longer be much of a risk at swimming facilities. Poor judgment, a lack of common sense, and alcohol consumption often contribute to neck injuries at swimming pools. This chapter stresses the value of effective signage and supervision in preventing theses accidents.

Chapter 17, Preventive Lifeguarding, offers a unique approach to lifeguarding. Rather than discussing skills and knowledge that lifeguards should possess, this chapter concentrates on supervision. This chapter should be beneficial to lifeguards wishing to improve their supervision of swimmers and to managers wishing to improve their supervision of lifeguards. An important distinction is made here between *saving* and *guarding*. Special topics such as the RID factor, the 10/20 rule, systematic scanning, high-risk patrons, and motivating lifeguards are also discussed.

Chapter 18, Legal Liability and Risk Management, is a special contribution to this book. This chapter is written by Annie Clement, who is an aquatic educator with a PhD who has also earned a law degree. She is a prolific writer and speaker who specializes in risk management. This chapter educates readers regarding the legal aspects of aquatics, how to safeguard guests, and how to prevent lawsuits.

Finally, Chapter 19 deals with routine operations. This discussion includes daily, weekly, and monthly procedures. Although checklists are a major part of routine operations, much information is offered concerning the philosophy of organized operations, the value of written records, and the importance of a common sense approach to pool safety and operations.

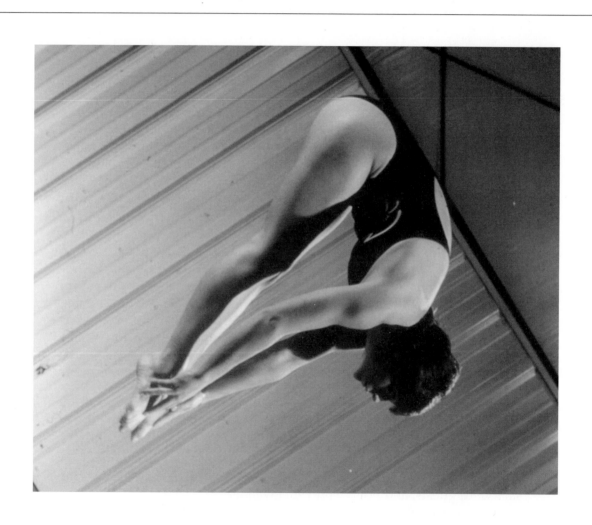

16

DIVING AND OTHER HEADFIRST ENTRIES

Key Concepts

• *Diving versus Headfirst*

• *The Spine*

• *The Diving Victim*

• *Safe Diving Envelope*

• *Residential Pools*

• *Public Pools*

• *Starting Blocks*

• *Diving Boards*

• *Signage*

• *Shallow Water*

Headfirst entries can cause catastrophic injury whenever shallow water is present. Traumatic spinal cord injuries often result in permanent paralysis. Nearly 70% of all sport-related spinal cord injuries are the result of headfirst entries into shallow water. Of these injuries, 95% occur in *less than 5 feet of water*, 5% occur between 5 and 8 feet, and virtually no injuries occur in water depths greater than 9 feet. Although spinal cord injuries most often occur in shallow water, they rarely occur from diving boards, particularly those placed in pools that meet competitive diving standards. Catastrophic neck injuries usually occur in the shallow end of the swimming pool rather than the deep end. Most headfirst entries injuries (approximately 50% to 60%) are alcohol related.[1]

Although many serious neck injuries occur in open water (beaches, lakes, and quarries), this discussion is limited to swimming pools only. Some pools present more of a risk than others when it comes to injuries because of inadequate dimensions and bottom contours, but lack of supervision and inadequate warnings also play a role in "diving" injuries. Safe "div-

ing" depths and distances is perhaps the most controversial topic in water safety circles. The purpose of this discussion is not to propose "diving" depths and distances that will guarantee safety but to reveal facts and opinions surrounding the "diving" controversy, which will assist pool professionals in developing safe "diving" and headfirst entry policies that will prevent accidents in their facilities.

Defintions

Before discussion of diving injuries, the term **diving** must be clearly defined. Too much blame is being placed on diving boards when **headfirst entries** into shallow water from decks, docks, and other platforms are the real culprits resulting in traumatic injuries.

Springboard diving is the act of entering the water headfirst from a diving board. Diving requires formal training from a qualified instructor or coach. Many springboard divers compete in springboard diving events, which is referred to as the **sport of competitive springboard diving**. All competitive diving should be supervised. Traumatic springboard diving injuries are extremely rare, particularly when it is supervised. As mentioned in Chapter 2, no catastrophic diving injuries have occured in the National Federation of State High School Associations (NFSHSA), the National Collegiate Athletic Association (NCAA), or U.S. Diving–sanctioned pools. This fact holds true for both competitive and recreational springboard divers. The high school organization (NFSHSA) does allow diving competitions in as little as 10 feet of water depth.

Headfirst entries closely resemble dives but are initiated by untrained, unsupervised individuals from decks, docks, or platforms other than diving boards. Some refer to this as *recreational diving*, but the term headfirst entries is preferred to clearly distinguish the

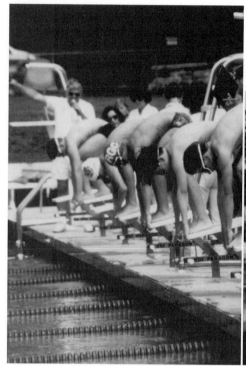
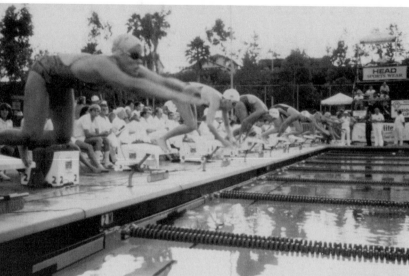

Fig. 16-1.   Competitive racing starts. (Courtesy KDI Paragon, Pleasantville, NY.)

two distinctly different activities. Headfirst entries may sometimes be referred to as "diving" in this text when they are not related to competitive springboard diving.

Racing starts are long, shallow, streamlined "dives" that are performed in competitive swimming from either blocks or decks (Fig. 16-1). Training and supervision should be required for all racing starts. Competitive swimmers use starts for water entries on both the front and the back. Improper racing starts *have* caused traumatic neck injuries. The NCAA regulations require a minimum of 4 feet for racing starts, but the National YMCA has moved to a 5-foot depth requirement. All racing starts should be supervised but especially when they are taught to swimmers. Other competitive swimming organizations allow racing starts in 4 feet of water when the starting platforms are 30 inches above the water and 3½ feet of water for starts when platforms are 18 inches tall. Because more individuals are experiencing catastrophic spinal injuries from competitive starting blocks than from competitive springboards, deeper depths are recommended for racing starts from platforms. Recommendations for the use of starting platforms are found later in this chapter.

These distinct features of diving, headfirst entries, and racing starts are important. Too often diving boards are removed from swimming pools after an intoxicated trespasser is injured entering the **shallow end** headfirst while showing off. Perhaps one of the most difficult issues in this area is determining what pool dimensions are required for safe springboard diving in private pools. Many residential pools simply do not have adequate depth or distance to permit safe springboard diving. It is impossible to determine safe diving depth and dimensions that will guarantee safety for everyone because most catastrophic injuries are the result of reckless, improper "diving." Conversely, it is easy to recommend very conservative numbers that would eliminate "diving" in many pools, but risk-taking individuals may continue to "dive," so this is also not a reasonable solution.

The Spine

The spine is a strong yet flexible column that supports the head and trunk and also protects the spinal cord. The spine is composed of individual vertebrae that are cushioned by a layer of cartilage called *inter-*

vertebral disks. The spinal cord is composed of a bundle of nerves and runs through the center of the vertebrae (Fig. 16-2).

Injuries to the spine include fractures, dislocations, sprains, and compressions. Any of these injuries can cause damage to the spinal cord resulting in temporary paralysis, permanent paralysis, or even death. Although these injuries can occur anywhere on the spine, most "diving" injuries damage the cervical region. Paralysis results from the point of trauma downward. Trauma to C7 downward usually results in paraplegia, whereas damage to C4 through C6 often results in quadraplegia. Many "diving" accidents result in complete quadriplegia.[2]

The Typical Diving Victim

Unlike drowning, which affects all ages, sizes, and ability levels, spinal injuries most often affect a certain group of swimmers. Although some females suffer severe spinal trauma, headfirst victims are more often male. Male victims of spinal injury are usually between 5' 7" and 6' tall and weigh between 145 and 185 lbs.[3] This group is at risk because they tend to be athletic and strike the bottom with great force. The victims are usually between 18 and 31 years of age and are generally athletic. Youths under the age of 13 years rarely suffer from severe headfirst accidents because they do not possess sufficient size and weight to strike the bottom forcefully enough to damage the spinal cord. Headfirst victims often injure themselves on their first entry during their first visit to the pool. When these accidents occur, supervision, "No Diving" signs, and warnings are usually missing, and the depth of water is less than 5 feet. Often when a severe spinal injury occurs, the water has poor visibility and the bottom lacks markings, making depth perception difficult. Many head-first accidents occur in the late evening or early morning hours during a pool party where alcohol is consumed.[4] Before discussing the types of pools and equipment most likely to be involved in spinal injuries, the safe diving envelope should first be discussed.

The Safe Diving Envelope

According to the American Red Cross, the **safe diving envelope** is the underwater area of a swimming pool into which a "diver" can enter headfirst safely without touching the sides, slope, or bottom. A depth of 9 feet should be encouraged whenever headfirst entries are allowed from a pool deck, unfortunately many pools allow headfirst entries in only 5 feet of water. Swimming pool staff and signage must encourage patrons to enter headfirst into deep water only and to use feet-first entries for shallow water. Underwater ledges, steps, and other obstructions must not be found in the diving envelope.

When a diving board is available, the safe diving depth must be present not only directly under the end of the board (plummet) but also in front of board and on either the side of the diving board. This text suggests a minimum diving depth of 11 feet, but between 12 and 12.5 feet is strongly preferred for 1-meter (low) competitive diving boards.. Deep, flat-bottom, constant-depth areas are safest for diving activities, but unfortunately these pools are not as common. Some pools that have diving boards are of the **hopper-bottom** or **spoon-shaped** variety. Although there may be sufficient depth for diving directly under the tip of the board, too often the shape of the pool bottom and sides does not allow for safe diving forward or to the sides of the plummet. The chance of hitting the upslope or sides of the pool is increased when diving into a hopper-bottom or spoon-shaped pool. In both types of pools, the bottom angles or slopes up sharply on all four sides from the deepest point to the breakpoint for shallow water[5] (see Fig. 1-6).

Unskilled, impromptu "dives" by untrained individuals into a spoon or hopper-bottom pool can be risky. The depth posted often refers to the plummet depth only. Some recreational "divers" travel forward rather than upward when attempting a dive. Conversely, competitive divers tend to achieve more height than distance from the board. Therefore a recreational "diver" diving into this facility may strike the upslope, which is significantly more shallow than the posted depth. Hopper-bottom and spoon-shaped bottoms are found in residential pools, hotel and motel pools, and even some older (more than 20 years) larger public pools.

Many residential and hotel and motel pools do not have sufficient size and depth to allow diving boards. Before a diving board is placed in a spoon-shaped or bottom-hopper pool, all conditions must be considered when evaluating whether a diver may hit the bottom. If there is any chance of a diver hitting the bottom or slopes from a diving board, diving equip-

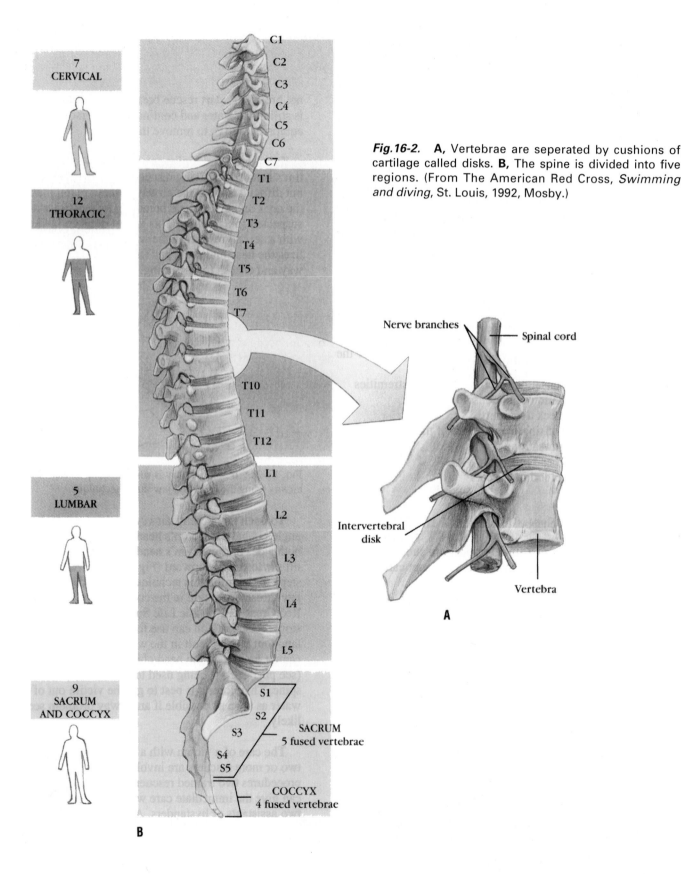

7 CERVICAL

12 THORACIC

5 LUMBAR

9 SACRUM AND COCCYX

C1
C2
C3
C4
C5
C6
C7
T1
T2
T3
T4
T5
T6
T7
T10
T11
T12
L1
L2
L3
L4
L5
S1
S2
S3
S4
S5

SACRUM
5 fused vertebrae

COCCYX
4 fused vertebrae

B

Fig.16-2. **A,** Vertebrae are seperated by cushions of cartilage called disks. **B,** The spine is divided into five regions. (From The American Red Cross, *Swimming and diving*, St. Louis, 1992, Mosby.)

Nerve branches

Spinal cord

Intervertebral disk

Vertebra

A

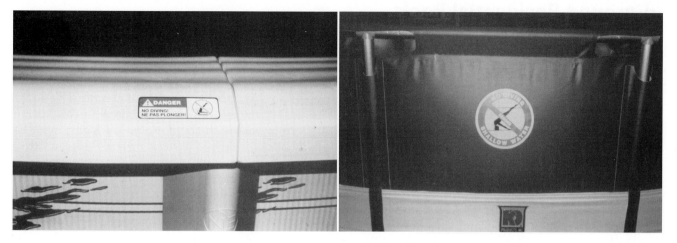

Fig. 16-3. "No Diving" signs on above-ground pools.

ment should be prohibited. When a diving board already exists in such a pool where depths and distances are marginal, a policy to consider may be to allow only children under the age of 12 to use the boards with direct supervision. But some consider diving boards to be an attractive nuisance for *all* age groups, so a lawyer should be consulted before establishing this policy. Also, the diving board must be low to the water and short and stiff. This rigid board is less likely to propel the diver as far out into the pool as longer, higher, or more flexible boards. In this case, a safe diving envelope would exist for children but not adults. If adults cannot be prevented from using the board in this case, even when they are trespassing, the diving board should be removed. These considerations *do not* guarantee headfirst injuries will not occur.

The National Spa and Pool Institute (NSPI), unlike some water safety experts and organizations that focus primarily on depth or profile of the pool, has published comprehensive residential swimming pool standards. The NSPI believes that no pool should be used for diving unless it meets all requirements of its standard, and even then, only well-executed, supervised dives in a forward direction be performed. The NSPI also recommends that only those participants who know how to "steer-up" safely be permitted to dive into the pool to avoid hitting the bottom. The terms *hopper bottom* or *spoon shaped* are not used in NSPI standards and do not indicate whether a pool meets NSPI standards.

Above-Ground Pools

Although not true in all cases, the smaller the pool, the more the likelihood of a neck injury. Above-ground pools are smaller, temporary pools that can be removed and stored and have average depths of 4 feet. Headfirst entries must *never* be allowed in above-ground pools.

Depths in an above-ground pool range from $3\frac{1}{2}$ to $4\frac{1}{2}$ feet, but the water depth in any particular above-ground pool is usually constant. The above-ground pool presents increased risks for headfirst entries not only because the water is shallow but also because in many instances headfirst entries can be performed from platforms or decks above the surface of the water. Pool ladders, decks, fences, and rooftops are all platforms from which the unwary have initiated "dives" resulting in catastrophic injury.

Above-ground pools are inexpensive and allow families to enjoy swimming in the privacy of their backyards. But when an above-ground pool is installed, every precaution must be taken to prevent any headfirst entries from taking place. Effective "No Diving" warnings must appear conspicuously on the pool itself, on the pool ladder, and anywhere else in close proximity to the pool (Fig. 16-3). Homeowners must warn all those visiting the pool that headfirst entries are strictly prohibited. Above-ground pools must never have diving boards or jump boards, and if they have a slide, only small children with supervision should use it. Adults should not use slides in an above-ground pool and all sliders must go down feet-first.

In-ground Residential Pools

Although many in-ground residential pools have diving boards, only some have a safe diving envelope into which a safe headfirst entry can be made. A 1-meter residential diving board should have sufficient depth (at least 10 feet) in any direction and must allow divers to manuever safely underwater without forcefully striking underwater surfaces. This is difficult to guarantee. Also, continuous depth in front of the board is more critical than more depth. The 10-foot NFSHSA requirement might be safe but only if this depth extends far enough forward to ensure that all divers will land in this depth. Again, many residential pools cannot safely accommodate diving from a springboard. The NSPI states that recreational diving can be safely accommodated only in a pool that meets all the requirements of its published residential swimming pool standard, depending on the classification of pool (Figs. 16-4 and 16-5).

If, however, a diving board already exists at an in-ground pool with marginal depths and distances and the decision has been made to leave it there, numerous precautions must be taken to regulate the use. Anyone older than 12 years of age should be banned from the board, and constant supervision is a must. A safety line with floats should also be installed on the surface that runs across the pool and parallel to the breakpoint line to give the diver a visual cue of where the shallow water begins. The safety line is also intended to prevent nonswimmers from entering the deep water. Depth markings, diving rules, regulations, and warnings must all be conspicuously placed around the pool and the diving board, but these alone do not guarantee diving safety.

As mentioned previously, only the shortest, lowest stiffest board should be used (10-foot length or less, 18 to 24 inches above the water). Placement of the diving board fulcrum and construction material of the board itself are also two important factors. When there is doubt about the appropriateness of diving from a springboard in a residential pool, the board should probably be removed. The precautions just mentioned do not guarantee injury prevention in pools that lack recommended diving depths and distances.

Serious neck injuries are not only caused when a diver hits a pool bottom. Several individuals have suffered paralyzing neck injuries while attempting to dive through an inner tube from a diving board in a backyard pool. Landing on other swimmers is also a serious problem. The results of these injuries are just as tragic as hitting the bottom of the pool. This illustrates that the water depth is not the only concern regarding diving boards.

Another way for adults to suffer a catastrophic neck injury is to go down a slide headfirst into the pool. This happens more than it should. The slider comes off the slide with tremendous force, causing severe impact with the bottom. The point must be emphasized that many neck injuries are caused in private and semipublic pools that try to offer "big pool" attractions in a small pool. To make matters worse, these pools often lack proper signage and supervision.

Public Pools

Many public pools offer springboard diving equipment, a safe diving envelope, and supervision. As a result, public pools should have fewer diving injuries than residential or semipublic pools. However, not all public pools have safe diving facilities.

Perhaps one of the greatest fears in a diving facility is of the patron hitting the board. Actually, springboards are quite flexible and forgiving when divers accidentally strike them. Hitting the board does happen occasionally, but this rarely results in serious injury. Hitting a springboard rarely if ever causes traumatic injuries, whereas striking the bottom of the pool or pool deck can be debilitating.

To prevent hitting the bottom during diving and other headfirst entries, children must be taught the concept of steering up to the surface after entering the water. Steering up to the surface is an important diving skill that should be emphasized in all water safety and learn-to-swim programs (Fig. 16-6).

Public pools should adhere to the standards of the one of several competitive diving organizations. The NCAA, Federation Internationale de Natation Amateur (FINA), U.S. Diving, or NFSHSA all provide recommended dimensions for safe springboard diving. The National YMCAs and the American Red Cross also offer instruction in safe diving techniques. Serious diving accidents have never occurred in facilities sanctioned by the competitive diving organizations listed above.

Public pools usually offer 1-meter springboards (low diving boards) and/or 3-meter diving boards (high diving boards). Although some pools have higher diving platforms (5, 7.5, and 10 meters), these are often closed to the public. If these platforms are

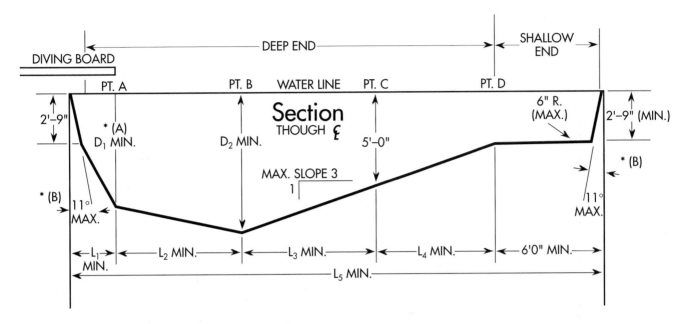

*IMPORTANT—A. MINIMUM DEPTH UNDER DIVING BOARD OR JUMP BOARD
B. TYPE I POOLS SHALL HAVE PLUMB WALLS AS SHOWN IN ARTICLE 3.6.5

POOL TYPE	MINIMUM DIMENSIONS							MINIMUM WIDTH OF POOL		
	D_1	D_2	L_1*	L_2	L_3	L_4	L_5	PT. A	PT. B	PT. C
0	See 3.5.5, 3.5.6		DIVING EQUIPMENT IS PROHIBITED							
I	6'-0"	7'-6"	1'-6"	7'-0"	7'-6"	6'-9"	28'-9"	10'-0"	12'-0"	10'-0"
II	6'-0"	7'-6"	1'-6"	7'-0"	7'-6"	6'-9"	28'-9"	12'-0"	15'-0"	12'-0"
III	6'-10"	8'-0"	2'-0"	7'-6"	9'-0"	6'-9"	31'-3"	12'-0"	15'-0"	12'-0"
IV	7'-8"	8'-6"	2'-6"	8'-0"	10'-6"	6'-9"	33'-9"	15'-0"	18'-0"	15'-0"
V	8'-6"	9'-0"	3'-0"	9'-0"	12'-0"	6'-9"	36'-9"	15'-0"	18'-0"	15'-0"

*See 3.5.2

Fig. 16-4. Reference chart of minimum deminsions for residential pools with manufactured diving equipment. The diagram shown is only a part of a complete, published standard for the type of pools indicated. It should not be used without reference to the entire published standard. The standard itself may be ordered from the National Spa and Pool Institute, 2111 Eisenhower Ave, Alexandria, Va 22314. (From NSPI-5: *Standard for residential swimming pools*, Alexandria, Va, 1987, The Institute.)

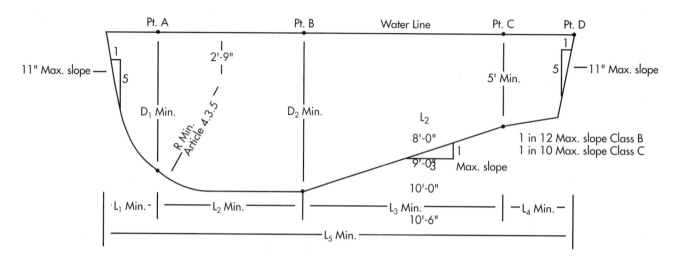

NOTE: L4 is a demension to allow sufficient length opposite the board. This may of coarse be lengthened to form the shallow portion of the pool.

POOL TYPE	RELATED DIVING EQUIPMENT		MINIMUM DEMINSIONS								MINIMUM WIDTH OF POOL AT:		
	MAX. DIVING BOARD LENGTH	MAX. BOARD HEIGHT OVER WATER	D_1	D_2	R	L_1		L_3	L_4	L_5	PT.A	PT.B	PT.C
VI	10'	26" (2/3 meter)	7'-0"	8'-6"	5'-6"	2'-6"		10'-6"	7'-0"	28'-0"	16'-0"	18'-0"	18'-0"
VII	12'	30" (3/4 meter)	7'-6"	9'-0"	6'-0"	3'-0"		12'-0"	4'-0"	28'-0"	18'-0"	20'-0"	20'-0"
VIII	16'	1 Meter	8'-6"	10'-0"	7'-0"	4'-0"		15'-0"	2'-0"	31'-0"	20'-0"	22'-0"	22'-0"
IX	16'	3 Meter	11'-0"	12'-0"	8'-0"	6'-0"		21'-0"	0	37'-6"	22'-0"	24'-0"	24'-0"

L_2, L_3 and L_4 combined represent the minimum distance from the tip of board to pool wall opposite diving equipment.

For board heights exceeding 3 meters 3 meters see Articles 4.5.2.

*NOTE: Placement of boards shall observe the following minimum deminsions. With multiple board installations minimum pool widths must be increased accordingly.

Deck Level Board to Pool Side	8'
1 Meter Board to Pool Side	10'
3 Meter Board to Pool Side	11'
1 Meter or Deck Level Board to 3 meter Board	10'
1 Meter or Deck Level Board to another 1 Meter or Deck Level Board	8'

Fig. 16-5. NSPI minimum demensions for diving in class B and C pools, public and semi-public pools. The diagram shown is only a part of a complete, published standard. It should not be used without reference to the entire published standard. The standard itself may be ordered from the National Spa and Pool Institute, 2111 Eisenhower Av, Alexandria, Va 22314 (From NSPI-5: *Standard for residential swimming pools*, Alexandria, Va, 1987, The Institute.)

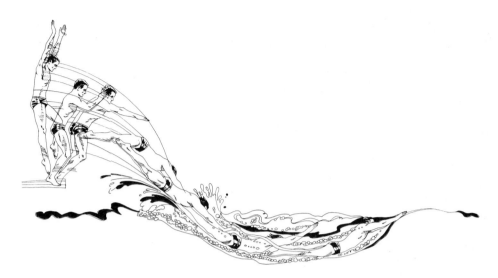

Fig. 16-6.   Steering up. (From NSPI: *The sensible way to enjoy your inground swimming pool*, Alexandria, Va, 1993, The Institute.)

open to the public, similar yet more stringent safety rules apply. The pool dimensions required for 1- and 3-meter diving boards are described. Although diving organizations provide a great deal of information on required depth and distances, the following information summarizes the most important figures:

Depth of water at plummet

1-meter board: minimum 11 feet, 12 to 12½ feet preferred

3-meter board: minimum 12½ feet, 13 feet preferred

Distance to the upslope 16½ feet to 20 feet

Distance to side wall

1-meter board: 8 feet

3-meter board: 10 feet

Pools with diving areas must display the rules on or near the diving equipment. Posting the rules alone is not sufficient; they must be strictly enforced. Typical rules include the following:

- Use handrails when climbing the stairs and while walking on the board.
- Only one diver is allowed on the diving board at a time.
- Only one bounce on the end of the board is allowed.

- Be certain the area is clear before diving or jumping.
- Dive or jump directly ahead.
- After each entry, exit quickly to the nearest ladder.
- Do not attempt new dives or tricks unless under the direct supervision of a teacher or coach.
- The hands must enter the water first on all headfirst dives.

When diving facilities are in use at a pool, a lifeguard should be specifically stationed there to manage the activity. In addition to enforcing all diving regulations, safety equipment for treatment of spinal injuries must be kept by the diving area. This includes a spine board, straps, and cervical collars. Lifeguards must also observe all diving rules when they are diving. All diving equipment, including the boards and the stands, should be checked daily. Diving boards should be used only when the proper facility dimensions are available.

Starting Platforms

Another area of potential for spinal injuries is the starting blocks or platforms. Both competitive and recreational swimmers have sustained traumatic neck

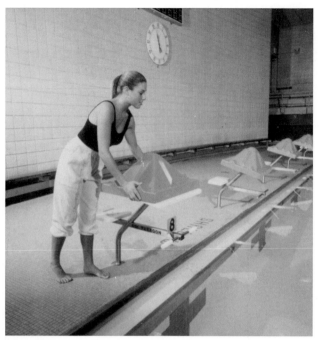

Fig. 16-7.   Starting platforms safety covers. (Courtesy KDI Paragon, Pleasantville, NY.)

injuries while performing racing starts from starting platforms. One explanation for the neck injuries to the competitive swimmers is the increased popularity of the pike or scoop racing dive that carries the swimmer deeper into the water. Poor teaching progression and unsupervised racing starts can also be blamed for these mishaps.

Every attempt should be made to locate starting blocks where there is a least 5 feet of water available, and 6 feet is now preferred by many. Most competitive swimming organizations require a minimum of 4 feet. Deeper water is preferred. When not in use by team members, diving platforms should either be removed or covered so that they cannot be used (Fig. 16-7). Signs warning swimmers of the danger associated with diving from these blocks should also be posted.

Signage

Proper signage is particularly important when attempting to safeguard patrons from injuring themselves by entering shallow water headfirst. Perhaps the most attention should be given to the shallow (less than 5 feet) areas of the pool. But patrons must also be warned of attempting headfirst entries in water depths between 6 and 9 feet. A variety of signs and warnings are available, but it is best to warn all patrons of dangerous diving areas as they enter the facility. This may be best accomplished be creating and illustrating no diving zones in the swimming pool. As guests enter the pool, graphics or statements should alert them as to where they can and cannot enter headfirst.

Signs and warnings must then be conspicuously placed around the facility so that patrons are sufficiently warned. "No Diving" signs and depth markers should be placed on the pool deck and on the pool wall just above the water line. Additional signs are needed on pool walls and fences. A new trend is to paint a stripe around the pool deck delineating the no diving zone. "No Diving" ceramic tiles are all available in letters as well as graphics. Graphic no diving signs may be more effective in multicultural, bilingual localities. Although "No Diving" signs should be used at pools, a totally effective diving warning has not been developed.

Summary

To prevent serious neck injuries at swimming pools, patrons must be warned of the serious consequences resulting from entering shallow water headfirst. This can be accomplished through effective signage and supervision. Water less than 5 feet deep must be particularly guarded from headfirst entries, but depths between 5 and 9 feet should also contain warnings. Special precautions must be taken to prevent headfirst entries at parties, in the evening, and when alcohol is served. Whenever possible, individuals should be encouraged to jump rather than dive, particularly the first time they enter a facility. Steering up to the surface immediately following each headfirst entire is a skill that must also be mastered.

Although most aquatic organizations concur that competitive diving should have a minimum depth of 11 feet and preferrably 121/2 feet, agreement is lacking on a safe diving depth for noncompetitive, recreational diving. The NSPI has published a suggested minimum standard for residential swimming pools since 1958. It has comprehensive design, dimensional, and safety requirements that NSPI says should be met for a noncompetitive diving board to be installed. Some water safety experts disagree with some of the minimum requirements in the NSPI standards and suggest that diving pools be deeper and longer than the minimum standards require.

Whenever pool patrons enter the water headfirst, they take a risk. All pool professionals must be aware of the risks associated with diving and other headfirst entries and develop a comprehensive plan to safeguard these individuals without eliminating the sport of springboard diving.

References

1. National Spinal Cord Injury Center, University of Alabama.
2. American Red Cross: *Lifeguarding*, Washington, DC, 1990, The Red Cross.
3. Wingfield JV: Ball State University, Muncie Ind, Jan 1993, personal communication.
4. Gabrielsen AM: *Diving injuries: a critical insight and recommendations*, Indianapolis, 1984, Council of the National Cooperation in Aquatics.
5. The American Red Cross: *Swimming and diving*, St Louis, 1992, Mosby.

Bibliography

The American Red Cross: *Swimming and diving*, St Louis, 1992, Mosby.
Gabriel J: *Diving safety: a position paper*, Indianapolis, 1992, US Diving.
Gabrielson AM: *Diving injuries: a critical insight and recommendations*, Indianapolis, 1984, Council fo the National Cooperation in Aquatics.
Gabrielson AM: *Swimming pools: a guide to their planning, design, and operation*, ed 4, Champaign, Ill, 1987, Human Kinetics.
Karmol D: The National Spa and Pool Institute, Sept 29 and 30, 1993, personal communication.
True S: The National Federations of High School Athletic Associations, Jan 26, 1993, personal communication.

Review Questions

1. Approximately what percent of all sport-related spinal injuries are the result of entering headfirst into shallow water?
2. What percent of all headfirst injuries occur in less than 5 feet of water?
3. Permanent paralysis often results from shallow water diving accidents caused by trauma to what specific body part?
4. Describe the type of person most likely to suffer a traumatic injury by entering headfirst into shallow water.
5. Briefly explain the safe diving envelope.
6. Headfirst entries must be completely prohibited in which type of pool?
7. At which end of the pool should the competitive starting blocks be located?

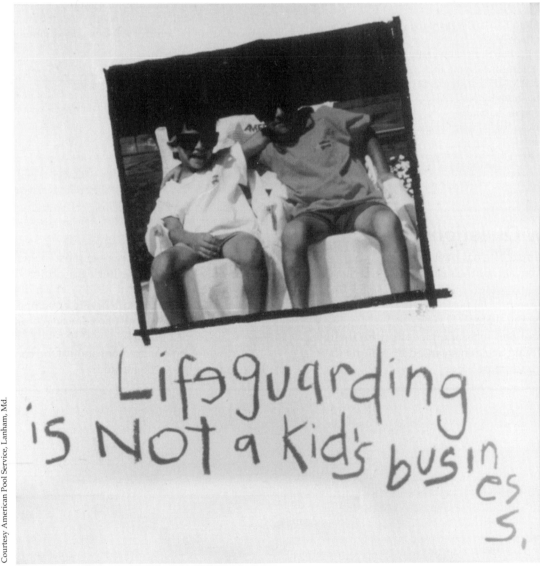

Lifeguarding is Not a kid's business.

17

PREVENTIVE LIFEGUARDING

In the early 1900s Commodore Wilbert E. Longfellow, concerned with the high number of drownings in the United States, began an aggressive crusade of water rescue and safety around the country. In 1910, he became the Commander in Chief of the U.S. Lifesaving Corps and established the nationwide American Red Cross Lifesaving Corps in 1914. The Commodore personally trained thousands of lifeguards and instructors throughout the country and convinced owners and operators of pools and beaches to staff their facility with his well-trained professionals. Largely through his efforts, the drowning rate in the United States began to drop dramatically.

In 1914 the drowning rate was 10.4 deaths per 100,000 participants. By 1947, this number was halved to 5.2 per 100,000 participants. By 1990, the drowning rate had been reduced to 1.9 per 100,000. This drastic reduction in drowning deaths is attributed to the "Commander" and the American Red Cross swimming and water safety courses that have been so popular in this country.[1] The YMCA of the United States has also had a rich and successful tradition of water safety and lifeguarding programs. The box shows a summary developed by the YMCA of aquatic safety developments.

Of all the drownings that do occur in the United States, less than 10% occur in guarded pools. But this number can also be drastically reduced by improving the training and supervision of lifeguards. This chapter is devoted to preventive lifeguarding techniques rather than water rescue techniques and procedures. In addition, this chapter concentrates on swimming pool guards rather than surf or beach lifeguards although concepts introduced here apply to both. Proper lifeguarding attitudes and philosophies are examined instead of specific training techniques and skills. The American Red Cross, the National YMCAs, and the National Recreation and Park Association (Ellis and Associates) have excellent books and courses available for the training of lifeguards. This chapter is intended as a supplement to those training texts and courses. Local lifeguarding requirements are available through the regulatory agencies in charge of pools in specific areas.

Lifeguarding: A Paradoxical Profession

Lifeguarding is a peculiar profession. Although much is required of lifeguards, for the most part they are underpaid and overworked. To be a lifeguard requires special training: first-aid certification, cardiopulmonary resuscitation (CPR) certification, and lifeguarding certification are usually minimal

---

Aquatic Safety Development

Royal Humane Society (1774)
Massachusetts Humane Society (1786)
U.S. Coast Guard Lifesaving Service (1871)
YMCA entrance into teaching (1885-1890)
Lifesaving Program, Springfield College (1911)
National YMCA Lifesaving Service (1912)
First American lifesaving text (1913)
Red Cross lifesaving training (1914)
YMCA Lifesaving & Swimming Manual (1929)
Cureton-Silvia test text (1939)
YMCA Lifesaving & Water Safety Instructor's Text (1940)
Silvia's *YMCA Lifesaving & Water Safety Today* (1965)
New YMCA Aquatic Safety & Lifesaving Text (1974)
YMCA Aquatic Safety & Lifesaving Program (1979)
On the Guard: YMCA Lifeguard Manual (1986)

---

requirements before potential lifeguards are even considered for employment. Rigorous skill tests and on-the-job training often begin once a lifeguard is hired. Most aquatic professionals agree that today's lifeguards are highly trained emergency care professionals, not babysitters. Lifeguarding has many responsibilities associated with it, although financial rewards are not great. Swimming pool lifeguards, possessing three certifications and being responsible for protecting and saving lives, often make less money than their peers working in fast food restaurants.

Compounding this situation is the fact that many lifeguards, although highly trained and extremely competent in water rescues, are distracted from watching swimmers in the water. One study of beach lifeguards found that lifeguards focused on swimmers only 51% of the time while on duty. Nearly half of the time on duty, the lifeguards in this study were found looking *away* from their areas of responsibility.[2] For the most part, lifeguarding is boring and tedious. Bored lifeguards often become mesmerized with one person or object in or out of the pool and ignore everyone else. This type of tunnel vision in lifeguards is not acceptable and jeopardizes safety of the pool patrons. Systematic scanning is just one of the defensive lifeguarding techniques that must be mastered to be an effective guard. Lifeguards must be trained to expect the unexpected and to make every attempt to prevent accidents instead of making rescues.

Lifeguard training in the past emphasized swimming rescues and water skills. In fact, over the years, even the names of the Red Cross courses have changed dramatically. The "Junior and Senior Lifesaving" course became the "Advanced Lifesaving" course which was eventually transformed into "Lifeguarding". Although today's lifeguards receive extensive training in the water, the emphasis is placed on water safety awareness and accident prevention. Before the 1970s it was felt that the lifeguards with the most rescues were the most competent. Today the trend has reversed. Many experts believe that those with the fewest rescues are the most vigilant in their supervision of swimmers.

The YMCA provides an excellent explanation describing the difference between lifesavers and lifeguards. They claim that although the words *lifesavers* and *lifeguards* share the same prefix, the areas of responsibility they share are quite dissimilar. A lifesaver is an amateur who stumbles on an aquatic emergency and accidentally becomes involved in the water rescue. Conversely, lifeguards are trained professionals who have accepted the responsibility of protecting swimmers at a specified place and time. Lifeguards have a moral, professional, and legal responsibility to prevent accidents by enforcing rules and regulations of the aquatic facility and to respond correctly to aquatic emergencies should they occur. Further, the box shows comparisons from the YMCA that distinguish lifesaving from lifeguarding.

The RID Factor

Frank Pia studied his films of hundreds of near-drowning victims at Orchard Beach on Long Island Sound to help develop the RID theory of unwitnessed drownings. He contends that unwitnessed drownings are caused by one or more of the following three factors:

Recognition

Pia claims that many drownings go unnoticed because lifeguards' perception of how a drowning victim acts on the surface is significantly different from what actually takes place. Victims hardly struggle. The arm stroke is similar to the breast stroke and may actually resemble play in the water. They cannot cry out for help because all their effort is spent on breathing in. The total "struggle" may last between 20 and 60 seconds.

Lifesaving versus Lifeguarding	
Lifesaver	*Lifeguard*
Reacts to an accident, acting after the fact	Acts to first prevent the accident, does react to emergency
Reacts from a moral principle only	Acts under a moral and legal duty
May be covered by the Good Samaritan Laws	Can be found liable and negligent in a court
Does not need certification	Must be certified by an accredited agency as required by law in some states or qualified and trained by an individual in that facility or setting
Has general training and is an amateur	Is a professional with specific training for specific locations, with specific procedures for emergencies
Usually has no special equipment available	Has specific rescue equipment for that aquatic setting

Despite these facts, many lifeguards expect troubled swimmers to display a frantic fight on the surface with plenty of splashing, "white water," and cries for help. True drowning takes place quickly and quietly. Films are available that can clearly illustrate to lifeguards how a truly distressed swimmer acts in the water. Knowing this, lifeguards are better able to detect swimmers in trouble.

Intrusion

Many lifeguards are not able to watch those in the water carefully because they are asked to perform additional tasks unrelated to preventive lifeguarding. This is particularly common at swimming pools. Their eyes are diverted because maintenance tasks such as water testing, backwashing, and deck cleaning are performed while lifeguards are on duty. If lifeguards are expected to safeguard those in the water, they cannot be given tasks that divert their attention away from these swimmers. Pool management often compromises good preventive lifeguarding by asking too much of the lifeguard unrelated to water safety.

Distraction

Perhaps more than any other factor, distractions play a major role in producing poor preventive lifeguarding. Boredom sets in easily for most guards and when this occurs, attention tends to drift away from the swimmers in the water. Socializing, horseplaying with peers, and just goofing off can occur in an attempt to cope with boredom. Lifeguards simply cannot afford to be distracted. To prevent distractions, lifeguards must use systematic scanning techniques to ensure that all patrons are being monitored. Lifeguards must also be supervised while on duty to be certain that they are scanning. Finally, all guards must adhere to the 10/20 rule.[3]

The 10/20 Rule

The 10/20 rule dictates that every lifeguard on duty must be able to detect a swimmer in distress within 10 seconds and make contact with the victim in the next 20 seconds.[4] To apply the 10/20 rule, lifeguards must be vigilant in their supervision, lifeguard stations must be appropriately placed for proper coverage, and lifeguards must be monitored continually to be certain that they are watching those in and around the water. Lifeguards must also receive instructions concerning which are the most hazardous areas within the swimming pool complex and which patrons are high-risk swimmers.

Systematic Scanning

To be effective in preventing accidents, lifeguards must develop systematic scanning techniques. Regardless of what scanning technique is chosen, each patron within the lifeguard's area of responsibility should be checked every 10 seconds. Many good lifeguards use individualized techniques they have personally developed.

Many lifeguards use a **circular scanning pattern** that requires them to visually scan the perimeter of their area of responsibility, and as the circle is completed, another smaller circle is begun inside the pool. These concentric circles keep decreasing in size until the center of the pool is reached. The circular scanning pattern is then reversed so that the circles become larger and move toward the perimeter where the scan began (Fig. 17-1).

Another scanning technique similar to circular

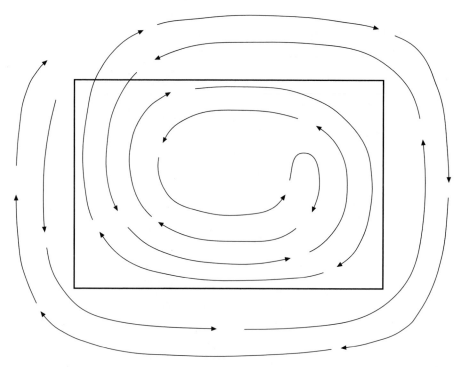

Fig. 17-1.   Circular scanning technique.

scanning calls for the **monitoring of hazardous areas** in an order of priority from most hazardous to least hazardous. The lifeguards prioritize the most dangerous facilities or equipment in their zone and then scan each item and the people around it before checking on the next area. For instance, a lifeguard may check the diving boards first, the pool decks second, the ladders third, under the lifeguard chairs fourth, and the lap swimming lanes last.

People watching is another technique whereby the lifeguards check all children first, senior citizens next, young adults next, and so on. Lifeguards should of course check on the high-risk patrons first. A helpful way of keeping track of all swimmers in a particular zone for the lifeguard is to periodically guess the number of patrons and then count them individually.

Preventive lifeguarding techniques require lifeguards to scan their areas of responsibility systematically so that boredom and distractions will not divert their attention. Lifeguards should be trained in scanning techniques, and they must also be monitored while on duty.

High-Risk Guests

Each facility should determine which patrons are high-risk guests. Once these individuals or groups are determined, the lifeguard must be made aware of these findings and then taught how to best safeguard these individuals. For example, a study conducted by Ellis and Associates determined the following groups to be at greater risk when they visited water-parks:

1. Children between the ages of 7 and 12 years of age
2. Minorities (Black, Hispanic, Asian, and others)
3. Parents with small children
4. Intoxicated guests
5. Overweight guests
6. Guests wearing personal flotation devices

Ellis and Associates also found the leading cause of accidents at water parks to be the following[6]:

1. Running
2. Collisions with equipment or others
3. Diving into shallow water
4. Heat exhaustion/stroke
5. Heart attacks

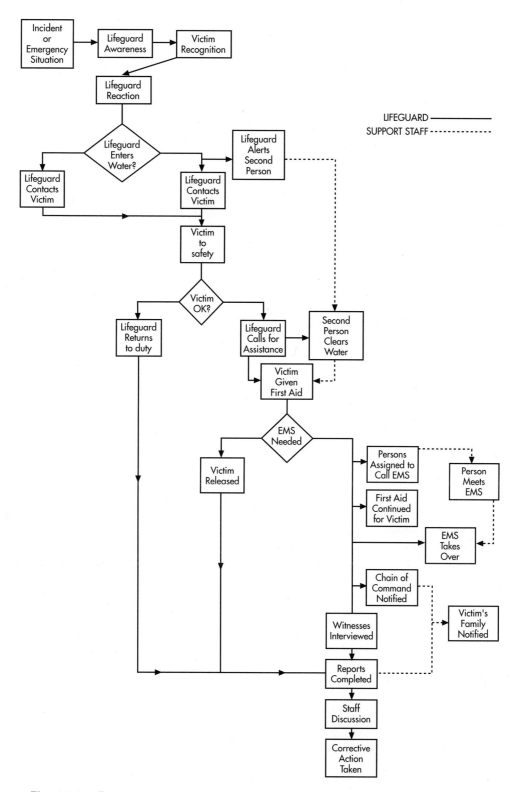

Fig. 17-2. Emergency action plan flowchart—single-lifeguard facility. (From American Red Cross: *Lifeguarding*, Washington, DC, 1990.)

Responding to Emergencies

Too often when lifeguards must respond to an emergency, they either do not respond properly or they injure themselves in the process. This happens because either the lifeguard panics or reacts quickly without thinking about what options are available. **Emergency action plans** must be established at every pool. Depending on the design of the pool and other factors such as proximity of the **emergency medical systems**, emergency action plans may vary. Lifeguards must know, understand, and practice the facility emergency action plan (Fig. 17-2).

When an aquatic emergency does arise, lifeguards must be trained to resist the temptation of overreacting by responding *too* quickly. Lifeguards are usually talented and gifted athletes. Quick reactions are a part of their training and within their capabilities. But too many react emotionally to a crisis and act before thinking. Every lifeguard should be trained to stop and think the situation through clearly before taking action. Reacting hurriedly to an emergency often leads to an inefficient rescue attempt or an injury.

Once an emergency is spotted, a predetermined emergency signal should be used to initiate the emergency action plan, but the first responder should stop and think clearly before taking action. If this process is followed, more lives would be saved and fewer injuries would occur to lifeguards.

Evaluating Lifeguards

One of the most significant contributions of Ellis and Associates to the lifeguarding profession is lifeguarding audits. Ellis and Associates trains, certifies, and supervises their lifeguards, most of whom work at water-parks. This lifeguard-training agency uses unannounced lifeguarding audits to spot-check facilities and guards. Audits not only check to see that lifeguards are doing what they are supposed to be doing on duty but also evaluate the guards on surprise, simulated emergency situations. Lifeguard audits and facility inspections are a portion of a total risk-management program[7].

Any pool can carry out its own lifeguard audit. This can be accomplished quite simply. A colored ball can be subtly placed into the water to determine how long it will take the lifeguard on duty to spot it or it may be helpful to record the lifeguard's behavior while on duty for objective data that can be used to constructively criticize the guard. Another supervisory technique is to record the amount of time spent looking *away* from the area of observation. Some pools make the use of a problem/incentive log that not only records lifeguard and facility deficiencies but also allows the supervisor to praise the lifeguard for a job well done (Fig. 17-3).

P.J. Heath recommends developing data-based evaluation methods at swimming pools so that lifeguard evaluations can be made accurately, consistently, and reliably. Too often, lifeguard supervisors criticize their staff in vague, opinionated, and emotional terms. Heath urges lifeguard supervisors to use coding sheets that analyze **on-task** and **off-task behaviors**. Off-task behaviors include such activities as social talking, nonattentive behavior, and insufficient scanning. By calculating the percentage of time spent on-task and off-task, the lifeguard can be easily rated. (See Fig. 17-4 and 17-5 for examples of Heath's coding sheets and summary reports[8].)

Job Description

Every lifeguard needs a job description to outline specific duties and responsibilities. Without a job description, confusion usually surrounds the pool employees. Lifeguards should be responsible for water safety and accident prevention *only* at the pool. If given other tasks, lifeguards must accomplish them when not stationed on duty. Whenever possible, personnel other than certified lifeguards should be assigned pool operation and maintenance tasks. Job expectations must be spelled out clearly in the job description. Behaviors that are not acceptable should also be highlighted in the job description. The chain of command is also very important and should be illustrated in the job description. A trend with some pool service companies is to have each lifeguard sign and date a lifeguard pledge, which can be customized for each pool (Fig. 17-6).

Rules and Regulations

Lifeguards must know, understand, and enforce all rules and regulations adopted by the pool. These rules should be posted conspicuously at the pool and passed out to the patrons if at all possible. When someone violates a swimming pool rule, the rule should be pointed out and the rationale for obeying the rule should be explained to the violator. Yelling

PROBLEM / INCENTIVE LOG

DAY; M T W T F S S	DATE:
POOL:	CODE:

POOL OPENED LATE	LIST TIME:
GUARD ARRIVED LATE	LIST TIME:
POOL CLOSED EARLY	LIST TIME:
HEALTH INSPECTION	PASS OR FAIL
GUARD NOT IN CHAIR/WATCHING POOL	
GUARD NOT IN UNIFORM	
FAIR OR POOR ON FIELD REPORT	
FAIR OR POOR ON EVALUATION	MIDSEASON END
FAILURE TO OBTAIN SUB FOR TIME OFF	
ASSISTED STAFFING	
OTHER / COMMENTS:	
EMP#:	NAME
EMP#:	NAME
EMP#:	NAME:
EMP#:	NAME:
COMPLETED BY:	ENTERED By:

Fig. 17-3. Lifeguard problem/incentive log. (Courtesy American Pool Service, Lanham, Md.)

SUMMARY REPORT

Employee: ___Dan Stevens_____ Location: ___WOSSC_____
Date: ___8-3-87_____ Position: ___P-3_____
Time Started: ___1:36____ Ended: ___1:48_____ Evaluator: ___PJH_____

Time/Task Analysis Results of Employee Behavior

Total Time ON-TASK	6:20-380 SEC	Comments:
Scanning Time	4:20-260 SEC	
Rescue Time	0:00	Total Time -
Discipline Time	1:10-70 SEC	8 - MIN
Managerial Time	:50-50 SEC	480 - SEC
Percent of Time ON-TASK	79 %	
Scanning Time	54 %	
Rescue Time	0 %	
Discipline Time	14 %	
Managerial Time	10 %	
Total Time OFF-TASK	1:10-100 SEC	Comments
Talking Time	:50-50 SEC	
Non-Attentive	:30-30 SEC	
Off Ready Position	0:00	
Poor Vantage Point	0:00	
Inappropriate Behavior	:20-20 SEC	
Percent of Time OFF-TASK	21 %	
Talking Time	10 %	
Non-Attentive	6 %	
Off Ready Position	0 %	
Poor Vantage Point	0 %	
Inappropriate Behavior	4 %	

ON-TASK - 79%
OFF-TASK - 21%

Fig. 17-4. Lifeguard summary report. (Courtesy P.J. Heath.)

and screaming at misbehaving patrons is often counterproductive. It must be remembered that rules and regulations are established to safeguard the swimmers by preventing accidents. Ignoring pool rules, either on the part of the swimmer or lifeguard, can lead to accidents.

Lifeguard Stations

Most states require lifeguards on duty to be in elevated lifeguard chairs. Ironically, numerous accidents are caused by the lifeguard getting in or out of the lifeguard stand, particularly during a crisis.

Some states require that a lifeguard be stationed "at pool side." Lifeguards and pool operators must be aware of the local ordinances concerning the lifeguarding requirement and the placement of these individuals. Lifeguard stations should be fully equipped with the recommended rescue and communication equipment. Although the required equipment varies with each state, the minimum equipment expected for a lifeguard would probably be the following:

1. A rescue tube or can (depending on which type is preferred)
2. A long, light reaching pole or shepherd's crook
3. A ring buoy with throwing line attached
4. Whistle and bullhorn

Lifeguards should be cautioned about the causes, symptoms, treatment, and prevention of heat stress and skin cancer. The lifeguard station is an ideal place to provide protection from the sun, including shade and cold water. Equipment to protect lifeguards from the hazards of bloodborne pathogens such as human immunodeficiency virus, hepatitis, and others as specified by the Occupational Safety and Health Association should also be accessible at the lifeguard stations. Some lifeguards carry protective equipment (pocket masks, shields, latex gloves)

LIFEGUARD EVALUATION CODING SHEET

LB	S	S	S	S	(NA)	(NA)	S	S	D	D	S	S	3 MIN.
PC	F/M/LO												

LB	S	S	D	D	S	S	(T)	(T)	(T)	(T)	(T)	(NA)	3 MIN.
PC	F/M/M												

LB	(IB)	(IB)	S	S	S	S	S	D	D	D	M	M	3 MIN.
PC	F/M/LO												

LB	M	S	S	S	S	S	S	S	S	S	M	M	3 MIN.
PC	F/M/LO												

POOL CLIMATE

Patron Load
Heavy (H)
Fair (F)
Light (L)

Type of Activity
Organized Play (OP)
Lap Swim (LS)
Free Play (FP)
Mixed (M)

Level of Activity
High (HI)
Medium (M)
Low (LO)

LIFEGUARD BEHAVIOR

On-Task Behaviors
Scanning (S)
Rescue (R)
Discipline (D)
Managerial (M)

Off-Task Behaviors
Talking (T)
Non-Attentive (NA)
Poor Vantage Point (PP)
Off Ready Position (RP)
Inappropriate Behavior (IB)

Fig. 17-5. Lifeguard evaluation coding sheet. (Courtesy P.J. Heath.)

in fanny packs so that they are never without this vital protection. Walking or standing at poolside, although not without drawbacks, is often an effective lifeguard station (Fig. 17-7).

Lifeguard Communications

There are many forms of communication for lifeguards. Clear communication becomes especially important during an aquatic emergency. Some forms of communications include the following:

- Whistles
- Flags
- Hand signals
- Bullhorns
- Telephones
- Walkie-talkies
- Other electronic devices

Regardless of what form of communication is selected for lifeguards, the language to be used for discipline and aquatic emergencies must be fully understood by lifeguards and patrons. Signals and their meanings should be posted near the entrance of the pool or the lifeguard stations.

Uniforms

Lifeguard uniforms are important not only to gain the attention and respect of the pool patrons but also to protect guards from the elements. Regardless of what type of apparel is chosen for the employee, "Lifeguard" should appear boldly on the front and back. Brightly colored lifeguard shirts, shorts, and hats are common at pools and beaches (Fig. 17-8). Pool managers and supervisors would be more successful getting their staff to wear uniforms if the staff

Today's Date_/_/_

"AS A PENN STATE LIFEGUARD AT THE McCOY NATA-
TORIUM INDOOR POOL, OUTDOOR POOL OR WHITE
BUILDING POOL, I WILL..."

• Continually scan the water so that everyone in my zone
  is checked every 10 seconds.
• Always guard the pool from the lifeguard chair or
  stand/walk at the pool's edge. Never anywhere else.
• Never leave the pool unattended, even for as little as 5
  seconds.
• Never read, study, write or sleep on duty.
• Always know and enforce all pool rules.
• Always be currently certified in lifeguarding and CPR.
• Always wear the Penn State lifeguard uniform (no
  sneakers or sweats).
• Always be punctual. On time at Penn State means
  reporting to the pool operator 15 minutes early.
• Always follow the emergency action plan described in
  the PSU lifeguard manual.
• Always watch out for "HIGH RISK" patrons (senior citi-
  zens, children, and minorities).
• Always report problems to Tom Griffiths or the pool
  operators.
• I have read and completely understand the lifeguard
  manual.

Print Your Name: _____

Sign Your Name: _____

Fig. 17-6. The Penn State lifeguard pledge.

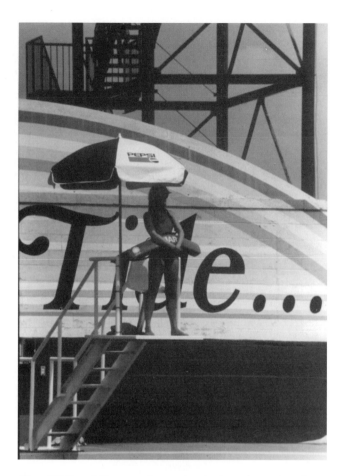

Fig. 17-7. Lifeguard: protected and protecting.
(Courtesy Water Safety Products, Melbourne Beach,
Fla.)

had input into the design and selection of the uniforms. Lifeguard hats and umbrellas should also be
supplied by the pool whenever possible. All staff
should be encouraged to wear hats and quality sunglasses that block ultraviolet rays and to apply gener-
ous amounts of sunscreen.

Motivating Lifeguards

Motivating lifeguards is often a problem because
lifeguarding is not as glamorous as many perceive
and it becomes boring and tedious rather quickly. In-
service training conducted periodically is highly recommended to prevent staffing problems and to keep
motivation high. In-service training should be
reserved not only for refining lifesaving water skills
but also for remotivating guards by rewarding the
good guards and improving communications in

weak areas. It is very important to allow the guards
to have input during in-service training and throughout the course of the season. Guards can also be beneficial in establishing policies, rules, and regulations.
As much as possible, lifeguards should be an important part of the decision making process at swimming
pools.

Lifeguard competitions are a good way of honing
swimming and rescue skills, improving camaraderie
and team spirit, and increasing fun at the workplace.
Lifeguard competitions are becoming increasingly
popular in this country.

In addition to in-service training, it is advisable to
offer continuing education whereby lifeguards can
obtain additional training beyond what they receive
at their facility. Providing release time for continuing
education and even paying for courses taken by lifeguards is very beneficial to and appreciated by lifeguards. Continuing education need not be an elabo-

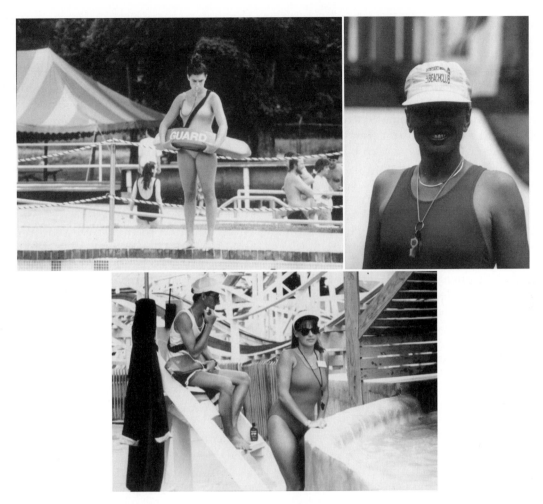

Fig. 17-8. Lifeguards on duty—clearly identifiable. (Courtesy Water Safety Products, Melbourne Beach, Fla.)

rate program. Simply setting a schedule for visiting other pools can be quite helpful to the staff.

Of course, lifeguard parties are a great way to show appreciation to the guards. If held at the pool, extreme caution must be exercised because lifeguards can injure themselves while showing off or competing. Awards can be given to guards who have given outstanding service to the pools.

Junior Lifeguarding Programs

In the past, junior lifesaving courses were taught to youngsters between the ages of 11 and 15 years. Because it was feared that many junior lifesavers would misuse their skills by attempting to make res-

cues, the program was changed to basic water safety courses.

However, many youngsters aspire to be lifeguards and have tremendous swimming ability, and it is no secret that the United States is experiencing a lifeguarding shortage. Junior lifeguard programs of today are a great way to recruit potential lifeguards, but more important, they provide another set of eyes and ears to help safeguard swimmers. After completing successful "internships" at local pools, they often have a job waiting for them when they attain lifeguarding age. Although junior lifeguards cannot make rescues, they can help with equipment and communications. Junior lifeguards can be invaluable during an emergency situation when the emergency medical services system must be activated. They can also provide supervision on decks, in wading pools, at slides, around obstructions, and inside buildings that lifeguards have trouble covering. Junior lifeguard programs are a great way to combat the lifeguarding shortage without incurring great expense.

Youngsters are not the only ones who can assist lifeguards at swimming pools. Senior citizens who enjoy the water and who have extra time can also provide another layer of supervision at pools. The senior citizens, like the junior lifeguards, are not trained to make water rescues, but they can assist. Senior citizens may even be more effective than lifeguards in enforcing rules and regulations and carrying disciplinary actions. Most pool lifeguards are between the ages of 17 and 21. For the most part, they are single and do not have children. Senior citizens, on the other hand are often grandparents. They have a lifetime of experience dealing with children and people in general. They can assist swimming pool staff in a variety of ways. Some senior citizens have been known to work for pool privileges rather than wages. Senior citizens are just another source to assist the lifeguards and safeguard the pool.

How many lifeguards?

Local bathing codes and swimming pool ordinances must be consulted to determine what type of lifeguards are required and how many should be on duty at any given time, but again, local bathing codes often offer minimal standards. Some states require 1 guard per 50 swimmers, other ordinances state that 1 guard must be on duty for every 2000 square feet of water surface area, and there are many other lifeguard standards. However, for busy public pools with a mixed clientele, you may want 1 lifeguard for every 25 swimmers.

More important, a pool staff must evaluate its swimming facilities and patron types to determine specific lifeguard requirements. Whenever the number of swimmers exceeds a predetermined limit placed on certain sections of the pool, additional guards should be added. For instance, in a diving well, two guards may be required when more than 10 people are using that specific facility. Having one criterion for all pools in the same geographical region is not a good idea because of the variety that exists among pools. Guarding 50 lap swimmers in a rectangular, shallow water pool without any obstructions is likely to be much safer and easier than guarding 50

people in a deep water wave pool with some obstructions. The 10/20 rule must be considered when determining lifeguard numbers.

There also may be minimum age and special certification requirements placed on lifeguards. For most public pools, the following lifeguard requirements may exceed local pool codes but are strongly recommended:

1. At least 17 years of age
2. *Current* lifeguarding certification from a nationally recognized agency
3. *Current* CPR certification
4. *Current* first aid certification
5. In addition to the above requirements, the employer should test each guard on rescue skills, lifeguarding knowledge, verbal skills, and situational problems that might arise.

Some risk managers state that at least two lifeguards must be on duty for all pools at all times. Although this is recommended for most public pools, it can be cost prohibitive for very small private or semi-public pools. Because the second lifeguard on the scene of an accident is responsible for calling 911 or other emergency numbers and clearing the pools of other swimmers, exceptions might be made for the small pool. These secondary tasks may be assigned to other staff personnel who are not lifeguards, provided they are mature and well trained in their jobs. This should only be done when it is certain that a minimum of two staff people are always on duty whenever the pool is opened (one lifeguard and one assistant to the lifeguard). This procedure must also be written into the job description and emergency action plan. Desk attendants are the most obvious candidates for assisting lifeguards in emergency procedures at small pools.

Some states require lifeguards to be in elevated lifeguard chairs, but others do not. In some cases, a roving guard is more effective than one who sits in an elevated chair. Perhaps the best combination is to have guards stationed in elevated chairs while one are more guards are roving. The keys to positioning lifeguards include the following:

1. Not being distracted by patrons
2. No sight obstructions or glare
3. Able to respond quickly to a distressed swimmer
4. Able to see all patrons and use the 10/20 rule

In determining the appropriate number and placement of lifeguards, common sense must be applied. Questions such as "Can I see everyone in my zone?"

and "Can I reach everyone in my zone quickly?" must be answered before deciding how many lifeguards must be on duty at a given time and where these guards should be placed. Lifeguards should rotate every 15 to 20 minutes to prevent boredom and should receive a rest break every 1 to 2 hours.

Summary

Certified lifeguards are most often well trained and highly competent. It must be emphasized, however, that the purpose of having lifeguards at poolside is first to prevent accidents and secondly to respond to emergencies promptly and properly. Lifeguards must be specifically trained for the facility that they will be working at and must be continually supervised. Motivating currently employed lifeguards and recruiting potential lifeguards is an important challenge that must be done continually. Many lifeguards are guilty of simply not watching the people in the water continuously.

References

1. American Red Cross, *Swimming and diving*, St Louis, 1992, Mosby.
2. Griffiths T: Do lifeguards do what they get paid to do?, *The New York Times*, Jul 19, 1987.
3. Pia F: *Parks & Recreation* June 1984, pp 52-67.
4. Ellis and Associates: *National pool & waterpark life guardtraining manual*, Houston, 1990.
5. Ellis and Associates, p 55.
6. Ellis and Associates, p 59.
7. Ellis and Associates, p15.
8. Heath PJ: *Splash* Jul/Aug 1991, pp 35-36.

Bibliography

American Red Cross, *Swimming and diving*, St Louis, 1992, Mosby.

American Red Cross, *Lifeguarding*, Washington, DC, 1990 The Red Cross.

Clayton, RD, Thomas, DG, *Professional Aquatic Management*, 2nd ed, Human Kinetics, Champaign, Illinois, 1989.

Ellis and Associates: *National pool & waterpark lifeguard training manual*, Houston, 1990.

Heath PJ: *Basic risk management for water parks*, San Antonio, 1992, Glynn Barclay.

The YMCA of the USA: *On the guard: the YMCA lifeguard manual*, Champaign, Ill, 1986, Human Kinetics.

Torney JA Clayton RD: *Aquatic instruction, coaching and management*, Minneapolis, 1970, Burgess.

Review Questions

1. Compare lifesaving to lifeguarding.

2. What are some systematic scanning techniques?

3. What is the RID factor?

4. What is the 10/20 rule?

5. Who are the high-risk guests at *your* pool?

6. Who initiated the American Red Cross Lifesaving program?

7. List three typical types of pool accidents.

8. List five methods of lifeguard communications.

18

LEGAL LIABILITY AND RISK MANAGEMENT

Annie Clement, PhD, JD

Aquatic activities involve risk. When risk exists, accidents will happen. In the few cases in which injuries resulting from accidents are severe, resources are required for medical, personal, and rehabilitation expenses. Under these circumstances, injured victims will usually look to anyone who the courts might decide was responsible for their injuries and who will thus participate in payment of expenses.

This chapter enables the aquatic specialist to become acquainted with the risks involved in aquatics, learn applicable legal theories and the results of contemporary court decisions, and develop risk management techniques for injury reduction and documentation of the high quality of care used in their work.

Risk in Aquatics

Aquatic activities are leisure sports and survival skills. Swimming, the most popular form of aquatics, is among the top participatory sports in the United States. The National Spa and Pool Institute (NSPI) listed 2,821,517 in-ground and 2,572,144 above-ground pools.[1] The more than 5 million pools are accompanied by a vast array of lakes, streams, and ponds: the Great Lakes; and surrounding oceans. An opportunity to enjoy water and water sports is available to most people in the United States. At the same time, *United States Swimming* reports that more than half of all Americans do not know how to swim, nor could they save themselves if thrown into the water. After examining the results of swim tests administered to new recruits at the United States Marine Corps Recruit Depot at Parris Island, South Carolina,

Lanctot noted that 70% were nonswimmers or swimmers with no knowledge of formal stroke mechanics.[2]

"Drowning is the third leading cause of accidental death to children under 5 years of age."[3] "In California, Florida, and Arizona, drowning is the leading cause of accidental death in this age group."[4] Present[4] examined the reports of drowning that occurred in four counties in Florida, Arizona, and California in a 6-month period in 1986. A total of 142 submersion accidents were reported, 40 victims died, 100 survived, and 2 could not be located for study. The typical victim was a male between 12 and 35 months of age. Often victims were last seen in the house, and more than two thirds were being supervised by one or both parents at the time of the accident. The swimming pool in which the submersion occurred was an in-ground pool, one that consumed a major portion of the owner's yard. Wintemute[5] confirms Present's work in concluding that 60% to 90% of preschool drownings occur in residential swimming pools.

Headfirst entry into pools accounts for a significant number of aquatic injuries and for approximately 10% of spinal cord injuries.[6] Present[7] reviewed all swimming injuries reported to hospital emergency rooms from May 1 to September 30, 1988. Approximately 83,000 pool injuries were treated in hospital emergency rooms in the 4-month period. A total of 28,500 injuries occurred as persons entered the pools. Of the 28,500 injuries, 15,600 resulted from performer's contact with the bottom or sides of the swimming pools, and 7700 were contacts with the bottom of the pools.

Among those reporting contact with the bottom of the pool on entry, 85% were entering in-ground pools. Of the in-ground pool body contacts, 68% of the victims entered from the deck, 23% from a diving board, and 9% from higher elevations or water slides. Of those hitting the bottom of the pool, 60% were entering water at a depth of less than 5 feet.[7]

Of those injured, two thirds sustained head, neck, and face injuries. Of all injuries reported, only 3% of the victims were hospitalized. Apparently, many people are hitting their heads on the bottom and sides of swimming pools and are not receiving serious injury. Another interesting comment was "almost three fourths of those reported to have been injured at in-ground pools and all of those reported to have been injured at above-ground pools believed they correctly judged the depth of the water they were entering."[7]

The injured person was male 62% of the time and female 38% of the time. Approximately 33% of the victims were under 15 years of age. When the victim was female, she was usually between 15 and 19 years of age; when the victim was male, he was usually between 10 and 14 years of age. Approximately 13% of the injured parties reported having consumed alcohol before the accident. This figure is less than that reported in earlier studies.[8]

In the middle 1980s, aquatic professionals experienced a series of accidents that involved coaches and teachers working with competitive athletes. The athletes were rendered quadriplegic as a result of hitting their heads on the bottom of 3- or 3 1/2-foot swimming pools after a shallow or stretch dive from a speed swimming racing block. Northeastern Universities' 6'5", 215-pound outstanding scholarship swimmer was the person to receive the most publicity and maybe the largest settlement—$7.25 million (*Tricarico v. Northeastern University*).[9] Five cases (*Day v. Visalia Unified School District*,[10] *Lloyd v. Jewish Community Center*,[11] *Collier v. Northland Swim Club*,[12] *O'Connell v. Continental Casualty Co.*,[13] and *Kozak v. Struth*[14]) received attention in the press; at least a dozen others have been settled and more are pending. These cases represent a first in litigation involving serious injuries in a sport in an *organized, supervised, and competitive atmosphere*. The use of the word *diving* rather than *racing block start* places an unfortunate penalty on the whole area of diving, an area that has had few accidents and very little if any litigation.

United States Diving[15] defines *diving* as "plunging headfirst into water" and *competitive diving* as a "sport involving head and feet first entries from 1 and 3 meter boards or 5, 7.5, and 10 meter platforms, whereby an athlete performs a list of dives according to the rules and regulations of a national and/or international governing body".

In the following, United states Diving[15] provides facts about injuries, litigation, and diving.

Competitive diving safety record

- Competitive diving suffers a poor image through association with accidents involving a dive into the water but with no connection to the sport itself.
- USD accident insurance claims indicate no record of a fatality or catastrophic injury.
- NCCA and NFSHSA report no record of fatalities or catastrophic injuries in competitive diving.
- In 80 years of competitive diving in the U.S., there is no record of a fatality or a catastrophic injury connected with a supervised training session or diving competition.
- Due to its exemplary safety record, USD is able to offer members affordable insurance.

Diving injury history

- Risk analysis studies indicate drowning and near-drowning accounts for 75% of the total risk for spas, pools, and associated equipment. Diving accounts for only 8% of the total risk.
- The majority of diving spinal cord injuries (SCI) are a result of no supervision.
- 75% of the diving SCI resulting in quadriplegia occurred in the natural aquatic environment (which are generally unsupervised sites).
- 25% of the diving SCI resulting in quadriplegia (approximately 63/year) occurred in swimming pools.
- 95% of the diving resulting in quadriplegia in pools occurred in the shallow rather than in the deep diving area of the pool.
- 89% of the diving SCI in pools occurred in residential, motel, hotel, or apartment pools (pools where there are usually no lifeguards on duty).
- 85% of the SCI in pools occurred with no qualified lifeguard, instructor, or coach present.

Aquatics present risk; injuries do occur. Injury statistics suggest that the two groups most often subject to injury and death are children under 2 years of age who drown and adults and juveniles who sustain spinal cord injuries after entering the water headfirst without checking water depth. People who fling their bodies into the water without checking the depth of the water and without an adequate understanding of the amount of water essential to successful headfirst entries make aquatics hazardous. This apparent hazard has been compounded by the accidents that have occurred under the direction of speed swimming coaches whose professional competence was insufficient to enable them to anticipate diving block injuries. Swimming and diving coaches should have sufficient knowledge of biomechanics to be able to avoid these injuries.

Why Would an Aquatic Professional be Sued?

Injury: serious debilitating injury

Most lawsuits in physical activities are the result of injuries, serious debilitating injuries. The cost of immediate care, expense of rehabilitation, and financial resources needed to enable a challenged person to lead a meaningful life are in most cases the reason for the suit.

Medical science's ability to maintain human life is phenomenal, but not without cost. When the injured victim is faced with no alternative but the taxpayer for support, the idea that someone might be liable for the injury and thus required to pay the bills is attractive.

Health insurance

As fewer participants have health insurance, the risk of lawsuits increases. Professionals must encourage and perhaps demand that participants maintain adequate health insurance.

Immunity statutes

Immunity means freedom from suit. Some federal, state, and local government employees have historically been immune from liability for acts for which a private agency would be held liable. Today, only a few government agencies have such immunity.

Federal Tort Claims Act

The Federal Tort Claims Act of 1946 permitted the "government to be sued when the government engaged in activities in competition to private enterprise. The act provides monetary recovery from the federal government where damages, loss of property, personal injury, or death are caused by the negligence or wrongful acts of federal employees acting within the scope of their employment, and where the United

States, if a private person, would be liable in accordance with the law of the place where the tort occurred. "[16] When the federal government engages in activities not engaged in by private entities, immunity continues to exist. Thus some acts of federal, state, and local government employees will be immune. An exemption to the Federal Torts Claims Act are claims arising out of intentional tort. Intentional torts, the responsibility of the employee, are discussed later.

An example of immunity is found in *Kitowski v. United States*.[17] The wrongful death suit was brought by the mother of Lee Mirecki, a Navy enlisted man, who died while participating in a sea rescue training program at the Naval Air Station in Pensacola, Florida:

> The recruits must participate in a drill known as "sharks and daisies," in which students, wearing only swim fins and no safety equipment, swim in a circle with their hands behind their backs. Instructors grab the students in either a front or rear headhold in an attempt to simulate panicking victims in need of rescue. If a student correctly performs the release procedure, he continues swimming in a circle and other instructors repeat the scenario. If a student fails to perform the maneuver correctly, he is given additional instruction.

> Mirecki had problems with the drill because of fear he had acquired in childhood. First, he withdrew from the sea rescue training program; later he agreed to return to the activity.[17]

> On the day of his death, March 2, 1988, he was once again undergoing the rigors of the sharks and daisies drill ... Mirecki had extreme difficulty with the drill and requested that he be dropped from the course and not be forced to re-enter the pool. Instead of honoring his request, the instructors seized him and forced him back into the water, and began "smurfing" him—holding him under the water until he was unconscious and had turned blue. At this time, other recruits were commanded to line up, turn their backs, and sing the national anthem. After being held under the water for a considerable length of time, Mirechi died from heart arrhythmia, ventricular fibrillation, and decreased oxygen.

The United States District Court dismissed the action, holding "that the Federal Tort claims Act (FTCA) does not permit claims from injuries to active military personnel that arise out of or are in the course of activity incident to service."[17] The United States Court of Appeals affirmed the decision. This case is an example of what can occur and be accepted under the limits of the FTCA. Most aquatic instructors are not covered under the FTCA. Aquatic instructors are discouraged from engaging in the activities mentioned even if the graduates of their programs will be expected to conduct rescues under extreme circumstances.

Recreational users statutes

Recreational users statutes exist in nearly every state. Originally designed to provide immunity to farmers who permitted the public to hunt, trap, and camp on their land, the statutes have been used to cover other properties used for recreational purposes. Recreational users statutes provide immunity for state, federal, and private property available with limited fees to the public. They seldom cover residential properties.

Examples of the use of recreational users statutes are *Midwestern, Inc. v. Northern Kentucky Community Center*[18] and *Lover v. Bucholtz*.[19] In the former case, a 17 year-old male became a quadriplegic after diving from a 3-meter board and hitting the bottom of a pool. Negligence was alleged on the part of the City of Covington and the community center. The court found both agencies immune under Kentucky's Recreational Statutes (KRS).

The following outlines pertinent parts of KRS 411.190:

(c) "Recreational" purpose: includes, but is not limited to, any of the following, or any combination thereof: hunting, fishing, swimming, boating, camping, picnicking, hiking, pleasure driving, nature study, water skiing, winter sports, and viewing or enjoying historical, archaeological, scenic, or scientific sites…

(d) "Charge" means the admission price or fee asked in return for invitation or permission to enter or go upon the land.

(2) The purpose of this section is to encourage owners of land to make land and water areas available to the public for recreational purposes by limiting their liability toward persons entering thereon for such purposes. "

The court concluded that according to KRS 411.190 the fact that the 17-year-old had not paid a fee, the City of Covington and the Northern Kentucky Community Center were immune from negligence.

In *Lover v. Buchholtz*, the Supreme Court of Ohio held that the Recreational Users Statute did not provide immunity to the owner of a residential swimming pool in which a social guest was injured.

Liability and the Professional

Instruction, supervision, and management create the organizing structure for the discussion of legal theories. Examples, including court cases, are explained. The instruction and supervision legal theories are those of importance to lifeguards and teachers; management theories play an important role in administrators' responsibilities.

Instruction/supervision
Negligence

Negligence occurs when a person does or fails to do an act that a reasonable person would be expected to do. It is behavior that falls beneath the standard established by law for the protection of others against harm. The elements of negligence are the following:

1. A legal duty of care
2. Breach of the legal duty
3. The breach of the legal duty was the cause of the injury
4. Substantial damage

The elements of negligence are a series of questions used by the court to determine liability. For liability to exist, all four elements must exist. Negligence is the form of litigation found most often in physical activity.

Legal duty of care. The legal duty of care is the level of care established by members of a profession. There are a number of ways in which aquatic professionals have established a legal duty or standard of care. They include the following:

1. State and federal statutes or specific laws
2. Certification programs provided by agencies such as Jeffrey Ellis Associates, the American Red Cross, and others
3. Guidelines and professional opinion (the standard established by an expert witness in a court of law)

Professionals are to identify the standard under which they plan to work and place that standard in writing. Once a complaint is filed, plaintiffs and defendants identify the standard or duty of the defendant. The duty may be established by a written statement, texts used in the field, or an expert witness. When the profession has a written statement, it is used. When a statement of the duty or standard does not exist, best professional thinking is used.

Breach of the legal duty. Breach of the legal duty means that the court, judge, and jury learn what the standard or duty of care should be and examine the facts to determine whether the defendant adhered to the standard.

Breach proximate cause of injury. If the defendant breached the established standard of care, the court then determines the relationship between the breach and the injury. Was the breach the cause of the injury? For liability to attach, the breach must be the cause of the injury.

Substantial damage. Significant physical or psychology damage should exist.

Degree of negligence. The seriousness of negligence is identified in degrees with negligence, gross negligence, and willful and wanton neglect as the categories:

Negligence—"an absence of that degree of care and vigilance which persons of extraordinary prudence and foresight are accustomed to use or... a failure to exercise great care."[20]

An example of negligence is the failure of a professional to inspect the deck of the pool for water and/or dirt.

Gross negligence—"failure to exercise even that care that a careless person would use."[20]

An example of gross negligence is failure to clean the deck when the instructor or lifeguard knew that water or dirt existed on the deck and that its presence could present danger to participants.

Willfull, Wanton, and Reckless Misconduct—"an intentional act of an unreasonable character in total disregard of human safety.[21]

An example is failure to prevent danger of which the professional was aware, such as allowing people to swim in a swimming pool containing water so cloudy that the bottom cannot be seen.

Defenses to negligence. Two defenses often used in response to a negligence claim are contributory negligence and assumption of risk. Contributory negligence means the injured person created, contributed to, or in some way was responsible for the injuries. Assumption of risk means that the injured victim consented to the risk involved in the activity. The consent may be expressed or in writing or inferred when an adult agreed to take part in an activity. When the consent is in writing, it may be drafted in contract terms and analyzed under contract law. A contract is the only method for transferring a risk. In light of the fact that minors cannot be held to a contract, the rights of minors cannot be signed away. "Assumption of risk can be used only when the parties know the risk exists, understand the nature of the risk, and freely choose to incur the risk."[22]

Comparative negligence. Comparative negligence is negligence based on percentages. It is a system in which the injured person's contributory negligence and assumption of risk reduce the injured person's recovery from the defendant in proportion to the injured person's relative fault. Vito v. State of New York[23] presents an example of comparative negligence. A 21-year-old college senior at the State University College of Brockport injured her back in executing a three-step approach front dive from a 3-meter board during a water safety instruction class. The court of claims or trial court found the state liable for the injuries but apportioned 80% of the fault to the student, who appealed the apportion.

The Supreme Court of New York, Appellate Division, Fourth Department stated the following[23]:

The Court of Claims properly found that the State was negligent through the acts of its instructor in permitting claimant to attempt the dive. The instructor's directive to claimant, which came at the close of a session dedicated to testing the swimming and diving competencies of the students, was correctly characterized by the trial court as being "fraught with danger." The instructor was aware of claimant's lack of control inasmuch as she had previously demonstrated considerable difficulty in executing the same dive from the lower 1-meter board. While the record is clear that the instructor gave the students the option to enter the water from the height of the 3-meter board either by diving or jumping, under these circumstances the instructor did not exercise reasonable care in affording claimant that option. There is ample evidence, however, to support a finding that affiant should bear a considerable share of the responsibility for the injuries. Indeed, she was in the best position to assess her own diving skills, or the lack thereof, and to consider whether one of the safer methods suggested by her instructor was more appropriate.

The Court of Claims apportioned liability equally between the parties.

The final decision on comparative negligence in this case is 50/50. This means that a dollar figure is placed on the judgment and that the defendant is liable for 50% of that figure. Had the trial court decision been affirmed by the court of appeals, the student would have received only 20% from the defendant.

Where negligence is found. Negligence is found most often in aquatics in the following areas:

1. Faulty equipment and facilities. Equipment and

facilities account for numerous injuries associated with aquatic accidents. Many of the early lawsuits dealt with cloudy water and chemical balance problems in pools. Today, facility and equipment suits tend to be "failure to warn" situations—failure to warn persons contemplating headfirst entries about the depth of the water in the pool or beach.

Three examples of failure to warn aquatic cases are *Murphy v. D'Youville Condominium Association, Inc,*[24] *Duda v. City of Philadelphia,*[25] and *Hampton v. Leisure Systems, Inc.*[26]

Murphy, an adult male, was seriously injured after striking bottom while diving into the shallow end of a swimming pool owned by defendants. Defendants contended that *Murphy* was contributorily negligent in failing to exercise ordinary care for his own safety. The court determined that *Murphy* was thoroughly familiar with the pool, had used it often the preceding year, and that the condition of the pool was normal on the day of the accident. The court made use of earlier law from *Simmons v. Classic City Beverages*[27] in stating "the plaintiff went into the situation with his eyes wide open. He saw the whole picture; he had the opportunity to measure the risks, if any, and was under no compulsion (to dive into 3 feet of water)…Every adult is presumed to be endowed with normal facilities, both mental and physical." The court granted summary judgment to the defendant (appellees) "on the ground that the uncontradicted evidence shows that the proximate cause of appellant's injury was his failure to exercise ordinary care for his own safety."

In *Duda,* a 9-year-old activated a preexisting spinal injury when she hit her head on the pool bottom after diving into 3 $\frac{1}{2}$ feet of water. Her parents sued the city, alleging failure to provide depth markings and failure to warn of the hazard of diving. Depth markings were required by state law. Although diving was prohibited in the pool, no warnings were posted. The jury awarded $709,700, allocating 80% liability to the city and 20% liability to *Duda's* parents for failure to supervise.

Hampton, a 19-year-old student on an approved high school outing, became a permanent quadriplegic after diving into the shallow end of a public park swimming pool. Hampton sued the park owner, franchisor of the park, and the school board. The park owner was sued in negligence for failure to warn of pool depth and for failure to prohibit diving. The franchisor was sued for the same theories and for negligent inspection and maintenance of the facility, whereas the school board was sued for lack of supervision. One teacher with no background in aquatics accompanied 80 students to the swimming event.

A structure settlement of $1.41 million included $762,000 from the park owner, $450,000 from the franchisor, and 200,000 from the school.

2. Failure to supervise. Failure to supervise is often listed as the form of negligence found in aquatic accidents. In *Walker v. Daniels,*[28] the surviving parents of a student who drowned in the Fort Valley State College pool while participating in recreational swimming sued the Georgia Board of Regents, State College lifeguards, an assistant professor and a chair of Health and Physical Education, and the director of campus safety. The trial court jury returned a verdict of $1,500,000 against all defendants. The defendants appealed. The Court of Appeals held that "neither professor of health and physical education nor director of campus safety breached any duty of care towards student which could be found to be proximate cause of his death." They affirmed the lower courts finding of liability of the Georgia Board of Regents and one of the lifeguards.

Two lifeguards were supervising a group of 50-60 participants the day of the incident. One guard was posted in a stationary position in a elevated chair with responsibility for the deep end of the pool.

One lifeguard "was posted at the shallow end of the pool but also should have been roving. However, he was inattentive; he was grabbing and touching female swimmers and generally engaging in horseplay. [The other lifeguard] … left his position and walked to the shallow end of the pool to ask [the lifeguard horsing around] … to change places with him because he was not fulfilling his responsibilities where he was. He then walked back to his chair but on the way received word that a body had been discovered at the bottom of the pool."

The importance of lifeguard training and continuous supervision is brought out in this case.

Patel v. Wet 'N Wild, Inc.[29] represents a new set of facts that are occurring more often in recent years. In *Patel*, a 28-year-old male slid headfirst down a water slide, suffering a depressed skull fracture and spinal fracture at C6 as he hit the bottom of the splash pool. *Patel* alleged negligence on the part of *Wet 'N Wild, Inc*, in allowing him to move down the slide headfirst. Defendants alleged that *Patel* failed to position himself properly on the slide. The jury awarded $740,000 to *Patel*; the trial court found *Patel* 15% liable for his injuries under comparative fault; *Wet 'N Wild* was found 85% liable.

In the first case the failure in supervision was a failure to systematically carry out a predetermined lifeguarding plan. The water slide incident reminds the professional of the need to provide easy-to-view signage with detailed instruction on the use of equipment and depth of specific areas of the pool. Even though warnings are posted, supervisors are expected to immediately stop participants who ignore or violate the written orders. Lifeguards who permit participants to move down water slides headfirst when written instruction warns of the danger of headfirst entry to the water are failing to maintain the agreed on standard of care.

3. Education malpractice. *Tricarico*,[9,30] described earlier, is the classic aquatic case in educational malpractice. Two other cases in which malpractice or faulty teaching were found to be the reason for the victim's injuries are *Small v. University System*[31] and *Perkins v. State Board of Education.*[32] *Small* herniated a disk while lifting a victim from a pool in a rescue procedure. She alleged that the instructor failed to teach the college course in a competent and safe manner and that students were not warned of the danger of executing such a procedure. The case was settled for $150,000.

A lifesaving surface dive that resulted in the victim sustaining head injury after hitting his head on the bottom of the pool were the facts of *Perkins*. *Perkins*, a 34-year-old male college student, was absent from class on the day the surface dive was taught. After the next lesson, he asked a member of the class to teach him the surface dive during the recreational swim period following the formal class instruction. His men-

tor described the skill but failed to emphasize the importance of maintaining the arms and hends above the head in executing the surface dive. *Perkin's* faulty execution of the surface dive resulted in his injuries.

The Twenty-First Judicial District Court, Parish of Tangipahoa, entered judgment for the State Board. Perkins appealed. The court of Appeals affirmed the lower courts decision saying that the instructor had not breached his duty of care for the student. Instructors are to be clear as to when instruction begins and ends in a class period. In this case the teacher's role was that of a lifeguard; no instruction was being provided at the time of the injury.

4. Failure to provide emergency care. Aquatic facilities are expected to have a detailed emergency rescue plan in effect whenever the pool is in use. This plan is to include immediate and temporary care in the water and on the deck and a system for swimming rescue. The system is to be in writing, known to employees, and rehearsed periodically. It is to be created in cooperation with local rescue authorities.

Intentional tort

An intentional tort is a deliberate act or failure to act. The person intended to do the act; they may not have intended to harm someone. When the court finds an intentional tort, the defendant is automatically liable. Administrators and insurance companies find it difficult to consider the commission of an intentional tort part of the learning process. Horseplay such as throwing someone into the pool at the completion of a competitive event is an intentional tort. Disciplining a person by demanding the swimming of an unreasonable number of laps of the pool is an intentional tort. Serious injuries resulting from horseplay could be intentional torts.

Although television often provides a picture of judges, officials, coaches, and swimmers being tossed into the pool at the completion of a meet, no lawsuits were found among these victims. Most of the horseplay lawsuits in aquatics have occurred in residential pool. *Smith v. Stark*[33] is an example of these cases. *Smith*, an 18-year-old college student, sustained serious injuries when he dove or was pushed into the shallow end of an in-ground residential pool. Smith had no recollection of how he entered the water. He sued, saying the pool was not properly marked. The

Supreme Court ruled for the defendant. In light of the fact that the plaintiff did not know how the injury occurred, the lack of depth warnings could not be considered the proximate cause of plaintiff's injuries. The plaintiff appealed. The Court of Appeals of New York affirmed the earlier decision.

Damages

Damages in tort cases are compensatory and punitive. Compensatory damages are expenses directly related to the injury that will make the person "whole." They include medical bills, lost wages, and permanent care necessary to maintain a challenged person. Punitive damages are assessed in an effort to deter the defendant from continuing to allow the unsafe environment to exist. Punitive damages may be awarded in negligence when the actions have been willfull and wanton neglect and in intentional tort cases.

Management

Aquatic administrators are to be aware of the legal theories relating to lifeguards and instructors and to those important to managers. Among the employer-employee relationships that are used in aquatics are regular employment and independent contractor status. Another management topic addressed in depth is the Americans With Disabilities Act.

Employment relationships

In the regular employer-employee relationship, the employee answers to the employer or to someone in the employer's chain of command. The employer dictates job duties, how the work will be performed, and the method of evaluation. In this relationship the employer is responsible for the torts of the employee. An *independent contractor* is an employment relationship in which the employer has only a contract right to the results to be achieved.

Regular employee

A regular employee is ensured an equitable hiring process, a safe working environment, and evaluation based on the identified job responsibilities. The employer dictates job tasks and controls the method of carrying out the tasks from hiring to termination. For a regular employment or an agency relationship to exist, the parties agree to the relationship, the employee knows that he or she is acting on behalf of the employer, and the employer assumes a fiduciary duty to pay the employee.

Vicarious liability. Under the legal theory *respondeat superior*, an employer is *vicariously liable* or responsible for torts committed by employees within the work environment. An administrator, for example, will be vicariously liable for the torts of their lifeguards and teachers. Also, the employer is personally responsible for hiring an incompetent employee. Aquatic administrators are responsible for checking applicants' backgrounds and credentials. Merely viewing a certification is insufficient; calls to the agency for verification are expected. Administrators are not responsible for employees' intentional torts or torts that are beyond the scope of their employment. If the administrator directs the employee to commit an intentional tort or to carry out a task beyond the job responsibilities, the administrator becomes liable. Insurance companies are often vigilant (and rightfully so) in determining whether a tort, intentional or negligent, was within the job responsibilities or was commanded or ratified by the employer. If the incident was beyond the scope of employment and neither commanded or ratified by the employer, it does not come under the employer insurance.

Volunteers working in administrative roles are held to the same vicarious liability as salaried employees are held. The expertise of the volunteer, not the wage of the employee, determines the liability. Some states have or are instituting immunity statutes for coaches who work without pay or for minimal fees. These statutes cover *only* negligence. The value of coaching immunity statutes are difficult to assess because they have not existed long enough to be challenged by the courts.

Safe working environment. Employees are expected to provide a safe working environment for their employees. Physical and psychological factors are considered in providing the safe work environment. When full safety cannot be ensured, a system of warnings about dangers that cannot be eliminated is to be provided. When possible, this information is provided to the prospective employee before the job is offered. Employers need to be sure that the employee knows of the risks, understands the magnitude of the risks, and then willingly accepts the job. If special safety equipment is mandated by law, it must be provided by the employer; if not mandated by law, employees should find it easy to purchase the equipment necessary to make them safe in the workplace. When risks become evident after a person is on the job, the employee is to be informed immediately.

Independent contractor. An independent contractor is an employment relationship in which the employer requests a certain service or product, specifies a level of performance and quality, agrees to pay the contractor in a lump sum, and possesses a contract right only to the results of the original agreement. The employee has no control over the workers who carry out the agreement and does not pay wages, insurance, compensation, or employee benefits. The employer is, however, liable for general working conditions. Independent contractors carry their own insurance; cover compensation, wages, and employee benefits; and withhold taxes.

Many sport specialists, including aquatic administrators, are making use of independent contractors in an effect to save the cost of record keeping and to avoid liability. When a manager chooses this form of employment, he or she must be aware that either a court or the Internal Revenue Service may put an independent contractor status to a rather tough set of tests, denying the status when an examination of the facts fails to warrant an independent contractor status. An employer using an independent contractor who is denied independent contractor status will automatically become liable for the torts of the independent contractor and his or her employees and will be subject to federal and state employee taxes and withholdings that have not been paid by the independent contractor. Such a ruling can place a thriving business into severe financial jeopardy.

Employees in sport and physical activity are signing independent contractor agreements without knowledge of what the agreement means. In some situations, employers are convinced that the signing of the agreement is all that is necessary to establish an independent contractor status. When such an agreement is challenged by a court or the Internal Revenue Service, the burden is on the employer to show that the employee fully understood the agreement.

The following provides assistance in determining the employment status. A finding of regular employee or independent contractor is based on the responses to the majority of questions. Failure to meet the majority of the tests will result in loss of status:

1. The agreement is in writing; both parties understand what an independent contractor status is and believe they are creating such a status. The use of employer identification and license numbers can be helpful in establishing that both parties understand the status. If possible, the agreement should be drafted and executed by an attorney with expertise in independent contractor agreements.

2. Control of the work environment. The independent contractor hires, evaluates, and terminates the employee. The independent contractor sets work schedules and methods of carrying out the task. The employer may periodically inspect the progress of the work, making suggestions for change only to the independent contractor.

3. Is the independent contractor engaged in a distinct occupation or business? When the task requires specific licensing or qualifications that prohibit the employer from evaluating employees, a case can be made for specialization.

4. Custom in the industry. Although an independent contractor is not the generally accepted custom in the aquatic industry, it is becoming popular in various sport and physical activity settings.

5. What skills are required? An employer hiring lifeguards under an independent contractor agreement can require certifications demanded by respective state statutes but cannot require a specific training program and certification when a number of programs exist for preparing lifeguards and aquatic instructors. Employers are not to provide any training other than a superficial orientation to the facility and agency. No in-service training or use of progressions and syllabi can be required. Aquatic administrators, in conjunction with their attorneys, may consider designating parameters for acceptable lifeguarding and teaching credentials. Aquatic administrators designating such parameters should look to independent contractor agreements in the trade industries for guidance.

6. Period of employment. Short-term employment raises less suspicion than long-term employment. Independent contractor agreements are often used to meet seasonal demands or to provide extra employees.

7. Method of payment. All payment is in a lump sum or periodic lump sum payments to the independent contractor.

In spite of the agreement, an employer may be personally liable for the following[34]:

1. Selecting a contractor with a history of carelessness.
2. Allowing a hazardous situation to exist.
3. Failing to perform a duty that they cannot delegate by law.
4. Allowing the party to do inherently dangerous work.

Grosso v. United State Navy is an example of litigation in aquatics under the theory of independent contractor. Darlene Grosso brought suit against the Bucks County Pool Service, Warrington Township, and the United States Navy for a shoulder injury she sustained while diving or swimming the backstroke during a swimming meet at Willow Grove Naval Air Station. The Township's motion for summary judgment was unopposed. United States Navy was granted "motion under Fed. R. Civ. P 12 (b)." The Bucks County Pool Service was denied summary judgment because it "had an independent contractor relationship with Warrington Township and therefore is not entitled to any of the immunities found in Pennsylvania's Political Subdivision Tort Claims Act." In reaching this decision the court used the following factors to establish Bucks County Pools (BCPS) independent contractor status[35]:

1. The written contract represented the entire agreement between the Township and BCPS...
2. The BCPS operated and managed the pool for three (3) years, the summers of 1982 to 1984. The 1983 contact was for a set term (May 28th through Labor Day), and fixed payment of $35,718.00 to be paid in three installments....
3. The contact required the BCPS to hire several people...No one from the Township supervised or otherwise reviewed...hiring or firing of the staff...
4. The only people (the lifeguard) reported to were the pool manager and Mr. Hughes.
5. The owner of BCPS was the sole person in charge of the operation and management of the pool and swim team.
6. The Township only got involved in the pool's operation if there was a problem.
7. The only task performed by the Township in the pool area on a regular basis was the cutting of the grass.
8. The BCPS completely took care of all the pool maintenance, and by contract, supplied any and all equipment necessary to operate and maintain the pools.
9. The contract specifically provided that any assistants hired by the BCPS were employees of the pool service and not the Township.
10. The Township, apparently based on residency, determined the pool's membership....
11. On some occasions the owner of BCPS—at his initiative—consulted with the maintenance man employed by the Township, regarding filtration or chlorination of the pool.

The clear picture, as sketched above, is one of an independent contractor.

For further information on independent contractor and employee concerns, note discussion generally of master/servant and vicarious liability. Section 220 of the Restatement of Agency, Second[36], current Internal Revenue Code, and others[22,34,37] provide additional information.

Americans with Disabilities Act of 1990

The American With Disabilities Act (ADA) of 1990[38] demands that challenged persons be mainstreamed and that the implementation of adapted programs and earlier statutes become reality. It is another form of civil rights legislation based on the following board general rights of the 14th Amendment to the Constitution:

No state shall make or enforce any law which shall abridge the privileges or immunities or citizens of the United States; nor shall any state deprive any person of life, liberty, or property, without due process of law; nor deny to any person within its jurisdiction the equal protection of the law.

The equal protection clause establishes that all people are equal and are to be treated as equals. ADA describes what that treatment should be for the challenged person. The following outlines parts of the act and the one court case relevant to aquatics. Also, recommendations are made for program change and evaluation. Assistance in employment can be obtained from many sources.

The purpose of the Act is the following[38]:

1. To provide a clear and comprehensive national mandate for the elimination of discrimination against individuals with disabilities

2. To provide clear, strong, consistent, enforceable standards addressing discrimination against individuals with disabilities

3. To ensure that the federal government plays a central role in enforcing the standards established in this act on behalf of individuals with disabilities

4. To invoke the sweep of congressional authority, including the power to enforce the fourteenth amendment and to regulate commerce, in order to address the major areas of discrimination faced day-to-day by people with disabilities.

The *term disability* for the purposes of the ADA means with respect to an individual the following[38]:

1. A physical or mental impairment that substantially limits one or more of the major life activities of such individuals

2. A record of such an impairment

3. Being regarded as having such an impairment

Title III of the ADA, Public Accommodations and Services Operated by Private Entities, Section 301, No. 7, I through L, specifically covers areas relating to aquatics. They are the following[38]:

I. A park, zoo, amusement park, or other place of recreation

J. A nursery; elementary, secondary, undergraduate, or postgraduate private school; or other place of education

K. A day care center, senior citizen center, homeless shelter, food bank, adoption agency, or other social service center establishment

L. A gymnasium, health spa, bowling alley, golf-course, or other place of exercise or recreation

All aquatic facilities open to the public are under the control of the act. Persons who make use of their residential pools for public swimming instruction will find their pools under the ADA.

"Readily achievable" is an important part of the ADA. It means easily accomplishable and able to be carried out without much difficulty or expense. In determining whether an action is readily achievable, factors to be considered include the following[38]:

1. The nature of cost of the action needed under this act

2. The overall financial resources of the facility or facilities involved in the action, the number of persons employed at such facility, the effect on expenses and resources, or the impact otherwise of such action upon the operation of the facility

3. The overall financial resources of the covered entity with respect to the number of its employees and the number, type, and location of its facilities

4. The type of operation or operations of the covered entity, including the composition, structure, and functions of the work force of such entity; the geographic separateness, and administrative or fiscal relationship of the facility or facilities in question to the covered entity

Specific prohibitions of discrimination under construction include the following[38]:

1. The imposition or application of eligibility criteria that screen out or tend to screen out an individual with disability or any class of individuals with disabilities from fully and equally enjoying any goods, services, facilities, privileges, advantages, or accommodation, unless such criteria can be shown to be necessary for the provision of the goods, services, facilities, privileges, advantages, or accommodations being offered

2. A failure to make reasonable modifications in policies, practices, or procedures, when such modifications are necessary to afford such goods, services, facilities, privileges, advantages, or accommodations to individuals with disabilities, unless the entity can demonstrate that making such modifications would fundamentally alter the nature of such goods, services, facilities, privileges, advantages, or accommodations

3. A failure to take such steps as may be necessary to ensure that no individual with a disability is excluded, denied services, segregated, or otherwise treated differently than other individuals because of the absence of auxiliary aids and services, unless the entity can demonstrate that taking such steps would fundamentally alter the nature of the goods, service, facility, privilege, advantage, or accommodation being offered or would result in an undue burden

4. A failure to remove architectural barriers and communication barriers that are structural in nature in existing facilities and transportation barriers in existing vehicles and rail passenger cars used by an establishment for transporting individuals (not including barriers that can only be removed through the retrofitting of vehicles or rail passenger cars by the installation of a hydraulic or other lift) where such removal is readily achievable

5. Where an entity can demonstrate that the removal of a carrier under clause (4) is not readily achievable, a failure to make such goods, services, facilities, privileges, or accommodations available through alternative methods if such methods are readily achievable

Enforcement

The ADA is enforced by the Attorney General of the United States. Among the ADA's provisions are the requirements of relief; auxiliary aid or service; modification of policy, practice, or procedure; and accessible facilities. Penalties are not to exceed $50,000 for the first violation and $100,000 for subsequent violations.

Whether litigation will become extensive under ADA is difficult to predict. The National Law Journal[39] noted 3358 alleged violations of employment standards and 1850 other alleged violations reported to the Justice Department over the past year. A number of the suits are against theaters for wheelchair access. *Anderson v. Little League*[40] is the first case in sport or physical activity. Mr. Anderson, a federal judge and a quadriplegic since a 1969 car accident, was denied an opportunity to coach his son's team in the Little League World Series. He wanted to coach the baseball team from the third base coaches's box. Little League officials said his location was a hazard. The Federal Court provided an injunction that allowed Mr. Anderson to coach from the third base box.

ADA concerns in aquatics have been identified.[41,42] Some of the researchers' suggestions are addressed in comments regarding reasonable accommodations, programming or instruction, staff education, and public relations.

Reasonable accommodations

Facilities are to be accessible on the exterior and interior. Areas to check accessibility are entrances and exits, parking lots, and locker rooms. Parking lots are to have adequate room for participants to enter and leave vans using either side or rear lifts. Side van exits require space between automobiles. Sidewalks and entrances to the building are to have ramps and doors that can be maneuvered from a sitting position. Locker rooms are to provide clean, individual, private, mixed-sex dressing quarters. Handheld showers and old wheelchairs are a must for bathing. Cleanliness is vital because many people are subject to infections.

Swimming pools are to have lifts, buddy systems in

operation, devices for the blind, and stair ramps. Above all, participants should expect comfortable, safe accommodations with privacy and no unwanted attention.

Programming and instruction

A comprehensive program will have integrated instruction using adaptations found in numerous programs. Specific flotation devices, aids, and buddy systems for the blind are integrated into the daily classes. When necessary, special programs are designed and provided for certain disabilities.

Staff education

For a program to be successful, staff are to be educated, activities and programs must be assessed to meet the needs of participants, and a willingness to change must exist. First, staff need to know the law and realize that the law will be enforced. Instruction on the ADA and other public laws enhances employees ability to implement the laws. Sensitivity in attitude and language to challenged participants enables employees to eliminate discriminatory remarks and feelings of insecurity they might possess. Opportunities are to be provided for practical experience in sign language, use of communication aids, wheelchairs, prosthetic devices, lifts, and transfers.

Public relations

An advisory committee is to be named to guide the agency in designing and carrying out their ADA risk management program. All publications, programs, protocols, releases, and health care statements are to be examined for prejudices.

Risk Management

Risk management is the identification, evaluation, and control of loss to property, clients, employees, and the public. Identification involves the creation of an audit in which all areas of risk are noted. An audit usually incudes a detailed analysis of local, state, and federal laws and professional guidelines; facilities; equipment; personnel; supervision; instruction; participants; and emergency and accident procedures. Each item in the audit is evaluated and a decision make to retain, alter, or eliminate. This system is unique to an agency and should be designed in conjunction with the insurance company and the attorney who will represent the agency in litigation. The risk management plan enables the professional to develop a paper record to document the quality of his or her work.

You cannot prevent a lawsuit. You can, however, build an effective defense. Professionals must recognize that a complaint could be filed against them at any time. If a person under their supervision is injured and if the injured party sustains considerable financial loss, a complaint may be filed. Persons engaged in teaching, coaching, supervision, or administration of aquatic activities need to prepare for a lawsuit with the same diligence that they would prepare for an accident. Professionals are to *rehearse, practice, and give attention* to the sequence of events that would occur should a legal complaint be filed.

Competent teaching, continuous inspection, and remediation of equipment and facilities, adequate records, and careful supervision should enhance a professional's chance of success in a court of law. You may be sued. If you are a good teacher and coach,competent administrator and supervisor, and effective leader and can document the quality of your work, you will succeed in a court of law.

Many agencies and nearly all risk management consultants recommend that a safety committee be created. The safety committee members play a role in the creation of the audit, assist in analyzing the results of the audit, and help establish the methods of control. Committee members meet periodically to consider the efficiency of the entire risk management plan, make recommendations, and monitor the results of implemented changes.

Audit

The following are suggestions to consider in preparing an audit in aquatics. They are not to be considered a comprehensive check sheet. They are merely examples of some of the topics that might be considered in creating an audit.

Local, state, and federal laws and professional guidelines

1. Identify local, state, and federal codes that affect aquatics in general and your agency in particular. They include specific codes for pools, water slides, lakes, and streams, and general health and maintenance standards.
2. Does the agency's status as "for profit" or "not for profit" affect its status under any of the above laws?

3. Does the state require that the pool operator be certified or tested? If so, what competencies are involved?
4. Retain all codes that directly affect the operation of the facility. Bring them up to date periodically.
5. Know the difference between a code and a guideline. A code must be followed; a guideline can be followed. Failure to follow a code can result in civil punishment: failure to follow a guideline will not result in civil punishment. A court may ask why you choose to ignore a guideline. When an agency chooses to ignore a popular guideline, they should document knowledge of the guideline and their reasons for choosing not to follow the guideline.
6. Be sure employees are aware of and follow codes.

Facilities

1. A system for routine inspection of all facilities exists. Identification of appropriate people to conduct the inspections are made. Time schedules are established for each element of the inspection. The system is checked periodically by an administrator.
2. Protocol for repair, follow-up, and the closing of a facility in need of immediate repair is created and used.
3. The general condition of facilities is compared with external agency guidelines.
4. Lighting and illumination meet National Electrical Code and state and local codes. Professional organizations' recommendation should be studied and implemented as feasible.
5. The facility meets the ADA standards; pools, water slides, entries, exits, and lockers rooms conform to standards.
6. Water depth markings are obvious and meet or exceed code. With the increase in international recreation, aquatic areas may need to be marked in meters and in feet and inches.
7. Headfirst entries into the water are controlled, and locations for entries are clearly marked.
8. Local health standards are maintained.

Equipment

1. Rescue equipment meets acceptable standards and is clean and ready to use.
2. Equipment for teaching, supervision, and res-

cue is inventoried and routinely inspected.

3. In-pool lifelines are installed according to specifications.

4. Lifeguard chairs and stations used in guarding permit full pool visibility.

5. Equipment is maintained, repaired, and used according to manufacturer's specifications

6. Instructions and warnings provided by the manufacturer are obvious to participants.

7. Emergency power for pool, locker rooms, halls, and stairways is available in the event of a power failure.

8. Diving blocks meet contemporary standards and are used only under supervision. Sleeves are available to cover blocks when not in use.

9. Diving boards are routinely inspected for wear.

Personnel

1. Employment guidelines appropriate for the agency are followed. Emphasis is placed on the avoidance of discrimination in hiring.

2. Complete job descriptions exist for each position.

3. Certifications and qualifications essential to success on the job are established and made known to applicants.

4. Applicants understand expectations made when they present certain credentials. They know what the literature and training guides have defined as their responsibilities.

5. Orientations are provided for personnel.

6. Policy manuals containing detailed information on emergencies and injury protocol are studied. Employees are asked to sign a statement that they have read, understand, and will comply with the policies and procedures contained in the manual.

7. Staff are informed on insurance coverage and legal responsibilities.

8. The work environment is safe for employees.

9. Employees are encouraged to report unsafe conditions.

Supervision

1. A recognized system for supervision is used. If a system other than a well-known system is used, the system in use is documented in detail.

2. The guarding system ensures that one or two

people are viewing each person in the water at all times.

3. Employees know their responsibilities.

4. Leasing with outside groups involves a contractual arrangement with all areas, including liability and insurance fully documented.

5. A system of crowd control exists and is rehearsed periodically.

6. Horseplay is prohibited.

7. Standards are maintained. Advertised standards and promises are keep.

8. When game play and water polo rules and officials are used, rules are documented. Rules are used as a means of identifying the risks involved in an activity.

Instruction

1. Content is selected with the needs of each individual in mind. The ADA legislation is given full consideration in content definition. The teacher is able to justify all aspects of the instruction. The goals and objectives of each test and certification are examined to be sure that the methods of satisfaction are appropriate for all learners. For example, the concept that a person is able to support their body in water over their head could be accomplished in various ways by people who are challenged. This area is open for creative ideas. Knowledge of biomechanics will become important to the extension of experiences for all learners.

2. Planning is to be documented. Courses of study, curricular plans, and learning sequences are on file.

3. Members of class are aware of the contents of each lesson and are able to verify that various instructions, particularly safety tips, were given.

4. Records of specific benchmark achievements exist and are available on request. Computer printouts are used when possible. Client progress and readiness for advanced work is documented and retained on file.

5. Documentation shows that clients were properly warmed up for the activity.

6. Documents demonstrate that appropriate safety techniques were used in the teaching of the activity.

7. Methodologies used by instructors meet the test of peer scrutiny.

8. Preassessment is used to qualify participants for certain activities.
9. If at all possible, individualized assessment and teaching is used.

Participants

1. Employees know participants and are prepared to work with routine concerns.
2. Participants understand risks involved in aquatics. Parents of minors are aware that their children are participating in the activity and are aware that the activity may have some inherent risks. Written statements may be required to ascertain this knowledge.
3. When appropriate, consent, warnings, and waivers are to be used. They serve to inform the public about the risks involved. Detailed information on these statements and contracts are available in other sources.
4. The use of arbitration to adjudicate fault in recreational injuries is becoming popular and should be investigated.
5. Established rules should be enforced. Participants failing to adhere to the rules are to be removed from the activity. These ejections are documented.
6. The facility provides an opportunity for participants to report unsafe conditions and register complaints.

Emergency accident plan

An accident that requires the calling of emergency services is serious and requires a full investigation. An accident that requires emergency room attention needs to trigger a comprehensive evaluation. When an aquatic specialist becomes aware of an accident within a week or two following the incident (such as an arm fracture identified 2 days later but believed to have occurred in the pool), the specialist should treat the incident as serious.

1. A plan exists. In addition to water rescue, the plan includes fire, tornado, and other hazards. Detailed written statements should exist; the plan should work effectively in a rehearsal.
2. Immediate and temporary care is identified. Appropriate people to execute the plan are selected. Practice sessions are conducted.
3. The system for obtaining additional help is planned in cooperation with local emergency medical agencies.

4. The role of the telephone in obtaining assistance is defined. Will cellular phones be used?
5. The system for obtaining emergency medical help is outlined and known to the Staff. Persons making the emergency calls are able to identify the address of the agency, the exact location of the injured party, and how best to get to the location. Information above the permanent phone is to be printed and easy to read; the same information is carried on a plastic card with the portable telephone. The caller should identify the victim by age, sex, injury, vital signs, and unique medical history. Instructors and lifeguards need to have information on unique characteristics of participants readily available.
6. A means of working with the media exists. Often the media come in response to the 911 call.
7. The system is known by all. It is rehearsed periodically and monitored for flaws at least once a year.
8. Emergency protocol is specific and is known.

Accident report

1. Freeze the incident. Make a snapshot of the entire situation, including witnesses. Did you observe anything before the accident? As soon as possible, place that image in writing. Only the care of the victim should be considered first.
2. Provide immediate and temporary care.
3. If possible, fill out an accident report as soon as immediate and temporary care is completed.
4. Obtain statement from witness. Record the names of all persons in the vicinity.
5. Be kind, but protect all parties. Do not admit anything.
6. Accident report forms should be readily available.
7. The retained attorney should be familiar with the form and believe it provides the best protection. Avoid after-the-fact descriptions of the accident.
8. Know when your insurance company will want a full-scale investigation.
9. Copies of completed accident reports are given to key administrators within 1 hour of the accident. They should be informed by telephone as soon as possible.

10. If a major accident occurs, debrief all people involved.

Suggestions made for categories and items in the audit above will hopefully trigger ideas for the audit to be used in your facility. Unique characteristics of your facility, special programs, and other situations may demand quite different categories and items. When the audit is complete, items are examined for potential risk. When the risk is found to be high, the agency may choose to remove the activity, retain the activity and reduce the risk by a change in the activity, or retain the activity and control the exposure to risk with insurance. These decisions are made with the guidance of the safety committee and retained counsel.

Competent aquatic professionals know aquatics, their roles in aquatics, and the legal theories that might affect their roles. They have a comprehensive risk management program that is reviewed yearly. If a serious accident occurs, they are able to meet the situation with the highest level of professional competence. Should a complaint be filed, professionals are able to document the high quality of their work.

References

1. National Spa and Pool Institute Market Survey, 1988.
2. Lanctot: Americans fail in swimming ability, *Aquatics International* Mar/Apr 1992, p 4.
3. Elder J: *Human factor analysis, child drowning study*. Bethesda, Md, 1987, US Consumer Product Safety Commission.
4. Present P: *Child drowning study: a report on the epidemiology of drowning in residential pools to children under age five*, Washington, DC, 1987, US Consumer Product Safety System.
5. Wintemute GJ: Childhood drowning and near-drowning in the United States, *Am J Dis Children* 144:663-669, 1990.
6. Samples P: Spinal cord injuries: the high cost of careless diving, *The Physician and Sports Medicine* Jul 1989, p 143.
7. Present P: *Diving study: report on injuries treated in hospital emergency rooms as result of diving into swimming pools*, Washington DC, 1989, US Consumer Product Safety Commission.
8. Gabrielson MA: *Diving injuries: a critical insight and recommendations*, Indianapolis, 1984, Council for National Cooperation in Aquatics.
9. *Tricarico v. Northeastern University*, Mass., reported in Association for Trial Lawyers of American Law Reporter, 31, Sept 1988.
10. *Day v. Visalia Unified School District*, Cal., Tulare County Superior Court, No. 116796, Mar 13, 1987.
11. *Lloyd v. Jewish Community Center, Md.*, Montgomery County Circuit Court, No. 0260, Oct 31, 1986.
12. *Collier v. Northland Swim Club*, 518 N.E. 2d 1226, 35 Ohio App. 3d 35 (1987).
13. *O'Connell v. Continental Casualty Co.*, Wisc., Ozaukee County Circuit Court, No. 81 C V 428, Jan 6, 1986.
14. *Kozak v. Struth*, 531 A. 2d 420 (1987).
15. Gabriel JL: *Diving safety: a position paper*, Indianapolis, 1988, United States Diving.
16. United States Code Annotated 2671-2680.
17. *Kitowski v. United States*, 931 F. 2d 1526 (1991).
18. *Midwestern, Inc. v. Northern Kentucky Community Center*, 736 S.W. 2d 348 (1987).
19. *Lover v. Buchholtz*, 526 N.E. 2d 300; 38 Ohio St. 3d 65 (1988).
20. Keeton WP, et al: *Prosser and Keeton on torts*, ed 5, St Paul, Minn, 1984, West.
21. Restatement of the Law of Torts (Second), 1965.
22. Clement A: *Law in sport and physical activity*, Dubuque, Ia, 1988, Brown.
23. *Vito v. State of New York*, 182 A.D. 2d 1070; 582 N.Y.S. 1992.
24. *Murphy v. D'Youville Condominium Association, Inc.*, 333 S.E. 2d 1 (Ga. App. 1985) 175 Ga. App. 156.
25. *Duda v. City of Philadelphia, Pa.*, Philadelphia County Court of Common Pleas, Mar Term 1984, No. 499, June 26, 1989.
26. *Hampton v. Leisure Systems, Inc.*, La., Tangipahoa Parish District Court, No. 85-414, Mar 2, 1990.
27. *Simmons v. Classic City Beverages*, 136 Ga. App. 150 (4), 220 S. E. 2d 734 (1975).
28. *Walker v. Daniels*, 407 S. E. 2d 70 1991.
29. *Patel v. Wet 'N Wild*, Inc., Fla., Orange County Circuit Court, No. 88-4107, Apr 25, 1991.
30. *Tricarico v. Northeastern University, Mass.*, Suffock County, Superior Court, No. 63949, May 2, 1988.
31. *Small v. University System*, N.H., Strafford County Superior Court, No. 85-C-240, Mar 23, 1990.
32. *Perkins v. State Board of Education*, La. App., 364 So. 2d 183 1979.
33. *Smith v. Stark*, 490 N.E. 2d 841 (N.Y. 1986).
34. Clement A: #7 and 14 Sport law: Product liability and employment relations. In Parkhouse (editor): *The management of sport*, St Louis, 1991, Mosby.
35. *Grosso v. United States Navy*, et al, United States District Court for the Eastern District of Pennsylvania, No. 85-0357, Slip Opinion, Oct 15, 1985.
36. Restatement of the Law of Agency (Second).
37. Urquhart JR, III: *Independent contract agreements*, Irvine, Calif, 1989, Fidelity.
38. *American With Disabilities Act of 1990*, Public Law 101-366, 104 Stat. 327, Jul 26, 1990 (Effective 1992).

39. Samborn R: A quiet birthday. *The National Law Journal*, 15:1, (1993).

40. *Anderson v. Little League Baseball, Inc.*, 794 E. Supp. 342 (1992).

41. Reynold GD: "Accessibility" means inclusive programs, *Aquatics International* 1993.

42. Priest L, Miller BB: Americans with disabilities—where are we today? *The National Aquatic Journal* 8:6-9, 1992.

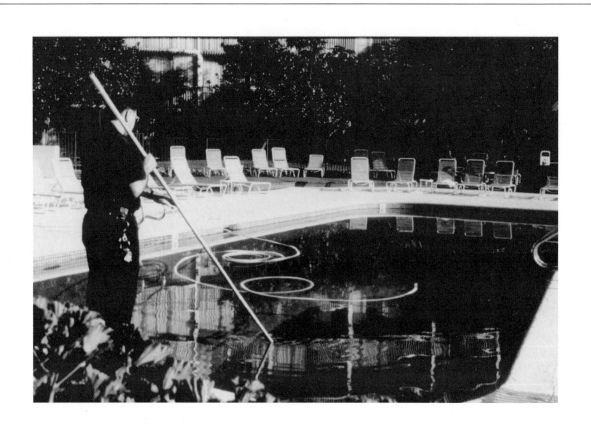

19

ROUTINE OPERATIONS: DAILY, WEEKLY, MONTHLY

Key Concepts

- *Record Keeping*
- *"Walk-Abouts"*
- *Opening Pools*
- *Closing Pools*
- *Maintenance*
- *Daily Routines*
- *Weekly Routines*
- *Monthly Routines*

Many important tasks must be performed by pool owners, operators, and managers. For experienced pool operators, many of these duties become habit and are an integral part of a daily, weekly, or monthly routine. It must be emphasized throughout this chapter, however, that check lists and records must be kept for up to 5 years on all operational tasks. In case a lawsuit is brought against the facility, facts and figures regarding the condition of the pool provide valuable information for the defense. Written procedures are also important because if the primary pool operator is unable to work due to illness or vacation, an assistant or lifeguard can perform these routines easily and correctly. (Written check lists are provided in Appendix. Whenever any of these procedures are completed, the date, time, and initials of the person completing the job should be recorded alongside the task on a check list.

The Pool "Walk-About"

Perhaps the most beneficial practice a pool owner or operator can perform is to evaluate the entire facility the first thing in the morning before the pool actu-

ally opens and the last thing at night after all patrons have left. This should be done slowly and carefully, without distractions. Carrying a clipboard to take notes at this time is helpful. Residential pool owners should also make this a practice. "Walk-abouts" should also be conducted during the day when the pool is in use but it is normally easier to spot deficiencies when the facility is quiet and calm. In addition, it allows the owner or operator more time to take corrective measures. Unfortunately, too many pool personnel rush through morning and evening procedures to simply open and close the pool on time. When this occurs, deficiencies often go unnoticed. The priorities when conducting the walk-about should be the pool water first, the filter room second, and the locker rooms and support facilities last.

Opening Procedures

Opening routines are critical, particularly at public pools. Bathing codes and local ordinances often supply lists of what must be done before opening and closing pools. Similar to the walk-abouts, when the pool is opened, the first to be checked is the pool water, followed by a trip to the filter room, and finally the locker rooms and other facilities.

The first priority when any swimming pool or spa is opened should be the condition of the water. "Is the water clear?" is the question all good pool operators ask themselves on arriving at the facility. If a 6-inch black disk or the main drain cannot be seen from everywhere on the pool deck, the pool or spa *must not* be opened. This particular water clarity standard is fairly consistent throughout the United States. If the water is not clear, corrective measures must be taken immediately so that clarity can be restored and the pool opened. The chemistry and filtration must both be checked in this case (Chapter 12).

Another priority is **water chemistry**. All chemical

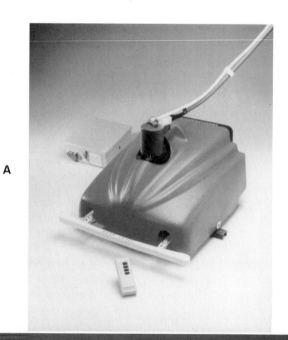

A

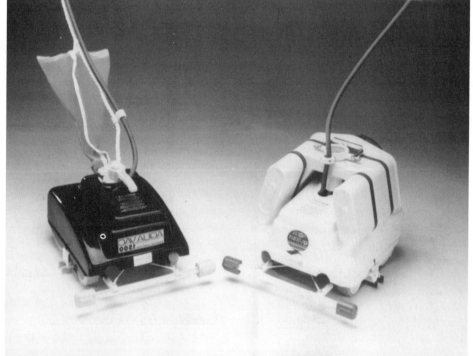

B

Fig. 19-1. **A,** remote control pool vacuum for large public pool. **B,** Electric pool vacuum for residential pools. (Courtesy Aqua Vac Systems, West Palm Beach, Fla.)

parameters should be within ideal ranges before the pool opens. If it is an outdoor pool and a hot, humid day is predicted, higher levels of free-available chlorinet (FAC) should be established earlier in the day so that when the sun and the swimmer loads are at their peaks, sufficient chlorine will be available. Particularly with chlorine and pH levels, it is important to get these readings where they should be before pools open, because once swimmers are in the pool, these levels are more difficult to control and adjust.

The **water level** is also an important factor when opening the pool. The level of the water should be sufficient to allow for a continuous skimming action either through skimmers or gutters. Water should be added immediately to ensure proper skimming action, and the amount of water should be recorded. This information is valuable when leaks are suspected. **Skimmer baskets** should be emptied before opening the pool or spa. The skimmer **weirs**, **baskets**, **equalizer lines**, and other associated parts should also be checked at this time.

All **drain covers** and **antivortex plates** must be in place. The general condition of the bottom is also important. Is **algae growth** visible? Is there any **debris** or **discoloration** in the water? The pool bottom should be checked for these concerns even though vacuuming may not be scheduled for that particular day.

One chore that must be completed before opening is **vacuuming** the pool bottom (Fig. 19-1). This task must be done after the water has been still for several hours so that particulate matter not oxidized or filtered can sink to the bottom. If performed in the evening shortly after the pool closes, dirt that has been disturbed by swimmers will still be suspended in the water. Although vacuuming is not required daily in many pools, it must be performed regularly and should follow a predetermined schedule. Many pools have a slow day, one in which the facility opens late or fewer patrons attend. This "off-day" or slow day, which is often Sunday, may allow sufficient time for proper vacuuming. Busy days may not provide adequate time for complete vacuuming.

Brushing the pool is almost as important as vacuuming and also should be done daily. Brushing is one of the best defenses against algae development in outdoor pools.

Once the pool water is monitored, the **filters** should then be checked. When the filter room is entered, the floor should be checked for standing water to ensure that filters and related equipment are not leaking. The **flow meter** should be checked and the flow rate recorded. If the **flow rate** is insufficient to provide the required **turnovers**, corrective measures should be taken immediately. When pressure filter systems are used, the pressure differential must be recorded daily, and this is best done before the pool opens. When the pool pump is checked, the noise and temperature of the pump are important. The **pump** should not be too hot or noisy. The pressure gauges on all pressure filters should then be checked to determine whether backwashing is needed. While backwashing, the **hair and lint strainer** should always be cleaned and checked. A clean, spare basket should always be immediately available, and the gasket and O-rings should always be checked during backwashing.

Cleaning or backwashing the filters should be done when swimmers are not in the water. It is best to perform this important function when the pool is closed so that distractions are not present. This is not always possible, however. Some experts prefer doing this chore in the evening. After the water filtration and chemistry is corrected or adjusted, the pool deck, lifeguard stands, pool equipment, and safety equipment should be readied for opening. The **pool deck** should be clear of water, obstructions, and other debris. Rescue equipment such as reaching poles, ring buoys, and rescue tubes, must be put into place before the pool opens.

Bathhouses, locker rooms, entrances, and other facilities also need special attention before opening the pool. These areas might be better prepared by a staff member who does not have water safety duties, although this might be financially imposing. These areas are best cleaned during the evening to allow adequate time for the floors to dry. Before the pool is opened, however, these areas must be carefully checked for standing water, debris, slippery spots, and adequate supplies.

Daily Routines

Once the pool is open, numerous tasks must be performed so that the pool and its equipment can be continually monitored. Of course, water chemistry must be checked diligently. Ideal ranges for any pool must agree with the swimming pool ordinances or bathing codes.

These ideal ranges should be posted and printed on

test kits, reports, and records so that anyone taking these readings will know whether they need to increase or decrease chemical levels. Typical chemical standards for swimming pools are as follows:

pH	7.2-7.8
FAC	1.0-3.0 ppm
Total available chlorinet (TAC)	No higher than 0.2 ppm above FAC
Combined available chlorine (CAC)	Less than 0.3 ppm
Oxygen reduction potential (ORP)	650-750 mv
Cyanuric acid (CYA)	20-30 ppm, no higher than 100 ppm (outdoor pools only)

The above readings should be taken hourly at busy public pools and perhaps every 2 hours at other pools. Water temperature, water clarity, weather conditions, and number of swimmers must also be recorded daily.

Although there are other chemical parameters that must be monitored, such as calcium hardness, total alkalinity, and the saturation index, they do not need to be measured daily because these values do not fluctuate as quickly. These measurements should be taken weekly at most pools.

Other daily tasks include the filtration process. The flow rate should be checked daily to ensure the proper turnovers. The filters must also be checked daily to see whether they require cleaning. Backwashing and other filter cleaning should be kept on the daily log along with the chemical readings.

Skimmers must be checked daily. However, depending on the season and geographical location of the pool, some skimmer baskets need to be emptied more frequently. When much organic debris is dropping into the pool, such as leaves or grass clippings, the skimmer baskets will need to be emptied several times each day.

The swimming pool deck should be cleaned daily. This may be done with a high-pressure washer or hose that not only does a superior job but also saves time. Decks are most often cleaned either before the pool opens or after the pool closes. Deck cleaning is performed at these times so that conflicts with swimmers and sunbathers can be avoided. Locker rooms, showers, and bathrooms must also be cleaned daily, but as mentioned earlier, these jobs are best performed before the pool opens. Deck furniture, lifesaving equipment, and any other associated apparatus must also be arranged before the opening of the pool.

Closing Routines

A walk-about is also strongly recommended shortly after the pool has closed for the day and all patrons have left. All rooms should be checked the doors are locked to be certain that no one is remaining in the facility. Bathroom stalls should be carefully checked to ensure that potential trespassers are not hiding there. Security lights must be turned on and all doors and gates must be locked. Both chemical readings and filtration readings should be taken for the last time. Chlorinators must be turned down or off, depending on the situation. All safety and programming equipment should be picked up and locked inside. Water temperature and clarity should also be recorded at this time, and the pool should be refilled with water as needed so that proper skimming action is maintained during the evening. All standing water, whether it be on the pool deck, in the locker rooms, or in the filter room, should be squeegeed off so that it does not create a problem for the morning shift. The flow rate should be recorded at this time, along with the pressure differential. Backwashing after the pool closes is a good idea. All debris including litter and lost and found articles must be removed after closing.

Weekly Routines

Water balancing should be a weekly routine. In addition to the daily chemical readings, total alkalinity and calcium hardness measurements must be taken each week. The **saturation index** should also be computed when these two values are found. The index should be recorded and corrective measures should be taken as soon as possible. The saturation index is perhaps one of the most overlooked tasks at pools (see Chapter 9).

In addition to balancing the water, most states require a **weekly bacteriological analysis** of the water. The water sample must be sent to a certified laboratory and may not exceed 200 bacteria/mm^3 in a standard plate count, and the total coliform count should not exceed 2.2/100 ml.

Another weekly duty is the sanitization of the pool deck and similar surfaces such as diving boards and locker room floors. Each of these surfaces can become very slippery if not disinfected regularly. When algae growth is a real problem, sanitizing these surfaces may be required more than once a week. However, if done well, weekly disinfecting should suffice.

In most pools, **shocking** should occur once a week, particularly if the pool is heavily used. This may be done either with a chlorine or nonchlorine shocking agent. It must be emphasized, however, that an accurate chloramine count is the only way to determine when shocking is needed. Shocking cannot take place with swimmers in the water.

A **scum line** or "bathtub" ring develops quickly around outdoor pools because of the large amounts of suntan lotion used. As a result, this line that occurs at the water level on the pool walls must be scrubbed cleaned regularly. The frequency of this chore varies with different pools, but typically, outdoor pools are scrubbed weekly, whereas indoor pools are scrubbed monthly. Spas and hot tubs, however, may have to be cleaned more often than once a week. Pool cleaners that will not scratch or destroy the finish of the pool must be used. Pool operators must be careful when selecting cleaners for this purpose; the cleaner must match the finish.

Any swimming pool apparatus that is secured to the deck or similar structure must be checked for sturdiness at least once a week. This includes **diving boards**, **ladders**, **lifeguard chairs**, and anything else that is bolted down. For instance, shaky ladders can easily cause accidents and lawsuits. At outdoor pools, umbrellas can become airborne during heavy winds. Because they can cause serious injuries, umbrellas must be tightly secured in place.

The filter room, guard room, first-aid room, front office, and similar facilities should be cleaned and organized at least once a week. Supplies that are missing and need to be replaced should also be noted. First-aid kits should also be replenished weekly. Lifeguard audits should also be conducted weekly.

Bulletin boards, phone recordings, and other information sources should be checked at least once a week to be certain that the data displayed are current.

Monthly

Unfortunately, many monthly tasks are often perceived as routines that should be done if time permits but in reality never get done. Monthly tasks should be assigned a specific date such as the first or fifteenth of every month or the first Monday of every month.

Chemical feeders should be cleaned monthly.

Particularly when pumping sodium hypochlorite or soda ash, chemical feeders tend to clog quickly. Gas chlorinators should also be checked. Manufacturer's recommendations for cleaning feeders must be followed. A common way of cleaning chemical feeders is as follows:

1. The feeder is turned off.
2. The foot valve and strainer are removed from the chemical solution it is pumping.
3. This assembly is placed in fresh water and pumped for 5 minutes to remove all chemicals.
4. The foot and strainer are placed in a 10% solution of muriatic acid, the pump is turned on, and at least a pint of the acid is run through the unit.
5. The assembly is removed from the acid solution and placed once again in fresh water to remove all acid from the unit. Pumping fresh water for at least 5 minutes should remove all acid before returning the unit to its original chemical solution.

Lighting should be checked at least once a month, as well as GFIs and fire extinguishers.

The **filter media** must also be checked monthly. If a sand filter is being used, the sand should be checked for mud balls or channeling or any other abnormality that may occur. Raking the sand clean and adding or replacing sand may also occur if the filter bed is inadequate. If a D.E. filter is used, the filter septa must be checked for tears or holes and repaired if necessary. When cartridge filters are used, they should be soaked at least once a month in a cleaner to remove excess oils.

Security checks of the facility are often conducted monthly. However, where security and vandalism are problems, this important routine may be done weekly or even daily. At outdoor pools, fences and gates are particularly important. Every barrier must be checked to be certain that trespassers cannot enter under or through gaps in the barrier. Doors, locks, and latches must also be checked regularly to ensure that they are in good working order. All security lights must be checked, as well as any electronic surveillance equipment.

Staff meetings, orientations, and review of emergency procedures should occur at least monthly. At crowded public pools, this important training procedure should be conducted more frequently. Whenever such a meeting takes place, attendance should be taken and a written record of the agenda should be kept for 5 years. This important information is critical during a lawsuit because it shows that the pool owner or operator kept the staff current with emergency procedures.

Typical topics to be covered during staff meetings are the following:

1. Problem areas that have recently arisen and review of customer complaints
2. Review of emergency procedures, which should include simulated rescues and back boarding procedures
3. Input from the staff regarding safety improvements and working conditions at the pool

MSDS sheets, first-aid kits, SCBA units, backboards, cervical collars, lifeguarding equipment, and similar safety apparatus should be checked between weekly and monthly depending on the type of pool.

Summary

This chapter has attempted to cover some of the more important routines that should be conducted at aquatic facilities. Not all operational procedures are covered in this section. Each pool is different. Therefore each pool needs specific routines that are customized. Using the check lists provided in the back of this book will help, but unique procedures and routines should be added. All records, logs, and check lists used at a pool should be kept for a minimum of 5 years in case an insurance claim or lawsuit is brought against the facility.

Bibliography

American Pool Service, *Pool operations manual*, Lanham, Md, 1990, The Service.

Clayton RD, Thomas DG: *Professional aquatic management*, ed 2, Champaign, Ill, 1989, Human Kinetics.

Gabrielson AM: *Swimming pools: a guide to their planning, design, and operation*, ed 4, Champaign, Ill, 1987 Human Kinetics.

Johnson R: *Swimming pool operations*, Harrisburg, Pa, Department of Community Affairs.

Kowalsky L (editor): *Pool/spa operators handbook*, San Antonio, Tex, 1991, National Swimming Pool Foundation.

NSPI: *The sensible way to enjoy your pool*, Alexandria, Va, 1983, The Institute.

Pope JR Jr: *Public swimming pool management*, I and II, Alexandria, Va, National Recreation and Park Association.

Williams KG: *The aquatic facility operator's manual*, Hoffman Estates, Ill, 1991, National Recreation and Park Association, National Aquatic Section.

Review Questions

1. What priority items must be checked before opening a pool?

2. What priority areas must be checked before closing a pool?

3. How often should a saturation index be calculated?

4. Why do chemical feeders need to be cleaned regularly?

SECTION VI
PESTICIDE SAFETY AND EDUCATION

In 1947 the Federal Insecticide, Fungicide, and Rodenticide Act (FIFRA) was enacted to regulate the use of pesticides. In 1977 FIFRA was amended, creating a certified pesticide applicator classification, and grouping pesticides into two categories, general and restricted use. General use pesticides are those that can be purchased and used by the general public. Restricted use pesticides may be purchased and used only by certified applicators or by someone under the supervision of a certified applicator. To become certified, a pesticide applicator must pass a training course approved by the Environmental Protection Agency (EPA). At the federal level FIFRA establishes *minimum* standards for pesticide use; individual states may mandate more stringent requirements.

In Pennsylvania pesticide use is regulated by the Pest Control Act. This Act was originally passed in 1973 and amended in 1990. As a result of the 1990 amendments the Department of Agriculture in the State of Pennsylvania requires all individuals who *commercially* apply pesticides, including algaecides, and chlorine, to have a pesticide applicator's license. Some states only require pesticide applicators to be licensed when making applications of restricted use pesticides, which are potentially more hazardous to humans and/or the environment than general use pesticides.

Pennsylvania, a leader in pesticide safety and education, requires that commercial applicators who are using both general use and restricted use pesticides must be licensed. If other states follow Pennsylvania's lead (and the District of Columbia already has), many pool operators will be required to have additional training in the safe handling and application of pesticides.

The information provided in this section is taken directly from the Penn State University *Pesticide Education Manual* developed in the College of Agriculture Sciences by Winand K. Hock and Cynthia L. Brown and received a Blue Ribbon Award from the American Society of Agricultural Engineers in its 1993 educational aids competition. Kerry Hoffman, Pesticide Education Coordinator, has provided valuable assistance and information to the author. The following chapters are merely a sample of available information that is most directly related to swimming pool applications. for more information regarding pesticide safety in your state, contact the State Department of Agriculture office.

20

FEDERAL AND PENNSYLVANIA PESTICIDE LAWS

Chemical pesticide use has increased sharply during the past 35 years, not only in the United States but worldwide. The benefits of pesticides to humans have been demonstrated. They have helped control malaria and other insect-vectored diseases; they have helped increase the yield and quality of numerous crops, resulting in more food and fiber for more people; and they have helped control nuisance pests. However, the wide scale use—and misuse—of pesticides is of worldwide concern because of associated human health and environmental problems.

Both the United States Congress and the Pennsylvania Legislature have enacted legislation that regulates the production, transportation, sale, use, and disposal of pesticides. The Federal Insecticide, Fungicide, and Rodenticide Act (FIFRA), first enacted in 1947, was amended significantly in 1972, then again in 1975, 1978, and 1988. This statute is administered by the U.S. Environmental Protection Agency (EPA). The Pennsylvania Pesticide Control Act of 1973 (Act 24) became law March 1, 1974, and became fully operational in October, 1977. This statute was amended significantly in December 1986 with the passage of Act 167.

Purpose of Pesticide Laws

In order to protect the public health and welfare and to prevent adverse effects on the environment, it is essential that pesticides be regulated. The purpose of the federal and state pesticide acts is to regulate in the best public interest, the labeling, sale and distribution, storage, transportation, use and application, and the disposal of pesticides. In essence, pesticides are under regulatory scrutiny from the time of their

From Hock WK, Brown CL (editors): *Pesticide education manual*, ed 2, University Park, Penn, Penn State University.

inception in the laboratory to their ultimate use in the field or their disposal in an approved manner. With the possible exception of human and veterinary drugs, no other class of chemicals receives such extensive testing in the United States prior to being registered and marketed.

Federal Insecticide, Fungicide, and Rodenticide Act (FIFRA), as Amended

The following are some of the major provisions of FIFRA and how they affect you.

The EPA can stop the sale or use of any hazardous pesticide. The EPA has the authority to issue removal orders and to seize products to keep them off the market.

State restrictions on pesticides cannot be more liberal than those of FIFRA. Individual states may impose stricter regulations on a pesticide, except the labeling and packaging must be uniform nationwide. Uniform packaging standards include container type, size, and color. Regulations provide for the disposal of pesticide containers and surplus or unwanted pesticides.

The applicator is not permitted to use any pesticide for any use other than that stated on the label, except those specific exemptions granted under regulations of the amended Pennsylvania Pesticide Control Act and Section 2 (ee) of FIFRA (described in the chapter, "The Pesticide Label"). No pesticide can be registered or offered for sale unless its labeling provides for reasonable safeguards to prevent injury to humans and adverse effects on the environment.

All pesticides are classified according to their potential hazards under those circumstances in which they are to be used. Two classifications are general use and restricted use.

General use pesticides generally have lower toxicity with less potential hazard to humans and the environment than restricted use chemicals. They can be bought and used by the general public without special permit or restriction. They must, however, always be used according to label directions.

Restricted use pesticides may be sold only to certified applicators and must be used only by those applicators or by persons working under their direct supervision. Restricted use pesticides and their uses are often quite hazardous to humans and/or the environment. Applicators must know how to use them properly.

It is important to note that under the amended state law, both commercial and public applicators must be certified, or work under the direct supervision of a certified applicator, to apply either general or restricted use pesticides to properties of another, and in some instances to their own property.

Some active ingredients in pesticides may be listed in both use categories, depending upon the formulation, the application method, and the intended uses. An emulsifiable concentrate formulation of a certain insecticide, for example, might be restricted use if applied by aircraft for a soybean pest. But, the same chemical with a lower percentage of active ingredient in a granular formulation could be general use if used as a soil treatment for turf pests.

The certification process by all the states and territories must be accomplished through EPA-approved programs. Each state is responsible for implementing the certification program. In Pennsylvania, the Department of Agriculture (PDA) is responsible for administering this program.

Although specific restrictions and circumstances may vary, pesticide manufacturers, dealers, transporters, and applicators are all subject to penalties for violations of FIFRA and the Pennsylvania Pesticide Control Act.

Pennsylvania Pesticide Control Act of 1973, as Amended

The amended Pennsylvania Pesticide Control Act is a companion bill to FIFRA. The state act defines how FIFRA and the state statute will be administered and regulated. Copies of the specific rules and regulations of the act can be obtained by contacting an office of the PDA. The major aspects of the act include the following:

Section 3: Declaration of purpose

"The legislature hereby finds that pesticides are valuable to our State's agriculture production and to the protection of man and the environment from insects, rodents, weeds, and other forms of life which may be pests; but it is essential to the public health and welfare that they be regulated to prevent adverse effects on human life and the environment. The purpose of this act is to regulate in the public interest, the labeling, distribution, storage, transportation, use, application, and disposal of pesticides. New pesticides are continually being discovered or synthesized which are valuable for the control of pests, and for use as defoliants, desiccants, plant regulators, and related purposes. The dissemination of accurate scientific information as to the proper use of any pesticide is vital to the public health and welfare and to the environment both immediate and future."

Section 4: Definitions

This section defines the terms used in this act including certified applicator, private applicator, commercial applicator, public applicator, pesticide application technician, and "under the direct supervision of a certified commercial or public applicator."

Section 5.1: Registration

Every pesticide used in Pennsylvania must first be registered with the PDA.

Section 6: Refusal to register, cancellation, suspension, legal recourse

- The Secretary (of Agriculture) may refuse to register a pesticide if it does not meet its proposed claims.
- The Secretary may cancel the registration of a pesticide following a judicial review if the registration does not comply with the act.
- A pesticide may be suspended from use if it presents an imminent hazard.

Section 7: Determinations: rules and regulations; classified for restricted use; and uniformity

The Secretary is authorized to adopt a list of restricted use pesticides for the Commonwealth. This list contains all those pesticides classified by the EPA for restricted use and those added by the Secretary to protect the health and welfare of the citizens of the Commonwealth.

Section 8: Prohibited acts

- No one shall deliver or transport within Pennsylvania any pesticide unless it is in a sound original container with a label attached.
- "No person shall use, or cause to be used, any pesticide inconsistent with its labelling. . . ."
- "No person shall handle, transport, store, display, or distribute pesticides in such manner as to endanger persons or the environment or endanger food, feed, or any other products that may be transported, stored, displayed or distributed with such pesticides." For example, do not transport bags of toxic insecticides on top of a load of livestock feed or store with bags of feed.
- "No person shall dispose of, discard, or store any pesticide or pesticide containers in such manner as to cause injury to humans, vegetation, crops, livestock, wildlife, or pollinating insects or pollute any water supply or waterway."
- "No person shall operate pesticide application equipment or devices in a faulty, careless or negligent manner."
- No individual shall purchase or attempt to purchase a pesticide classified for restricted use, unless the individual is a certified applicator.
- No one shall refuse to keep and maintain required records on the transportation, sale, and use of pesticides.
- No person shall engage in the business of applying pesticides on the lands of another without first obtaining a current, valid license pursuant to the provisions of this act.

Section 9: Denial, suspension, and revocation of licenses, permits, and certificates

Persons found in violation of the Act or its regulations may have their applicator's certification suspended or revoked after being given an opportunity to present their views to the Secretary.

Section 10: Stop sale, use, or removal order

If there is reasonable cause to believe that a pesticide is being used in violation of the act, the Secretary is authorized to stop the sale and use of such material.

Section 12: Pesticide dealer license

All pesticide dealers who sell restricted use pesticides must be licensed and maintain required records of sales.

Section 13: Pest management consultant license

All pest management consultants must be licensed.

Section 14: Examination for pest management consultant license

Pest management consultants are required to pass a written examination.

Section 15.1: Pesticide application license

Each business, public utility, government agency, etc. applying or contracting for the application of pesticides, which meets the definition of a commercial applicator, must obtain a pesticide application license (business license) for those categories in which it is doing business. A certified applicator must be employed by the business, utility, or agency at all times. Furthermore, the business, utility, or agency must provide evidence of financial responsibility to PDA before a license may be issued.

Section 16.1: Standards of qualifications for certification of commercial applicators

Individuals shall become certified upon the successful completion of a written examination in basic core knowledge and in each category in which the individual desires to become certified. A fee will be charged for the examinations. Attendance at PDA approved courses will result in the accumulation of credits which will be applied to recertification requirements.

Section 16.2: Procedures to register pesticide application technicians with PDA

Noncertified employees of any business or public agency must be registered as pesticide application technicians when these employees apply pesticides without a certified applicator physically present at the application site.

Section 17.1: Public applicators

Persons applying pesticides as employees of any unit of a federal, state, or local government agency must comply with Section 16.1 and 16.2 of this act. A certification will be charged.

Section 17.2: Private applicators

This section affects almost every Pennsylvania farmer. A private applicator is defined as "a certified applicator who uses or supervises the use of any pesticide which is classified as restricted use for purposes of producing any agricultural commodity on property owned or rented by him or his employer or (if applied without compensation other than trading of personal services between producers of agricultural commodities) on the property of another person." A private applicator must pass a proctored, written examination administered by the PDA to become certified and issued a permit. The permit shall remain valid for three years and recertification can be accomplished by attending approved update training programs and accumulating the required recertification credits.

Section 20: Reports of pesticide accidents, incidents, or loss

Significant pesticide accidents or incidents must be reported. A significant pesticide accident or incident is one which creates danger to human beings or results in damage to plant or animal life.

Section 21: Inspection of equipment

Equipment used for application of pesticides may be inspected.

Section 22: Reciprocal agreement

Certification of applicators may be on a reciprocal basis with other states.

Section 23.1: Temporary suspensions

The Secretary may temporarily suspend a license or certificate for just cause issued under Act 24 as amended.

Section 24: Storage and disposal of cancelled pesticides

Pennsylvania will use the procedures and regulations of the EPA for the safe disposal or storage of any pesticide that has had its registration cancelled.

Section 25: Pesticide advisory board

The Governor will appoint members to a Pesticide Advisory Board to advise the Secretary on problems relating to the use and application of pesticides in the Commonwealth.

Section 25.1: Additional regulatory authority

The Secretary shall prepare regulations for the following application situations:
- Prior public notification for the aerial application of restricted use pesticides to rights-of-way.
- Prior notification by commercial applicators to individuals residing in dwellings on lands imme-

diately adjacent to a restricted use pesticide application site.
- The prohibition of the application of restricted use pesticides within 100 feet of certain publicly owned or designated environmentally sensitive lands.

Section 27: Information

For the purpose of dispensing information needed in certification and other areas, the Secretary may cooperate with The Pennsylvania State University or any other public educational institution and industry association.

Section 29: Criminal penalties

This section discusses criminal penalties for unlawful conduct under the act.

Section 30.1: Civil penalties

This section discusses the civil penalties the Secretary may assess upon an individual or business.

Section 33: Enforcement

Pesticide inspectors are authorized to sample and examine pesticides or devices on any public or private premises. They may also:
- Have access to inspect pesticide application equipment
- Inspect lands exposed to pesticides
- Inspect storage and disposal areas
- Inspect or investigate complaints of injury to humans and land
- Sample pesticides being applied or to be applied

Section 35: Records

The Secretary may require records to be kept by persons issued a license, certificate, or permit under the act.

Section 37: Delegation of duties; exclusion of local laws and regulations

This act and all its various provisions are of statewide concern and, therefore, involve the whole field of regulation, distribution, notification of use, and use of pesticides to the exclusion of all local regulations and ordinances.

Additional Federal and State Laws

The following federal and state laws also regulate pesticides. The Resource Conservation and Recovery

SETTLEMENTS OF ACTUAL LEGAL CASES

Under the amended Pennsylvania Pesticide Control Act, the Pennsylvania Department of Agriculture has the responsibility to investigate pesticide incidents. This requires the determination of causes, remedies, and whether regulatory action should be taken. The following are summaries of some actual incidents. Each was a violation of a prohibited act in Section 8 and resulted in an enforcement action.

Case 1

Several cases of herbicide and bags of insecticide were being transported on a flatbed truck. The cases were stacked higher than the truck sideboards and approximately ten cases of liquid herbicide fell from the truck, resulting in a herbicide spill on a public highway. The responsible party was cited for "transporting pesticides in such a manner as to endanger the environment."

Case 2

An application of a nonselective, root absorbed herbicide was made to brush and woody weeds along a utility right-of-way. There was root uptake by several large spruce trees on a neighboring property outside the right-of-way border. The products label warns the user not to apply the herbicide where desirable species of vegetation may have root systems in the treated areas. This violation of the label resulted in severe injury or death of the affected trees. The applicator was cited for use of a pesticide "inconsistent with its labeling."

Case 3

A private residence was treated by an exterminator with a rodenticide. Two dogs belonging to the homeowner died soon after the treatment. Tissue analyses did not reveal any pesticide residues in the animals so the cause of their deaths remained unknown. The applicator, however, was cited for handling a pesticide "in such a manner as to endanger man or his environment." The bait had not been placed in tamper-proof bait stations and was found in locations easily accessible to children and pets.

Case 4

A termiticide was sprayed by an exterminator on the interior surfaces of a root cellar. Label instructions permit the termiticide to be used only for subterranean injection into soil or foundation walls. The applicator was cited for using a product "inconsistent with the labelling," and "in such a manner as to endanger persons or food."

Case 5

Following an application of an agricultural herbicide, a tractor drawn spray rig was hosed down behind a farm building. The farm building was located uphill and bordering a neighbor's property. Injury to the neighbor's lawn resulted from surface runoff of the rinse solution. The applicator was cited for "disposing of a pesticide in such a manner as to cause injury to vegetation."

Act (RCRA) regulates the disposal of hazardous wastes. It is administered by the EPA nationally and the Pennsylvania Department of Environmental Resources.

The Superfund Amendments and Reauthorization Act of 1986 (SARA) of which Title III is commonly known as the Emergency Planning and Community Right-to-Know Act of 1986 establishes procedures for emergency planning preparedness and reporting of specific quantities of stored or spilled hazardous chemicals, including pesticides. It is administered by the EPA nationally and the Pennsylvania Emergency Management Agency in Pennsylvania. Each county also has an emergency planning committee.

The Transportation Safety Act of 1974 regulates the transport of hazardous materials, and establishes rules for packing, handling, labeling, placarding, and routing. It is administered by the Pennsylvania Department of Transportation.

The Pennsylvania Worker and Community Right to Know Law requires that employers provide employees and other interested parties with certain pesticide use and safety information. It is administered by the Pennsylvania Department of Labor and Industry.

The Clean Streams Law and the Fish Laws regulate the use of pesticides in any aquatic environment and are administered by the Pennsylvania Fish and Boat Commission.

Bibliography

See end of Chapter 24.

21

THE PESTICIDE LABEL

One of the more important tools for the safe and effective use of pesticides is the product label. Pesticide manufactures are required by law to put certain information on the label, information which when not heeded and followed can result in a pesticide accident and legal action against the violator. *Labels are legal documents* providing directions on how to mix, apply, store, and dispose of a pesticide product.

Labels are not exclusive to pesticide chemicals. Most products purchased and used daily (including breakfast cereal, furniture polish, mouthwash, laundry detergent, paints and food items) bear labels which identify the product, its purpose, details on use, the manufacturer, and other information.

The label is the main means available to the manufacturer to communicate information about the product to the user.

The Background of the Label

To appreciate the value of the information on a pesticide label, consider the time, effort, and money spent in gathering it. The information on a product label is the result of years of research by scientists from both laboratory and field tests. This information takes a minimum of six years to obtain and costs a chemical company millions of dollars. Chemical companies continually make new compounds and then screen them in the laboratory and greenhouse for possible pesticide use. For each material that finally meets the standards of a potential pesticide, thou-

From Hock WK, Brown CL (editors): Pesticide education manual, ed 2, University Park, Penn, Penn State University.

sands of other compounds are screened and discarded for various reasons. When a promising pesticide is discovered, its potential use must be evaluated. If the company believes it has a worthwhile product and there is a strong possibility for a significant sales market, wide-scale testing and label registration procedures are begun. In the development and labeling of a pesticide, scientists and registration specialists are interested in not only proving that the chemical will control pests, but also that it will not cause unreasonable adverse effects.

Many kinds of carefully controlled tests must be done to determine the effectiveness and safety of each pesticide under a wide range of environmental conditions.

Toxicity and toxicological tests

How poisonous or dangerous is a pesticide to humans, wildlife, and other organisms? Does the chemical cause any long term or chronic effects? Will the test chemical cause any skin or dermal reactions? To determine these and other health effects, the pesticide is administered at different dosages to test animals, usually rats and mice. These toxicological tests alone often will cost the company several million dollars to complete.

Efficacy or performance tests

Does the pesticide control the target pest? The company must have performance data to show that the pesticide will control a particular pest or group of pests on one or more hosts or sites, including plants, animals, soil, and structures. Data must show that the pesticide, when used for its intended purpose and according to directions, is a useful product.

Information is also needed on crop varieties, soil

types, application methods and rates, and number of required applications. Tests must show that the pests are controlled, crops or animals are not injured, yield and/or quality has been improved, and that the pesticide definitely provides a worthwhile benefit.

Degradation, mobility, and residue tests

What happens to the pesticide after it is applied? A series of studies is needed to show how long it takes for the compound to break down (degrade) into harmless materials under various conditions. Does it move through soil to groundwater? Does it move into the plant from the treated soil?

Residue studies are conducted for each method of application on each treated crop or animal. These tests determine how much, if any, of the pesticide residue (or its breakdown product) remains on or in the crop or animal. From these data, the number of days from the last pesticide application until harvest or slaughter is determined. A residue *tolerance* or the maximum amount of a pesticide residue that may legally remain on or in food or feed at harvest or slaughter, is established by the United States Environmental Protection Agency (EPA).

A residue tolerance is set for a pesticide on each crop or commodity. Tolerances are expressed in "parts per million" (PPM).

For example, the tolerance for carbaryl (Sevin) insecticide on blackberries is 12.0 ppm; on blueberries 10.0 ppm.; while in poultry the tolerance is only 5.0 ppm. Pesticide residues on or in food or feed commodities must not exceed the residue tolerance limits when the crop or animal (including meat, milk, and eggs) is ready for market or livestock feeding. If a residue is over the tolerance limit, the commodity can be condemned and destroyed.

Effects on wildlife and environment

The chemical company must determine the effects of field applications of the pesticide on wildlife and the environment. Any potentially harmful effects on wildlife and the environment that are recognized during these studies must be included in the environmental impact statement submitted to the EPA.

EPA label review

The chemical company is now ready to take these data to the EPA for review. The chemical company asks for pesticide "use registrations" on as many crops, animals, or other application sites as it has pest management test data to support its claims. The label must be approved by EPA before a product can be marketed.

Parts of the Label

Some labels are easy to understand; others are complicated. It is the user's responsibility to read and understand the label before buying, using, storing, or disposing of a pesticide. Each of the label components will be discussed in this section.

Trade, brand, or product names

Every manufacturer has trade names for its products. Most companies register each trade name as a trademark and will not allow any other company to use that name without permission. Different trade names are used by different manufacturers, even though the products contain the same active ingredient. The brand or trade name shows up plainly on the front panel of the label and is the one used in advertisements and by company salespersons.

The brand name often indicates the type of formulation and the percentage of active ingredient present. For example, Sevin 50WP is a brand name. Sevin is the registered trade name and the formulation is a wettable powder containing 50 percent active ingredient.

Ingredient statement

Every pesticide label must list every active ingredient and its percentage in the container. Inert ingredients are not usually named, but the label must show what percentage of the total contents they comprise. The ingredient statement must list the official chemical names and/or common names of the active ingredients. Let's look at the following Sevin insecticide example:

Sevin 50WP
Active ingredient:
carbaryl (1-naphthyl N-methyl carbamate)—50%
Inert ingredients—50%

The *chemical name* is the complex name that identifies the chemical components and structure of the pesticide. This name must be listed in the ingredient statement on the label. For example, the chemical name of Sevin is 1-naphthyl N-methyl carbamate.

Because chemical names are usually complex, many are given a shorter *common name*. Only those common names officially accepted by the EPA may be used in the ingredient statement on the pesticide label. The official common name is usually followed by the chemical name in the list of active ingredients. The common name for Sevin is carbaryl. By purchasing pesticides according to the common or chemical names, you will be certain of getting the right active ingredient, no matter what the brand name or formulation.

Use classification statement

Every pesticide product is classified by the EPA as either *Restricted Use* or *Unclassified/General Use*. Every pesticide product that is federally classified as restricted use must include the following statement in a prominent place on the front panel of the pesticide label:

Restricted use pesticide

For retail sale to and use only by certified applicators or persons under their direct supervision and only for those uses covered by the certified applicator's certification.

Pesticides labeled for restricted use warrant special attention. Many pesticides are designated as restricted use products if there is reason to believe they could harm humans, livestock, wildlife, or the environment, even when used according to label directions. Persons using these products need special training and a certain level of competence to ensure they can handle these pesticides properly. The restricted use statement may indicate why the pesticide has been classified as such.

Type of pesticide

The type of pesticide is usually listed on the front panel of the pesticide label. This short statement indicates in general terms what the product will control. Examples:

- insecticide for control of certain insects on fruits, nuts, and ornamentals
- herbicide for the control of woody brush and weeds

Net contents

The front panel of the pesticide label shows how much product is in the container. This is expressed as pounds or ounces for dry formulations or as gallons, quarts, or pints for liquids. Liquid formulations may also list the pounds of active ingredient per gallon of product. Many labels now also include metric units (grams, kilograms, liters) as part of the contents information.

Name and address of manufacturer

The law requires that the manufacturer or formulator of a product put the name and address of the company on the label. This is so you will know who made or sold the product.

Emergency telephone number

Many pesticide manufacturers include an emergency telephone number on their product labels. These companies are ready to assist anyone in the event of an emergency (poisoning, spill, fire) involving their products.

Registration number

An EPA registration number (for example, EPA Reg. No. 3120-280) must appear on all pesticide labels. This indicates that the pesticide product has been registered and its label approved by the EPA. In cases of special local needs, pesticide products may be approved for use in a specific state. An example of such a registration is EPA SLN No. PA-910002. In this case, SLN indicates "special local need" and PA means that the product is registered for use in Pennsylvania.

Establishment numbers

An EPA establishment number (for example, EPA Est. No. 5840-AZ-1) must also appear on the pesticide label to identify the facility that produced the product. This is necessary in case a problem arises or the product is adulterated in any way.

Signal words and symbols

Every pesticide label must include a signal word. This important designation gives the user an indication of the relative acute toxicity of the product to humans and animals.

The signal word must appear in large letters on the front panel of the pesticide label along with the statement, "Keep Out of Reach of Children." The following signal words may be found on pesticide labels:

- **DANGER-POISON**, skull and crossbones symbol—These words and symbol must appear on all products that are highly toxic by any route of entry into the body. Peligro, the Spanish word for danger, must also appear on the label.
- **DANGER**—Products with this signal word can cause severe eye damage or skin irritation.
- **WARNING**—This word signals that the product is moderately toxic either orally, dermally, or through inhalation; or causes moderate eye and

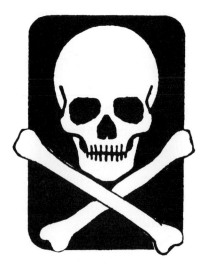

skin irritation. Aviso, the Spanish word for warning, must also appear on the label.

- **CAUTION**—This word signals that the product is slightly toxic either orally, dermally, or through inhalation; or causes slight eye and skin irritation.

Signal words can be used to choose the least toxic chemical that will give the desired level of pest control. The chapter "Toxicity and Health" also provides information about signal words.

Precautionary statements

All pesticide labels contain additional statements to help applicators decide what precautions to take to protect themselves, their employees, and other persons (or animals) that could be exposed. Sometimes these statements are listed under the heading, "Hazards to Humans and Domestic Animals." They may be composed of several sections.

Routes of entry statements

These statements indicate which route or routes of entry (mouth, skin, lungs) are particularly hazardous. Many pesticide products are hazardous by more than one route, so study these statements carefully. A DANGER signal word followed by "May be fatal if swallowed or inhaled" gives you a far different warning than, DANGER followed by "Corrosive—Causes eye damage and severe skin burns."

Typical DANGER label statements include:
- Fatal if swallowed
- Poisonous if inhaled
- Extremely hazardous by skin contact—rapidly absorbed through skin

- Corrosive—causes eye damage and severe skin burns Routes of entry statements are not uniform on all labels and many variations are found. More than one or even all four precautions may be stated on a label.

Typical WARNING label statements include:
- Harmful or fatal if swallowed
- Harmful or fatal if absorbed through the skin
- Harmful or fatal if inhaled
- Causes skin and eye irritation

Typical CAUTION label statements include:
- Harmful if swallowed
- May be harmful if inhaled
- May irritate eyes, nose, throat, and skin

Specific action statements

These statements usually follow the route of entry statements. The specific action statements recommend specific precautions to take and protective clothing and equipment to wear to reduce exposure to the pesticide. These statements are directly related to the toxicity of the pesticide product (signal word) and the routes of entry. DANGER labels typically contain statements such as:
- Do not breathe vapors or spray mist
- Do not get on skin or clothing
- Do not get in eyes

Typical WARNING labels combine specific action statements from DANGER and CAUTION labels.

CAUTION labels generally contain specific action statements which are less threatening than those on the DANGER label, indicating that the toxicity hazard is not as great:
- Avoid contact with skin or clothing
- Avoid breathing dust, vapors, or spray mists
- Avoid getting in eyes

Protective clothing and equipment statements

Pesticide labels vary in the type of information they contain on protective clothing and equipment. Some labels carry no such statement at all. Other pesticide labels fully describe appropriate protective clothing and equipment. A few list the kinds of respirators which should be worn when handling and applying the product; others require the use of a respirator but do not specify a type or model. Follow all advice on protective clothing or equipment which appears on the label. However, the lack of such a statement or the mention of only one piece of equipment does not rule out the need for additional protection. To determine the proper type of protective clothing and equipment needed, consider the signal word, the route of entry statements, and the specific action statements Read the basic guidelines described in the chapters "Toxicity and Health" and "Using Pesticides Safely."

Other precautionary statements

Labels often list other precautions that should always be followed when handling the product. These are self-explanatory:

- Do not contaminate food or feed
- Remove and wash contaminated clothing before reuse
- Wash thoroughly after handling and before eating or smoking
- Wear clean clothes daily
- Not for use or storage in and around a house
- Do not allow children or domestic animals into the treated area

These are common sense statements. The absence from the label of such statements does not indicate that these precautions should be ignored.

Statement of practical treatment

This section lists first-aid treatments recommended in case of poisoning. Typical statements include:

- In case of contact with skin, wash immediately with plenty of soap and water
- In case of contact with eyes, flush with water for 15 minutes and get medical attention
- In case of inhalation exposure, remove victim from contaminated area and give artificial respiration, if necessary
- If swallowed, induce vomiting

All DANGER labels and some WARNING and CAUTION labels contain a note to physicians describing the appropriate medical procedures and antidotes for poisoning emergencies. The label should always be available in emergencies.

Environmental hazards

Pesticides can be harmful to the environment. Some products are classified restricted use because of their environmental hazards. Watch for special warning statements on the label concerning hazards to the environment.

Special toxicity statements

If a particular pesticide is especially hazardous to wildlife, it will be stated on the label. For example:

- This product is highly toxic to bees

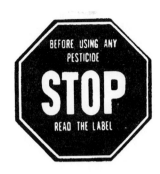

- This product is toxic to fish
- This product is toxic to birds and other wildlife

These statements alert pesticide users to the special hazards posed by a product. They should help applicators choose the safest product for a particular job and remind them to take extra precautions.

General environmental statements

Some of these statements appear on virtually every pesticide label. They are reminders to follow certain common sense procedures to avoid contaminating the environment. The absence of any or all of these statements does not indicate that you do not need to take adequate precautions. Sometimes these statements follow a "specific toxicity statement" and provide practical steps to avoid harm to wildlife. Examples of general environmental statements include:

- Do not apply when runoff is likely to occur
- Do not apply when weather conditions favor drift from treated areas
- Do not contaminate water by improperly disposing of rinsewater and other pesticide wastes
- Do not apply when bees are likely to be in the area

Physical or chemical hazards

This section of the label describes any special fire, explosion, or chemical hazards the product may pose. For example:

- Flammable—Do not use, pour, spill, or store near heat or open flame. Do not cut or weld container.
- Corrosive—Store only in a corrosion-resistant tank.

Hazard statements (hazards to humans and domestic animals, environmental hazards, and physical or chemical hazards) are not located in the same place on all pesticide labels. Some labels group them under the headings listed above. Other labels list them on the front panel beneath the signal word. Still other labels list the hazards in paragraph form somewhere else on the label under headings such as "Note" or "Important." Prior to use, the label should be examined carefully for these statements to ensure that the product is handled properly and safely.

Reentry statement

Some pesticide labels contain a reentry interval statement. The information tells how much time must pass between the last application of a pesticide and when people can reenter a treated area without wearing appropriate protective clothing and equipment. Reentry intervals are set by both the EPA and some states. Reentry intervals set by states are not always listed on the label; it is your responsibility to determine if one has been established by state pesticide regulatory officials. It is illegal to ignore these reentry intervals.

The reentry statement may be printed in a box under the heading "Reentry" or it may be in a section with a title such as "Important," or "Note," or "General Information."

For field applications—if no reentry statement appears on the label or none has been set by your state, then all unprotected persons must wait at least until sprays have dried or dusts have settled before reentering without protective equipment.

For all other types of pesticide applications—be sure to follow label directions regarding reentry.

Storage and disposal

All pesticide labels contain general instructions for the appropriate storage and disposal of the pesticide and its container. State and local laws may vary considerably, so specific instructions usually are not included. One or more statements may appear in a special section of the label titled "Storage and Disposal" or under headings such as "Important," "Note," or "General Instructions."
These include:
- Store herbicides away from fertilizers, insecticides, fungicides, and seeds.
- Store at temperatures above 32°F (0°C).
- Do not reuse container; render unusable, then burn or bury in a safe place.
- Do not contaminate water, food, or feed by storage or disposal.
- Triple-rinse and dispose in an approved landfill or bury in a safe place.

Seek sound advice if needed to determine the best storage and disposal procedures for your operation and location. Read this section before you purchase the product to be sure you can meet the requirements.

Directions for use

These instructions provide the directions on how to use the product. The use instructions will tell you:
- The pests which the manufacturer claims the product will control
- The crop, animal, or site the product is intended to protect
- The proper mixing instructions
- How much to use (rate) and how often
- How close to harvest the product can be applied
- Phytotoxicity and other possible injury
- Where and when the material should be applied

It is illegal and considered a misuse to use any registered pesticide in a manner inconsistent with its labeling. Examples of pesticide misuse include applying a pesticide to a site that is not listed on the label, applying a pesticide at a higher-than-labeled rate, and handling a pesticide in a manner that is in violation of specific label instructions (i.e., storage near food or water, improper container disposal.) In some instances, however, use of a pesticide in a manner that is not described by the label directions is allowable and not considered a violation of the label.

The Federal Insecticide, Fungicide, and Rodenticide Act, as amended, and certain rules and regulations under the authority of the amended Pennsylvania Pesticide Control Act of 1973 have been modified to exclude the following application procedures from "use inconsistent with product labeling." In other words,

1. a pesticide may be applied to control a target pest not specified on the label, provided the pesticide is applied to a crop, animal, or site specifically listed on the label.
2. any method of application may be used which is not prohibited by the label.
3. a pesticide may be applied at a dosage, concentration, or frequency less than that specified on the label.
4. a pesticide-fertilizer mixture may be used if the mixture is not prohibited by the label.

Labels for agricultural pesticides often list *preharvest intervals* (days to harvest) and/or *preslaughter intervals*. These are the minimum number of days which must pass between the last application of a pesticide and harvest of crops or the slaughter or grazing of livestock. Intervals are set by EPA to allow time for the pesticide to break down on or in the crop or in the meat of livestock. Adhering to these intervals prevents possible poisoning of grazing animals and prevents residues greater than the EPA approved tolerance on food, feed, or animal products.

Many terms are used on labels to describe when and how to use pesticides. Many technical terms are also found in leaflets and bulletins that you may get from your local cooperative extension office, land-grant university, or other agencies. Your understanding of these terms (i.e., preplant vs. postemergence, band vs. basal) will help you obtain maximum results from pesticide applications. Refer to the glossary in the manual. If you do not understand the directions on a label, check with your pesticide dealer or salesperson, a county extension agent, or a vocational agriculture instructor. The label provides a wealth of information. Failure to follow the instructions on a pesticide label can result in a serious pesticide accident and constitutes a legal violation subject to civil or criminal prosecution. Remember, the label is a legal document. The user is liable for personal injury, crop damage, or pollution incurred through misuse of a pesticide.

When to Read the Label

Before you buy a pesticide, read the label to determine:
- Whether it is the pesticide you need for the job
- Whether the pesticide can be used safely under the application conditions
- Whether you have the proper application equipment for the job
- Whether you have the necessary protective equipment
- How much pesticide is needed
- Whether there are any restrictions for use of the pesticide

Before you mix the pesticide, read the label to determine:

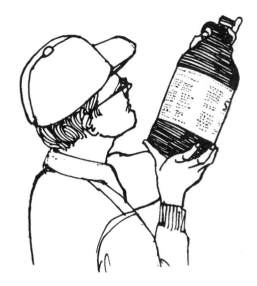

- What protective equipment you should use
- What the pesticide can be mixed with (compatibility)
- How much pesticide to use
- The mixing procedure

Before you apply the pesticide, read the label to determine:
- What safety measures you should follow
- Where the pesticide can be used (livestock, crops, structures, etc.)
- When to apply the pesticide (including the waiting period for crops and animals)
- How to apply the pesticide

Before you store or dispose of the pesticide or pesticide container, read the label to determine:
- Where and how to store the pesticide
- How to dispose of the pesticide container
- Where and how to dispose of surplus pesticide

In addition to the pesticide label, manufacturers often provide supplemental labeling information. These materials (e.g. pamphlets, brochures, information sheets and advertising) complement the product label, but do not legally substitute for the label.

CHEMCO NO PEST INSECTICIDE

Restricted use pesticide. For retail sale to and use only by Certified Applicators, or persons under their direct supervision, and only for those uses covered by the Certified Applicator's certification.

ACTIVE INGREDIENT: **BY WEIGHT**

deltathion (1,2 phospho-(5)-4 chloromethane)...............................50%
INERT INGREDIENTS...............<u>50%</u>
                 TOTAL 100%

HAZARDS TO HUMANS AND DOMESTIC ANIMALS

Wear long-sleeved clothing, full length trousers, eye protection, and protective gloves when handling. Wash hands and face before eating or using tobacco. Bathe at the end of work day, washing entire body and hair with soap and water. Change clothing daily. Wash contaminated clothing thoroughly before reusing.

STATEMENT OF PRACTICAL TREATMENT

If Swallowed: Do not induce vomiting. Contains aromatic petroleum solvent. Call a physician or poison control center immediately. **If In Eyes:** Flush with plenty of water for at least 15 minutes. Get medical attention. **If On Skin:** Wash with plenty of soap and water. Get medical attention if irritation persists. **If Inhaled:** Remove to fresh air immediately. Get medical attention.

NOTE TO PHYSICIANS: "No Pest" is a cholinesterase inhibitor. Treat symptomatically. If exposed, plasma and red blood cell cholinesterase tests may indicate significance of exposure (baseline data are useful). Atropine, only by injection, is the preferable antidote. Oximes, such as 2-PAM/protopam, may be therapeutic if used early; however, use only in conjunction with atropine. In case of severe acute poisoning, use antidote immediately after establishing an open airway and respiration.

ENVIRONMENTAL HAZARDS

This pesticide is toxic to birds and extremely toxic to fish. Do not apply directly to water. Do not contaminate water by cleaning of equipment or disposal of waste. This product is highly toxic to bees exposed to direct treatment or residues on blooming crops or weeds. Avoid use when bees are actively foraging.

"No Pest" is a pesticide which can move (sleep or travel) through soil and can contaminate groundwater which may be used as drinking water. "No Pest" has been found in groundwater as a result of agricultural use. Users are advised not to apply "No Pest" where the water table (groundwater) is close to the surface and where the soils are very permeable (i.e., well drained soils such as loamy sands). Your local agricultural agencies can provide further information on the type of soil in your area and the location of groundwater.

REENTRY STATEMENTS

Do not apply this product in such a manner as to directly or through drift expose workers or other persons. The area being treated must be vacated by unprotected persons.

Do not enter treated areas without protective clothing until sprays have dried.

Written or oral warnings must be given to workers who are expected to be in a treated area or in an area about to be treated with this product. When oral warnings are given, warnings shall be given in a language customarily understood by workers. Oral warnings must be given if there is reason to believe that written warnings cannot be understood by workers. Written warnings must include the following information: "WARNING! Area treated with "No Pest" Insecticide on (date of application). Do not enter without appropriate protective clothing until sprays have dried. If accidental exposure occurs, follow the instructions below." (Written warnings must include the STATEMENT OF PRACTICAL TREATMENT given at the beginning of this label.)

STORAGE AND DISPOSAL

PROHIBITIONS: Do not contaminate water, food or feed by storage or disposal. Open dumping is prohibited. Do not reuse empty container.

STORAGE: Store in original container only. Keep container closed when not in use. Store "No Pest" in a well ventilated clean dry area out of reach of children and animals. Do not store in areas where temperature averages 115°F (46°C) or greater. Do not store in or around the home or home garden. Do not store near food or feed. In case of spill or leak on floor or paved surfaces, soak up with sand, earth or synthetic absorbent. Remove to chemical waste area.

PESTICIDE DISPOSAL: Pesticide wastes are toxic. Improper disposal of excess pesticide, spray mixture or rinsate is a violation of federal law. If these wastes cannot be disposed of by use according to label instructions, contact your State Pesticide or Environmental Control Agency or the Hazardous Waste Representative at the nearest EPA Regional Office for guidance.

CONTAINER DISPOSAL: Metal Containers: Triple rinse (or equivalent). Then offer for recycling or reconditioning, or puncture and dis-

Continued

CHEMCO NO PEST INSECTICIDE—cont'd

pose of in a sanitary landfill, or by other procedures approved by state and local authorities. **Plastic Containers:** Triple rinse (or equivalent). Then offer for recycling or reconditioning, or puncture and dispose of in a sanitary landfill, or incineration, or, if allowed by state and local authorities, by open burning. If burned, stay out of smoke. **Glass Containers:** Triple rinse (or equivalent). Then dispose of in a sanitary landfill or by other approved state and local procedures.

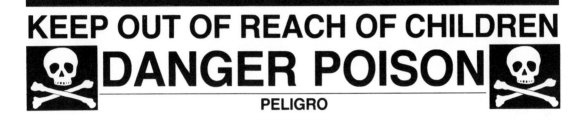

22

TOXICITY AND HEALTH

Many pesticide accidents can be traced to applicator carelessness or misuse. These accidents can damage plants, injure livestock or wildlife, and more importantly, endanger the health of the user or other people. Pesticides need to be biologically active, or toxic, to be effective against the pests they are intended to control. Toxicity is a measure of their capacity to cause injury; it is a property of the chemical itself. Hazard, or risk, on the other hand, is the potential for injury, or the degree of danger involved in using a pesticide under a given set of circumstances. Hazard depends on both the toxicity of the pesticide and the risk of exposure to harmful amounts of the chemical.

The best way to avoid or minimize the hazards of pesticide use is to know what you are using and how to use it. This means you must read the label carefully and follow instructions. The attitude of the user is of utmost importance. If users mistakenly think they know exactly how to use a pesticide, or do not care what precautions should be taken, accidents are more likely to occur. People must realize both their legal and moral obligations when using pesticides. By taking adequate precautions and practicing good management—with safety in mind—there should be few accidents from the use of pesticides.

In this chapter we will review the many facets of pesticide toxicity and health. We will look at how pesticides enter our bodies, what symptoms they can induce, and what treatments are available if an accident should occur. Pesticide injuries involving humans occur because chemicals can be absorbed by the body, can cause skin or eye damage (topical effects), or can induce allergic responses. Any chemical can be poisonous or toxic if absorbed in excessive

amounts, even common table salt if too much is consumed. The toxic effects of a pesticide depend on both the toxicity of the chemical and the amount the body absorbs following exposure.

Exposure: How Pesticides Enter the Body

Four ways a pesticide can enter the human body are through: (1) the skin (dermal), (2) the lungs (inhalation), (3) the mouth (oral), and (4) the eyes.

Dermal

In most pesticide exposure situations, the skin is the most important route of entry into the body. Evidence indicates that about 97 percent of all body exposure to pesticides during an application is through skin contact. Dermal absorption may occur as the result of a splash, spill, or drift when mixing, loading, applying, or disposing of pesticides. It may also result from exposure to crop residues or treated animals or when cleaning or repairing contaminated application equipment.

Even if only a small amount of chemical is allowed to remain on the skin it can be absorbed into the body, and the person can be poisoned. Different parts of the body vary in their abilities to absorb pesticides. Research with certain pesticides has found that the scrotal area and the head are quite absorptive, although cuts, abrasions, and skin rashes can enhance absorption in other parts of the body. Pesticide formulations vary in their ability to be absorbed through the skin. In general, wettable powders, dusts, and granular pesticides are not as readily absorbed as are oil-based liquid formulations such as emulsifiable concentrates.

From Hock WK, Brown CL (editors): Pesticide education manual, ed 2, University Park, Penn, Penn State University.

Dermal

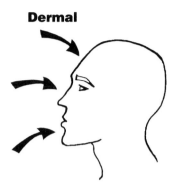

Inhalation

Protection of the lungs is especially important when pesticide powders, dusts, gases, vapors, or very small spray droplets can be inhaled during mixing, loading, or application. If breathed into the lungs, pesticides can enter the bloodstream rapidly and completely. If inhaled in sufficient amounts, pesticides can also cause damage to nose, throat, and lung tissue.

Inhalation

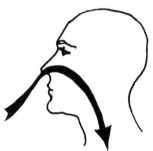

Oral

Accidental oral exposure occurs most frequently when pesticides have been taken from the original labeled container and put into an unlabeled bottle or food container. Unfortunately, children are the most common victims in these situations.

Oral exposure also occurs when liquid concentrates splash into the mouth during mixing or while cleaning equipment. The mouth must never be used to clear a spray line or to begin siphoning a pesticide from a tank or container. Chemicals can also be swallowed when eating, drinking, smoking, or even licking one's lips. Since many pesticides are rapidly and completely absorbed by the intestinal tract, it is essential to always wash hands and face thoroughly before eating, drinking, or smoking.

Eyes

Under certain conditions and with certain pesticides, absorption through the eyes can be significant and particularly hazardous. Eyes are very sensitive to many pesticides and considering their size are able to absorb surprisingly large amounts of chemical. Serious eye exposure can result from a splash or spill, drift, or by rubbing the eyes with contaminated hands or clothing.

Avoiding exposure is the key to safe pesticide use. Proper protective equipment (described in the chapter "Using Pesticides Safely"), when worn correctly, helps avoid exposure.

Toxicity and Potential Health Effects of Pesticides

As we discussed earlier, the toxicity of a pesticide is its capacity or ability to cause injury or illness. The toxicity of a pesticide is determined by subjecting test animals (usually rats, mice, rabbits, and dogs) to different dosages of the active ingredient and each of its formulated products. Two types of toxicity are acute and chronic.

Acute toxicity

Acute toxicity, based on a single, short-term exposure, is determined by at least three methods: (1) dermal toxicity is determined by exposing the skin to the chemical; (2) inhalation toxicity is determined by the test animals breathing vapors of the chemical; and (3) oral toxicity is determined by feeding the chemical to test animals. Any harmful effects that occur from a single exposure by any route of entry are termed acute effects. The effects of acute pesticide poisoning usually occur within minutes or hours after exposure. In addition, the effect of the chemical as an irritant to the eyes and skin is examined under laboratory conditions.

Acute toxicity is usually expressed as LD_{50} (lethal dose 50) or LC_{50} (lethal concentration 50). This is the amount or concentration of a toxicant (i.e. pesticide) required to kill 50 percent of a test population of animals under a standard set of conditions. LD_{50} values of pesticides are recorded in milligrams of pesticide per kilogram of body weight of the test animal (mg/kg), or in parts per million (ppm). For example, a LD_{50} of 135 means that it would take approximately 135 milligrams of a chemical for each kilogram of an animal's body weight to kill one-half of the test

Table 22-1. Acute toxicity categories for pesticides

Category	LD^{50} Oral (mg/kg)	LD^{50} Dermal (mg/kg)	LC^{50} Inhalation (mg/l)	Eyes	Skin	Required Signal Word
I. Highly toxic	Trace to 50	Trace to 200	Trace to 0.2	Corrosive; corneal opacity not reversible within 7 days	Corrosive	DANGER—POISON, skull and crossbones except DANGER only for severe eye or skin hazard
II. Moderately toxic	50 to 500	200 to 2,000	0.2 to 2	Corneal opacity reversible within 7 days; irritation persisting for 7 days	Severe irritation at 72 hours	WARNING
III. Slightly toxic	500 to 5,000	2,000 to 20,000	2 to 20	No corneal opacity; irritation reversible within 7 days	Moderate irritation at 72 hours	CAUTION
IV. Relatively nontoxic	Greater than 5,000	Greater than 20,000	Greater than 20	No irritation	Mild or slight irritation at 72 hours	CAUTION

animals in a population. LC$_{50}$ values of pesticides are recorded in milligrams of pesticide per volume of air or water (ppm). To put these units into perspective, 1 ppm is analogous to 1 inch in 16 miles or 1 minute in 2 years.

LD$_{50}$ and LC$_{50}$ values are useful in comparing the toxicity of different active ingredients as well as different formulations of the same active ingredient. The lower the LD$_{50}$ value of a pesticide, and therefore the greater the acute toxicity of the chemical. Pesticides with high LD$_{50}$ values are considered the least acutely toxic to humans when used according to the directions on the product label.

Acute toxicities are the basis for assigning pesticides to a toxicity category and selecting the appropriate signal word for the product label.

Signal words

Those pesticides that are classified as "highly toxic," on the basis of either oral, dermal, or inhalation toxicity, must have the signal words DANGER and POISON (in red letters) and a skull and crossbones prominently displayed on the package label. PELIGRO, the Spanish word for danger, must also appear on the labels of highly toxic chemicals. Acute oral LD$_{50}$ values for pesticide products in this group range from a trace to 50 mg/kg. As little as a few drops of such a material taken orally could be fatal to a 150-pound person.

Some pesticides products have the signal word DANGER without the skull and crossbones symbol. This is done because possible skin or eye effects are more severe than suggested by the acute toxicity (LD$_{50}$) of the product.

Pesticide products considered "moderately toxic" must have the signal words WARNING and AVISO (Spanish) displayed on the label. Acute oral LD$_{50}$ values range from 50 to 500 mg/kg. From 1 teaspoon to 1 ounce of this material could be fatal to a 150-pound person.

Pesticide products classified as either "slightly toxic or relatively nontoxic" are required to have the signal word CAUTION on the pesticide label. Acute oral LD$_{50}$ values are greater than 500 mg/kg.

Chronic toxicity

The chronic toxicity of a pesticide is determined by subjecting test animals to long-term exposure to the active ingredient. Any harmful effects that occur from small doses repeated over a period of time are termed chronic effects. Some of the suspected chronic effects from exposure to certain pesticides include birth defects (teratogenesis); fetal toxicity (fetotoxic effects); production of tumors (oncogenesis), either benign (noncancerous) or malignant (cancerous/carcinogenesis); genetic changes (mutagenesis); blood disorders (hemotoxic effects) nerve disorders (neurotoxic effects); and reproductive effects. As a consequence, a number of pesticides include chronic toxicity warning statements on the product label. The chronic toxicity of a pesticide is more difficult to determine through laboratory analysis than is acute toxicity.

Pesticide poisoning

The symptoms of pesticide poisoning can range from a mild skin irritation to coma or even death. It is important that pesticide users and handlers learn to recognize the common signs and symptoms of pesticide poisoning.

The effects, or symptoms, of pesticide poisoning can be broadly defined as being either topical or systemic. Topical effects generally develop at the site of pesticide contact. Topical effects from exposure to pesticides are a result of either the irritant properties of a chemical in a pesticide formulation (an active or inert ingredient), or an allergic response by the victim. Dermatitis, or inflammation of the skin, general-

ly is accepted as the most commonly reported topical effect associated with pesticide exposure. Symptoms of dermatitis range from reddening of the skin to blisters or rashes. Some persons may be allergic to pesticide chemicals. Symptoms of an allergic reaction range from reddening and itching of the eyes and skin to respiratory discomfort often resembling an asthmatic condition.

Systemic effects are quite different from topical effects. They often occur away from the original point of contact as a result of the pesticide being absorbed into and distributed throughout the body. Systemic effects often include nausea, vomiting, fatigue, headache, and intestinal disorders.

Different classes or families of chemicals cause different types of symptoms. Individuals also vary in their sensitivity to different levels of these chemicals. Some people may show no reaction to a dose that causes severe illness in others. Be alert for the early symptoms of pesticide poisoning. Early recognition of symptoms and an immediate appropriate response may save a life. Remember, however, that the development of certain symptoms is not always the result of exposure to a pesticide. Common illnesses such as the flu, heat exhaustion or heat stroke, pneumonia, asthma, respiratory and intestinal infections, and even a hangover from overindulgence can cause similar symptoms. Some individuals exhibit allergic reactions when using pesticides or when these materials are applied in or around their homes or places of work. When symptoms appear after contact with a pesticide, seek medical attention immediately. *Take the label with you* or, if need be the container, but do not put it in the passenger section of a vehicle. The doctor needs to know what the product ingredients are, and an antidote is often listed on the label. If the Material Safety Data Sheet (MSDS) is available, take this with you too as it frequently contains information for the doctor in the event of an emergency.

If you use or handle pesticides or reside near areas where they are used, have the name and number of the nearest Poison Control Center readily available. These centers are staffed on a twenty-four-hour basis. Their numbers are available from your local hospital, physician, or county cooperative extension office. However, do not wait until an emergency arises to obtain the number of the Poison Control Center nearest you.

For pesticide emergencies, the National Pesticide Telecommunications Network (NPTC) located in Lubbock, Texas, is also available. The NPTC toll free telephone number, 1-800-858-7378, provides a variety of information about pesticides to anyone in the United States, twenty-four hours a day, 365 days a year.

All emergency numbers should be readily available by the telephone, and in service vehicles involved in transporting pesticides. Warehouses and retail outlets should list these numbers along with other emergency numbers near telephones to enable any employee to use them in the event of an emergency.

First Aid for Pesticide Poisoning

Immediate and appropriate action may be necessary to prevent serious injury to a victim of pesticide poisoning. It could indeed be a life-or-death matter. Someone may need to administer first aid to the victim. The product label should be a first source of information in a pesticide exposure emergency. Call you poison control center or a physician. *First aid is only the "first response" and is not a substitute for professional medical help.*

General first aid instructions

- Have current labels and Material Safety Data Sheets (MSDS) available. Obtain these at time of purchase.
- Have emergency response telephone numbers readily available.
- Assemble a first aid kit with all of the necessary supplies.
- Always have a source of clean water available. In an extreme emergency, even water from a farm pond, irrigation system, or watering trough could be used to dilute the pesticide.
- If oral or dermal exposure has occurred, the first objective is usually to dilute the pesticide and prevent absorption.
- If inhalation exposure occurs, get the victim to fresh air immediately.
- Never try to give anything by mouth to an unconscious person.
- Become familiar with the proper techniques of artificial respiration; it may be necessary if a person's breathing has stopped or become impaired.
- If there is a likelihood of being directly exposed to a pesticide while administering first-aid, or removing the victim from an enclosed area, be sure to wear appropriate protective clothing and equipment. Remember, one breathe of some poisons is enough to incapacitate a person.

Specific first aid instructions

If you are the only person available to deal with the victim, do the following:

FIRST—See if the victim is breathing; if not, administer artificial respiration.

SECOND—Decontaminate the victim immediately; wash thoroughly. Speed is essential.

THIRD—Call the doctor or hospital.

If more than one person is available to help the victim, do the following:
- One person should check that the victim is breathing; if not, give artificial respiration, then begin to decontaminate the victim.
- Another person should call the hospital or doctor immediately, then assist with the decontamination of the victim.

If the pesticide has been spilled on the skin or clothing, remove the clothing immediately if it has been contaminated and thoroughly wash the skin with soap and water. Avoid harsh scrubbing as this enhances pesticide absorption. Rinse the affected area with water; wash again and rinse. Gently dry the affected area and wrap it in loose cloth or a blanket, if necessary. If chemical burns of the skin have occurred, cover the area loosely with a clean, soft cloth. Avoid the use of ointments, greases, powders, and other medications unless instructed by a medical authority.

It may be best to dispose of contaminated clothing. But if you decide to keep it, wash it before reuse. Store and wash all contaminated clothing separately from any other laundry.

If the pesticide has entered into the eyes, hold the eyelid open and immediately begin gently washing the eye with clean running water. Do not use chemicals or drugs in the wash water unless instructed by a

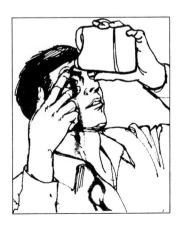

physician or poison control center. Continue washing for 15 minutes. Avoid contamination of the other eye if only one eye is involved. Flush under the eyelids with water to remove debris. Cover the eye with a clean piece of cloth and seek medical attention immediately.

If the pesticide has been inhaled, get the victim to fresh air immediately. Carry the victim, do not allow the victim to walk. Have the victim lie down and loosen clothing. Keep the victim warm and quiet. If the victim is convulsing, watch the breathing and protect the victim's head. Keep the chin up to keep air passages free for breathing. If breathing stops or is irregular, give artificial respiration. Do not attempt to rescue someone who is in a closed contaminated area unless you are wearing appropriate protective equipment.

If the pesticide has been swallowed, the most important decision to be made is whether or not to induce vomiting. The decision must be made quickly and accurately; the victim's life may depend on it. Where specific instructions are given, always follow the label directions. If the pesticide has entered the mouth but has not been swallowed, the mouth should be rinsed with large amounts of water. If the pesticide has been swallowed it should usually be voided fast, but NEVER induce vomiting if the victim is unconscious or convulsing. The victim could choke to death on the vomitus.

Never induce vomiting if the victim has swallowed petroleum products (kerosene, gasoline, oil, lighter fluid, EC pesticides) unless directed to do so by the label, a physician, or a poison control center. Many pesticides which are formulated as emulsifiable concentrates are dissolved in petroleum products. The letters EC or words "Emulsifiable Concentrate" on the pesticide label are signals NOT to induce vomiting of a concentrated material without first consulting the product label or a physician. Petroleum products aspirated (inhaled) into the lungs can cause serious respiratory disorders. If you are certain the victim has swallowed a dilute preparation, have the person vomit immediately.

Never induce vomiting if the victim has swallowed a corrosive poison—a strong acid or alkali (base). A corrosive poison will burn the throat and mouth as severely coming up as it did going down. Determine what poison the person has ingested. The victim may experience severe pain and have extensive mouth and throat burns. Fortunately, most commonly used pesticides are not corrosive. However, some household disinfectants and germicides fall into this category.

The best first aid is to dilute the poison as quickly as possible. For acids or alkalis, give the patient plenty of water or milk. It is very important that the victim get to a hospital without delay.

To neutralize acids—If you are sure the poison is an acid, give the victim milk of magnesia (1 tablespoon in 1 cup of water). In an extreme emergency, if milk of magnesia is not available give the victim baking soda in water. Exercise extreme caution, however, because baking soda reacts with acids to form carbon dioxide (CO_2) gas. Some doctors report that large amounts of CO_2 can induce perforation of the intestines or stomach wall.

To neutralize alkalis—If you are sure the poison is an alkali, give the victim lemon juice or dilute vinegar. Whatever the circumstances, contact a poison control center or a physician as quickly as possible.

How to induce vomiting

Induce vomiting only as first aid until you can get the victim to a hospital. Do not waste a lot of time attempting to induce vomiting. Make sure the victim is kneeling forward or lying on their side to prevent vomitus from entering the lungs and causing additional damage.

- First give the patient at least two glasses of water to dilute the poison. Do not use carbonated beverages.
- If possible, use ipecac syrup to induce vomiting. Ipecac is extremely effective in emptying the stomach contents and is available in small quantities on a nonprescription basis from most drug stores.
- If ipecac syrup is not available, put your finger or the blunt end of a spoon at the back of the throat to induce vomiting. Do not use anything sharp or pointed! Do not use salt water to induce vomiting.
- Collect some of the vomitus for the doctor. A chemical analysis may be necessary in some cases.
- After vomiting has occurred, give the patient 2 to 4 tablespoons of activated charcoal in water. Activated charcoal acts as a sponge to adsorb many poisons. Pharmaceutical grade activated charcoal is available from most drug stores; activate charcoal prepared for cleaning up pesticide spills may be substituted in an emergency.
- Never administer activated charcoal at the same time as ipecac syrup, because the ipecac will bind to the charcoal and be deactivated before it can induce vomiting.

Only first aid has been discussed here. Obtain the assistance of a physician or poison control center. Get the victim to a doctor or hospital if necessary and take the pesticide label with you.

How Pesticides Poison

Symptoms of poisoning from exposure to pesticides can range from minor skin and eye irritation to severe difficulty in breathing and convulsions depending on the toxicological characteristics of the specific pesticide. Different classes of pesticides affect different systems in the body, but, in general, the insecticides/nematicides are the most toxic and cause more poisonings than any other class of compounds. The following sections highlight the cholinesterase inhibitors, testing procedures and antidotes, and other groups of pesticides that can affect the health of humans.

Cholinesterase inhibitors

The most serious poisonings usually result from acute exposure to organophosphate and N-methyl carbamate insecticides/nematicides. The symptoms of systemic poisoning from exposure to these pesticides begin as fatigue, headache, giddiness, sweating, dizziness or blurred vision, cramps, nausea, vomiting, and diarrhea. Moderate symptoms that may develop include numbness, changes in heart rate, general muscle weakness, difficulty in breathing and walking, pinpoint pupils, excessive salivation, and an increase in the severity of the earlier symptoms. In advanced poisoning cases there may be convulsions and coma which could ultimately lead to death.

Organophosphate insecticides include such chemicals as methyl and ethyl parathion, chlorpyrifos, diazinon, azinphos-methyl, malathion, dimethoate, and trichlorfon. The N-methyl carbamates include carbaryl, carbofuran, methomyl, and aldicarb.

Organophosphates and N-methyl carbamates inhibit the enzyme cholinesterase (ChE), thereby interfering with the normal function of the nervous system. All living animals with cholinesterase in their nervous system, such as insects, fish, birds, humans, and other mammals, can be poisoned by these chemicals.

In order to understand how the organophosphate and carbamate pesticides affect the nervous system, one needs to understand how the nervous system actually works. The nervous system, which includes the brain, is the most complex system in the body. It consists of millions of cells in an extensive communications network throughout the organism. Messages or electrical impulses (stimuli) travel along this complex network of cells. Nerve cells or neurons do not physically touch each other; rather there is a gap or synapse between cells. The impulses must therefore cross or "bridge" the synapse between nerve cells in order to keep a message moving along the entire network.

When an impulse reaches the synapse, a chemical, acetylcholine, is released to carry the message on to the next cell. Acetylcholine is the primary chemical responsible for the transmission of nerve stimuli across the synapse of two neurons. After the impulse is transmitted across the synapse, the acetylcholine is broken down by the enzyme, acetyl cholinesterase. Now the synapse is "cleared" and ready to receive a new transmission.

Organophosphate and carbamate insecticides/nematicides inhibit the activity of cholinesterase (hence the name cholinesterase inhibitors), resulting in a build up of acetylcholine at the nerve endings. An increase in acetylcholine, for whatever reason, results in the uncontrolled flow of nerve transmissions between nerve cells. The nervous system is therefore "poisoned" by the accumulation of acetylcholine, which results in the continual transmission of impulses across the synapses. High concentrations of acetylcholine causes muscle contractions and twitching, glandular secretions, sensory and behavioral disturbances, and respiratory depression which can lead to death.

The effects of organophosphate or carbamate poisoning can result in both systemic and topical symptoms. Direct exposure of the eye, for example, can cause localized symptoms such as constriction of the pupils, blurring of vision, an eyebrow headache, and severe irritation and reddening of the eyes. Symptoms and signs of systemic poisoning are almost entirely due to cholinesterase inhibition and the subsequent accumulation of acetylcholine at the nerve endings. Early symptoms depend on the route of absorption and the severity of the intoxication. Gastric symptoms such as stomach cramps, nausea, vomiting, and diarrhea appear early if the material has been ingested. Similarly, salivation, headache, dizziness, and excessive secretions which cause breathing difficulties are initial symptoms/signs if the material has been inhaled. Involvement of the respiratory muscles can result in respiratory failure. Stomach/intestinal, and respiratory symptoms appear at the same time if the pesticide is absorbed

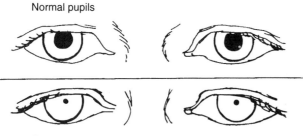

Normal pupils

Constricted (pinpoint) pupils

through the skin. In children, the first sign of poisoning may be a convulsion. Miosis (constricted pupils) may not occur initially; in fact, just the opposite, excessive dilation, may be present as an early sign.

In advanced poisoning, the victim is pale, sweating, and frothing at the mouth. The pupils of the eyes are constricted and unresponsive to light. Other symptoms include changes in heart rate, muscle weakness, mental confusion, convulsions and/or coma. The victim may die if not treated.

Cholinesterase testing

Persons who regularly work with organophosphates or carbamates should consider having periodic cholinesterase tests. The blood cholinesterase test can measure the effect of exposure to organophosphate and carbamate pesticides well below the level that causes symptoms in people. Since cholinesterase levels can vary considerably between individuals, a "baseline" must be established for each person. In fact, a small percentage of the population has a genetically-determined low level of cholinesterase. Even minimal exposure to cholinesterase inhibitors can present a substantial risk to these people. Baseline testing should always be done during the time of year when pesticides are not being used or at least 30 days from the most recent exposure. Establishing a baseline value requires at least two tests performed at least 72 hours but not more than 14 days apart. If these two tests differ by as much as 20 percent, a third test is often recommended.

Cholinesterase tests can be repeated at regular intervals during times when organophosphate and carbamate pesticides are being used and then compared with the baseline level. Cholinesterase tests for the organophosphates are more reliable than for the N-methyl carbamates. Unless a substantial amount of carbamate has been absorbed and a blood sample taken within two hours of the suspected exposure, it is unlikely that cholinesterase levels will be found

depressed. In such cases, a urine analysis may be necessary to detect the presence of certain metabolites. The purpose of routine cholinesterase monitoring is to enable a physician to recognize the occurrence of excessive exposure to organophosphates and carbamates. If a laboratory test shows a cholinesterase drop of 30 percent below the established baseline, the worker should be retested immediately. If a second test confirms the drop in cholinesterase, the person should be removed from further contact with organophosphates and carbamates until cholinesterase levels return to the pre-exposure baseline range.

Antidotes

Antidotes for organophosphate or carbamate insecticide/nematicide poisoning should be prescribed and administered only by a physician. They can be extremely dangerous if misused. Doctors and hospitals should be advised which pesticides are used locally, and encouraged to have appropriate antidotes available for treating pesticide poisonings.

Atropine sulfate

This antidote is given intravenously to counteract the effects of excessive acetylcholine at the nerve endings. It can be given repeatedly as symptoms occur, the need and dosage based on the body weight of the victim. Atropine can be used for both organophosphate and carbamate poisoning. Atropine should never be used to prevent poisoning.

Protopam chloride (2-PAM)

This antidote, used in conjunction with atropine, helps to reactivate cholinesterase in organophosphate poisoning. Protopam chloride is never used where carbamates are involved in the poisoning.

Other pesticides

Organochlorine insecticides such as Kelthane, lindane, methoxychlor and Thiodan can affect the nervous system of mammals. The initial signs and symptoms of organochlorine poisoning depend in part on the route of entry of the pesticide into the body. Nausea and vomiting commonly occur soon after ingestion, whereas apprehension, twitching, tremors, confusion, and convulsions are often associated with dermal absorption.

The chlorophenoxy herbicides include 2,4-D, 2,4-DB, MCPA, mecoprop, and dichlorprop. These chemicals can be moderately irritating to the skin and eyes.

Inhalation of spray mist may cause coughing and a burning sensation in the nasal passages and chest. Prolonged inhalation sometimes causes dizziness. Ingestion will usually cause vomiting, a burning sensation in the stomach, diarrhea, and muscle twitching.

The herbicides paraquat and diquat can be very injurious if poisoning occurs. Exposure of the hands to concentrates can result in irritation and cracking of the skin, as well as discoloration, abnormal growth, and even loss of nails. When splashed in the eye, paraquat concentrate causes conjunctivitis (membrane inflammation). Inhalation of spray mist may irritate the respiratory passages, causing a scratchy throat and a nosebleed. The most serious poisonings from these herbicides have usually resulted from accidental or intentional ingestion of the concentrate. The pulmonary (lung) reaction which follows ingestion of paraquat is often fatal.

The thiocarbamates include a wide variety of fungicides (for example, zineb, mancozeb, ferbam, thiram, and maneb) and herbicides (for example, butylate and EPTC). Their acute toxicity to humans is generally considered to be low, but they can be irritating to skin and eyes. Inhalation of spray mist or dust from these pesticides may cause throat irritation, sneezing, and coughing.

Pyrethroids or synthetic pyrethrins include such insecticides as fenvalerate, permethrin, cypermethrin, and cyfluthrin. Salivation, vomiting, diarrhea, lack of coordination, and tremors can result if very large doses are absorbed. The pyrethroids can cause irritation of the eyes, skin, and mucous membranes of the nose, mouth, and throat. Pyrethrum, derived from the flowers of certain chrysanthemum species, is still used in many home and garden products. It can cause eye, respiratory, and skin irritation in sensitive individuals.

Bibliography

See end of Chapter 24.

23

Using Pesticides Safely

There are many reasons for using pesticides properly and safely. The misuse of pesticides can have immediate, as well as long-term effects upon humans, pets and wildlife, structures and the environment. Misapplication can also waste considerable time and resources, and can lead to injury to crops and livestock, and failure to control the pest.

Pesticides must be used correctly to ensure the continued availability of a full range of products in the future. Every time an incident occurs through either misuse or carelessness, the future availability of crop and livestock protection chemicals is jeopardized. Prudent and safe use will help to minimize any adverse regulatory actions.

There are important common sense principles for the safe and effective use of pesticides. Some of the principles discussed throughout this chapter are listed below:

- Use pesticides only when necessary, and, as far as practicable, as part of an integrated pest management program.
- Be familiar with all current federal, state, and local pesticide laws and regulations.
- Always read the label to be sure you are treating a labeled crop or site at the proper time and application rate.
- Do not allow children to play around pesticide application equipment, or the mixing, storage, and disposal areas.
- Lock pesticides in their original labelled containers inside a properly marked cabinet or storeroom, away from food and feed.
- Where possible, work in pairs when applying highly toxic pesticides.
- Mix only as much pesticide as you intend to use.

- Wear appropriate protective clothing and equipment.
- Never eat, drink, or smoke while handling pesticides.
- Properly maintain and calibrate pesticide application equipment.
- Avoid drift to nontarget areas. Dusts drift more than sprays; airblast sprayers usually create more drift than boom sprayers.
- Avoid spilling pesticides on skin or clothing. Should an accident occur, wash immediately with soap and water. Have ready access to a clean water source and first aid supplies at all times.
- If pesticide poisoning is suspected, contact your nearest Poison Control Center, hospital emergency room, or physician. Take the product label with you.
- Stay out of recently sprayed areas until the spray has dried. Observe reentry intervals specified on the label.
- Dispose of empty containers according to the label, in a manner that does not endanger humans, animals, or the environment.
- Bathe or shower after handling pesticides or pesticide contaminated equipment. Wash clothing after applying pesticides, keeping in mind that, until laundered, such clothing must be handled with the same caution as the pesticides themselves. Keep pesticide contaminated clothing separate from the family wash.

Protect Yourself from Pesticides

The chapter on toxicity and health identified the hazards to humans that can be posed by pesticides.

From Hock WK, Brown CL (editors): Pesticide education manual, ed 2, University Park, Penn, Penn State University.

The greatest risks arise in handling concentrates, especially when mixing, loading or applying them. Although a dilute chemical is generally less hazardous than a concentrate, the hazard increases when there is significant drift or when appropriate safety and application procedures are not followed. Danger of exposure also exists when cleaning up spills or repairing equipment or entering treated areas prematurely.

Even though it can be uncomfortable and cumbersome to wear, appropriate protective clothing and/or equipment should always be worn by anyone working with pesticides. The type of protective clothing and equipment needed depends on the job being done and the type of chemical being used. Some farm chemicals require full protection, including a respirator, during mixing, application, and disposal. Some fumigants require special equipment to be worn such as a selfcontained breathing system.

Read the label on the pesticide container carefully and follow all directions concerning necessary protective clothing and equipment. The instructions on a label may include such statements as:
• Avoid skin contact
• Keep from breathing dust or vapors
• Keep out of eyes

Even if protective clothing is not specifically mentioned on the label, protection may be needed to reduce the risk of chemical contact. Similarly, a statement specifying only one piece of safety equipment does not rule out the need for additional protection. Minimum protection should consist of a long-sleeved shirt and long trousers or overalls, gloves, proper footwear, and a hat.

Clothing

Protective clothing includes a clean, long-sleeved shirt and long trousers make of a tightly woven fabric or a water repellent material. Wearing an undershirt adds protection. Additional layers of clothing help to absorb pesticide and reduce the amount that reaches the skin. Avoid pants with cuffs to prevent collecting granules or powder in the cuff. When a granular pesticide is used, shake clothing and empty pockets and cuffs outdoors.

A cotton T-shirt and shorts do not provide adequate protection when applying pesticides.

Alternatively, coveralls, whether disposable or reusable, may be worn. Different brands vary in their comfort, durability, and the degree of protection they provide. Disposable coverall garments are available

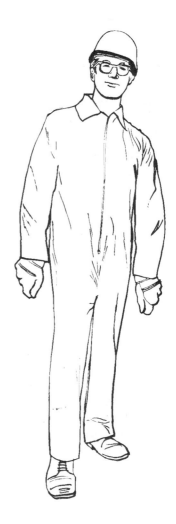

that are laminated or bonded with other fabrics or substances to increase wearer protection from chemicals. Be sure the sleeves and the legs of the suit are sufficiently tight to prevent pesticides from reaching exposed arms and legs. Suits that are elasticized at the wrists and ankles are helpful.

A liquid-proof apron, raincoat, or rainsuit should be worn when pouring and mixing concentrates and when using the more toxic products because coveralls usually do not provide adequate protection against spills and splashes. An apron should cover the body from your chest to your boots. Water-proof clothing should be worn whenever mist or spray drift could substantially wet your work clothes. Aprons and rainsuits should be made of rubber or a synthetic material resistant to the solvents in pesticide formulations.

Gloves

Wear unlined, waterproof gloves when handling or applying pesticides. Gloves should be long enough to cover the wrist and should not have a fabric wristband. Gloves are made from many materials, but current information indicates that nitrile, butyl, and neoprene provide the best protection for both liquid and dry pesticide formulations. Natural rubber gloves are recommended only for dry formulations. Never use leather or fabric gloves because they tend to absorb pesticides and transfer them to the skin. Decontamination is virtually impossible once leather and fabric gloves have become saturated; disposal is the only option. Be certain gloves are approved for use with the chemicals you intend to use. Some rubber products react with certain solvents and become sticky as the rubber dissolves. If this occurs, dispose of these gloves and use gloves approved for use with pesticides. Check gloves frequently to be sure there are no holes—fill them with water and squeeze; discard any damaged or leaking golves.

For most jobs, shirt sleeves should be worn on the outside of the gloves to keep pesticides from running down the sleeves into the gloves. But, when working with hands and arms overhead, sleeves should be tucked into the gloves with the cuff of the gloves turned up to catch any material that might run down the gloves. Wash off chemicals with soap and water, before removing the gloves, to avoid contaminating your hands while removing the gloves.

Hats

A waterproof head covering should be worn when handling pesticides. A hood, hard hat, or wide-brimmed rain hat will help to protect the head, face, and neck. Hats should be either disposable or easy to clean with soap and water. They should not contain absorbent materials such as leather, straw, or cloth.

Shoes and boots

Boots should be unlined and made of rubber. Because of their absorbency, boots of leather, canvas, or cloth materials should never be worn when handling pesticides. Trouser bottoms shoud be worn outside the boots to prevent pesticides from running down the leg and into the boot.

Goggles or face shield

Tightly fitting, nonfogging goggles, or a full-face shield should be worn when there is any chance of getting pesticide in the eyes. This is especially important when pouring or mixing concentrates or handling dusts or toxic sprays. Those who wear contact lenses may want to consult an eye doctor prior to using pesticides.

Goggles and face shields should be kept clean at all times. They can be washed with soap and water, and sanitized by soaking equipment for two minutes in a mixture of 2 tablespoons chlorine bleach in a gallon of water. Then rinse them thoroughly with clean water to remove soap and sanitizer; wipe with a clean cloth and allow to air dry. Pay particular attention to the goggle headbands. They are often made of absorbent material that requires regular replacement.

Respirators

For many toxic chemicals, the respiratory (breathing) system is the quickest and most direct rout of entry into the circulatory system. From the blood capillaries of the lungs, these toxic substances are rapidly transported throughout the body.

Respiratory protective devices vary in design, use, and protective capability. In selecting a respiratory protective device, the user must first consider the degree of hazard associated with breathing the toxic substance, and then understand the specific uses and limitations of the available equipment. Select a respiratory that is designed for the intended use, and always follow the manufacturer's instructions concerning the use and maintenance of that particular respirator. Different respirators may be needed for application of different chemicals or groups of chemicals. Select only equipment approved by the National Institute of Occupational Safety and Health (NIOSH), and the Mine Safety and Health Administration (MSHA). The NIOSH/MSHA approval numbers begin with the letters TC.

Types of respirators

Respiratory protective devices can be categorized into three classes: air-purifying, supplied-air, and self-contained. Since most pesticide contaminants can be removed from the atmosphere by air-purifying devices, we will look at these in greatest detail.

Air-purifying devices include chemical cartridge respirators, mechanical filters, gas masks (also referred to as canister filter respirators), and battery powered respirators. They can be used only in atmospheres containing sufficient oxygen to sustain life.

• Chemical cartridge respirators provide respiratory protection against certain gases and vapors in concentrations not greater than 0.1 percent by volume,

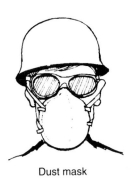

Dust mask

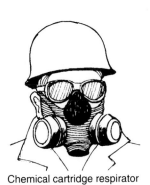

Chemical cartridge respirator

provided that this concentration does not exceed an amount that is immediately dangerous to life and health. They are for use only when exposure to high, continual concentrations of pesticide is unlikely, such as when mixing pesticides outdoors. They are available either as half-masks covering only the nose and mouth, or as full-face shields for both respiratory and eye protection.

- Mechanical filter respirators (dust masks) provide respiratory protection against particulate matter such as mists, metal fumes, and nonvolatile dusts. They are available as either disposable or reusable half masks that cover the nose and mouth, or as reusable full facepieces. Dust masks should never be used when mixing or applying liquids because splashed or spilled liquids or pesticide vapors can be absorbed by the mask, creating an exposure hazard to the user.

- Many respiratory protective devices are combinations of chemical cartridge and mechanical filter (a prefilter) respirators. These can provide respiratory protection against both gases and particulate matter.

- Full face respirators provide respiratory protection against particulate matter, and/or against certain specific gases and vapors, provided that their concentration does not exceed an amount that is immediately dangerous to life and health. Gas masks, like full facepieces, cover the eyes, nose, and mouth, but will last longer than cartridges when continuously exposed to some pesticides. A gas mask will not, however, provide protection when the air supply is low. A special respirator with a self-contained air supply should be worn in these situations.

- Battery powered air-purifying respirators equipped with pesticide filters/cartridges are also effective in filtering out pesticides particle and vapors. They

are available as halfmasks, full- face masks, hoods, andprotective helmets, and are connected by a breathing hose to a battery powered filtration system. This type of filtration system has the additionnal advantage of cooling the person wearing it. But, like other air-purifying devices, this system does not supply oxygen and must be worn only when the oxygen supply is not limited.

Chemical cartridge respirators protect against light concentrations of certain organic vapors. However, no single type of cartridge is able to remove all kinds of chemical vapors. A different type of chemical cartridge (or canister) must be used for different contaminants. For example, cartridges and canisters that protect against certain organic vapors differ chemically from those that protect against ammonia gases. Be sure that the cartridge or canister is approved for the pesticide you intend to use. Cartridge respirators are not recommended for use against chemicals which possess poor warning properties. Thus, the user's senses (smell, taste, irritation) must be able to detect the substance at a safe level if cartridge respirators are to be used correctly.

The effective life of a respirator cartridge or canister depends on the conditions associated with its use—such as the type and concentration of the contaminants, the user's breathing rate, and the humidity. Cartridge longevity is dependent on its gas and vapor sorption capacity. When the chemical cartridge becomes saturated, a contaminant can pass through the catridge, usually allowing the user to smell it. At this point, the cartridge must be changed immediately. There are times when the mechanical prefilter also needs to be changed. A prefilter should be replaced whenever the respirator user feels that breathing is becoming difficult. Dispose of all spent cartridges to avoid their being used inadvertently by another applicator who is unaware of their contaminated condition.

Chemical cartridge respirators cannot provide protection against extremely toxic gases such as hydrogen cyanide, methyl bromide, or other fumigants. Masks with a self-contained air supply are necessary for these purposes.

Use and care of respirators

Respirators are worn as needed for protection when handling certain pesticides. Prior to using a respirator, read and understand the instructions on the cartridge or canister and all supplemental information about its proper use and care. Be sure the filter is approved for protection against the pesticide you intend to use. Respirators labeled only for protection against particulates must not be used for gases and vapors. Similarly, respirators labeled only for protection against gases and vapors should not be used for particulates. Remember, cartridges and filters do not supply oxygen. Do not use them where oxygen may be limited.

All respirators must be inspected for wear and deterioration of their components before and after each use. Special attention should be given to rubber or plastic parts which can deteriorate. The facepiece, valves, connecting tubes or hoses, fittings, and filters must be maintained in good condition.

All valves, mechanical filters, and chemical filters (cartridges or canisters) should be properly positioned and sealed. Fit the respirator on your face to ensure a tight but comfortable seal. A beard or large sideburns may prevent a good face seal. Two tests can be done to check the fit of most chemical cartridge respirators. The first test requires that you place your hand tightly over the outside exhaust valve. If there is a good seal, exhalation should cause slight pressure inside the facepiece. If air escapes between the face and facepiece, readjust the headbands until a tight seal is obtained. Readjusting the headbands may at times not be sufficient to obtain a good seal. It may be necessary to reposition the facepiece to prevent air from escaping between the face and facepiece. The second test involves covering the inhalation valve(s) by placing your hand over the cartridge(s). If there is a good seal, inhalation should cause the facepiece to collapse. If air enters, adjust the headbands or reposition the facepiece until a good seal is obtained.

Get to fresh air immediately if you sense any of the following danger signals:
- You begin to smell or taste contaminants.
- Your eyes, nose, or throat become irritated.
- Breathing becomes difficult.
- The air you are breathing becomes uncomfortably warm.
- You become nauseous or dizzy.

The cartridges or filters may be used up or abnormal conditions may be creating contaminant concentrations which exceed the capacity of the respirator to remove the contamination.

After each use of the respirator, remove all mechanical and chemical filters. Wash the facepiece with soap and warm water, and then immerse it in a sanitizing solution such as chlorine bleach (two table-spoons per gallon of water) for two minutes, followed by a thorough rinsing with clean water to remove all traces of soap and bleach. Wipe the facepiece with a clean cloth and allow to air dry.

Store the respirator facepiece, cartridges, canisters, and mechanical filters in a clean, dry place, preferably in a tightly sealed plastic bag. Do not store respirators with pesticides or other agricultural chemicals.

Handle respirators with the same care that you give your other protective equipment and clothing.

Consult the label and MSDS for instructions about protective equipment and clothing. And remember that protective equipment has limitations. A person is never completely protected and must still use caution and common sense to prevent pesticides from contacting the body.

Many different brands and styles of protective equipment are available. It may take several tries before the right equipment is found. Farm supply stores, chemical dealerships, and local hardware stores may stock some types. A wide selection is also available from a variety of mail order companies.

Laundering pesticide contaminated clothing

All protective clothing and equipment should be washed at the end of each day's use because the concentration of pesticide in the fabric tends to build with successive exposures. The more concentrated the pesticide in the fabric, the more difficult it is to remove during laundering. Contaminated clothing should be stored and washed separately from the family laundry. Pesticides can be transferred from one garment to another in the wash water. Cases have been reported in which several family members developed skin rashes after wearing clothes that were washed in the same water as pesticide contaminated clothing. Remember to wear waterproof gloves when handling contaminated clothing, and be sure to check the product label for any specific laundering instruction. Clothing that has become saturated with a product concentrate should be discarded.

Some residues may be removed by presoaking the contaminated clothing in an appropriate container, or by using a prewash cycle on the washing machine.

Always use a prewash product in any pretreatment process. Washing in hot water at full water level removes more pesticide from clothing than washing in colder water temperatures. The hotter the better; cold water might save energy, but it is relatively ineffective in removing pesticides from clothing.

Washing clothes more than once should increase the amount of pesticide removed, but it may not remove all residue.

Most laundry detergents are effective in removing pesticides from fabric. However, heavy duty liquid detergents typically have better oil removing ability and, therefore, are more effective than other detergents in removing emulsifiable concentrates. The ease of pesticide removal through laundering does not depend on toxicity, but on the formulation of the pesticide. Bleach or ammonia may possibly help in the removal or break down of certain pesticides, but never mix them together because they react to form chlorine gas which can be fatal.

After washing, be sure to rinse the washing machine with an empty load, using hot water and the same detergent. Line drying of clothing is recommended for two reasons. First, it eliminates the possibility of residues collecting in the dryer. Second, residues of many pesticides will break down when exposed to sunlight.

Finally, wash gloves, hands, and arms after the laundering process.

Store Pesticides Safely

Proper pesticide storage helps prolong chemical shelf life while protecting the health of people, animals, and the environment. Consult the pesticide product label for specific storage information. Basic guidelines that are essential for safe pesticide storage are presented in the following sections.

Storage area

All pesticides should be kept out of reach of pets, livestock, children, and irresponsible people. A storage facility must be secured against theft, vandalism, and unauthorized access. Store pesticides in a locked place such as a separate building, room, or cabinet. For storage outdoors, a security fence should be erected.

The storage facility should be located where water damage is unlikely to occur. Soil and land surface characteristics should be considered when selecting a storage area or constructing a storage facility to prevent contamination of surface water or groundwater from runoff, leaching, or drainage. The floor in a storage facility should be free of cracks and have an impermeable surface that can be cleaned and decontaminated in the event of a spill. A floor that is sloped

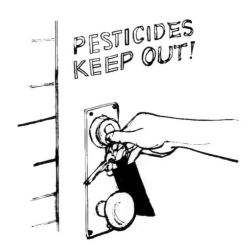

into a containment system or recessed below the level of the doors will help to keep pesticides whithin the restricted area. In certain situations, diking or some other containment structure may need to be constructed around the storage facility. In addition, the following guidelines should be observed:

- Place highly visible warning signs on walls, doors, and/or windows to indicate to anyone attempting to enter the facility that pesticides are stored there. "No Smoking" signs should be displayed. Fireproof construction is best.
- Store pesticides in an area away from food, feed, potable water supplies, veterinary supplies, seeds, and protective equipment. This prevents contamination from vapors, dusts, or spills, and reduces the likelihood of accidental human or animal exposure.
- Maintain a well ventilated storage area to prevent the accumulation and movement of vapors and dust into work areas. Avoid temperature extremes. Very high or low temperatures can cause pesticide deterioration. Exhaust fans directed to the outside will help to reduce temperatures and remove dust and vapors from the storage facility.
- Keep pesticide containers out of direct sunlight to prevent overheating.

Pesticide containers

- Store pesticides only in their original containers. Never use soft drink bottles, fruit jars, fuel cans, or other types of nonpesticide containers. Besides being illegal, serious poisonings could result from using the wrong container because children as well as most adults associate the shape of container with its contents.

- Keep the original label attached to the container. To keep a label legible, protect it with transparent tape or lacquer. Remember, the label is the most important safety factor in the use of pesticides. Do not let it become damaged or destroyed.
- Bulk or mini-bulk tanks should be placed on a reinforced concrete pad or other impermeable suface. Diking around a tank will keep spilled or leaking pesticide inside a restricted area and will also help to prevent damage to the tanks from vehicles and equipment. A dike should be large enough to contain the volume of the liquid in the tank plus at least an additial 10 percent. Valves and pumps should be within the diked area. All drains within the dike should be connected to a holding tank.
- Never lend any pesticide product in an unmarked or unlabelled container. Pesticide users should not rely on verbal directions.
- Close containers securely when not in use. Dry formulations tend to cake when wet or subjected to high humidity. Opened bags of wettable and soluble powders, dusts, and granules can be placed into sealable plastic bags or other suitable containers. This reduces moisture absorption by the material, and prevents a spill should a tear or break occur.
- Store liquid formulations and small containers of dry formulations on metal shelving. Metal shelving will not absorb spilled chemicals and is easier to clean than other surfaces.
- Store liquids and heavier containers on the lower shelves. Containers should not extend beyond shelving where they could be bumped or knocked off. Be sure the shelving wil be able to handle the quantity and weight involved.
- Place larger metal drums and nonmetalic containers on pallets.
- Store volatile herbicides separately to avoid possible cross contamination of other pesticides, fertilizers, and seeds.
- Check containers regularly for leaks, breaks, rust, and corrosion. If a leak or break occurs, place the container inside another container, or transfer the contents to an empty container which originally held the same material and has the same label attached.

Safety

- Have duplicate copies of labels available for the products currently being used. These will be need-

Pesticide kills cows

Joe was helping his neighbor Sam plant corn. When Joe finished planting, he had a little corn rootworm insecticide left in the hopper. Joe looked for a container to dump the granules into. There it was, an empty feed mineral bag blowing around the barnyard. Hoppers emptied, Joe sat the bag over by the shed intending to "take care of it later."

In the meantime, Frank, a hired hand, saw the bag by the shed and because it was a feed mineral bag, he carried it over and put it in the feed shed. After all, Frank was just doing his job, and he was going that way anyway. He had no reason to suspect the bag did not contian feed minerals. Besides, Joe had moved the planter so why should Frank be suspicious.

When Bob, another farm hand, went to the feed shed, he noticed that it was time to mix some more feed. Logic told him to use the opened bag before opening another, so he unknowingly poured the pesticide granules into the feed mixer. the granules and mineral feed supplement were so similar in appearance that Bob didn't notice anything peculiar. Also, pesticides are "never" stored in the feed shed. The result was more than 60 dead dairy cows.

Keep pesticides in original containers.

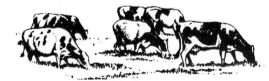

Pesticide kills cows

ed in case of an emergency. A Material Safety Data Sheet should also be available for every hazardous chemical in the storage facility.

- Wear the appropriate protective clothing when handling pesticide containers.
- Label all items used for handling pesticides (measuring utensils, protective equipment, etc.) to prevent their use for other purposes.
- Clay, pet litter, fine sand, activated charcoal, vermiculite, or similar commercially available absorbents can be used to clean up spills or leaks. Hydrated lime and bleach should be available for decontamination of spill surfaces, but never use these two materials together. A shovel, broom, and heavy-duty plastic bags are also needed for spill containment and cleanup.

• Treated seed presents a potential hazard if not stored properly. Such seed is usually treated with a brightly colored dye to serve as a warning that the seed has been treated with a pesticide. Unfortunately, the bright colors may be attractive to children. Treated seed should never be used for feed or mixed with untreated seed. It should be handled with the same care as the pesticide itself and stored in a locked storage facility away from feed, veterinary supplies, pesticides, other chemicals, equipment, pets, and children.

• Keep plenty of soap and water available in or close to the storage facility. A fire extinguisher, first aid equipment, and emergency telephone numbers should all be readily available.

Shelf life of pesticides

Keep an inventory of all pesticides in storage and mark each container with the purchase date. If a product has an effective shelf life recorded on the label, you will know how long the product should remain usable. If there are questions about the shelf life of a product, contact the dealer or manufacturer. Pesticide deterioration may be indicated during mixing by excessive clumping, poor suspension, layering, or abnormal coloration. Sometimes, however, pesticide deterioration from age or poor storage conditions may be apparent only after application as indicated by poor pest control and/or damage to the treated crop or surface.

To minimize storage problems, avoid storing large quantities of pesticides for long periods. Keep records of previous usage to make good estimates of future needs. Buy only as much as you will need for the season; recommendations may change by next season.

Reporting requirements

Title III of the Federal Superfund Amendments and Reauthorization Act of 1986 (SARA Title III) is also called the Emergency Planning and Community Right-to-Know Act. The Act requires among other things the reporting of inventories of certain pesticides if the amount stored is greater than a "threshold planning quantity (TPQ)". Facilities that produce, use, or store, at anytime, a designated substance above a specific TPQ must notify the State Emergency Response Commission (SERC) and, in Pennsylvania, the county Local Emergency Planning Committee (LEPC).

It is also a good idea to inform your local fire department if you store any agricultural chemicals, including fertilizers. Chemical fires often cannot be extinguished by ordinary means, and the smoke from the fire can be extremely hazardous to fire fighters. The fire department must be properly prepared in the event of an agricultural chemical fire.

More discussion on minimizing fire hazards is provided in the chapter on "Pesticide Emergencies."

Mix and Load Pesticides Safely

The most hazardous activities involving pesticides are mixing and loading of concentrates. Always have adequate protective clothing and equipment available and put them on before handling or opening a pesticide container. Remember that a respirator or appropriate form of eye protection should be worn if there is any chance of pesticide inhalation or eye exposure. Never eat, drink, or smoke while handling pesticides. Before opening the container read the label so you are familiar with mixing and usage directions.

Carefully choose the pesticide mixing and loading area. It should be located outside, away from other people, livestock, and pets. Pesticides should not be mixed in areas where a spill or overflow could contaminate a water supply. If the mixing area is unavoidably near a well, pond, or stream bank, the area should be graded to slope away from the water. Also, lengthen the water hose to permit filling and mixing as far away from the water source as possible. Mixing chemicals on a concrete pad facilitates cleanup and prevents spilled pesticides from contaminating the soil.

If you must work indoors, or at night, be sure there is adequate ventilation and light. Have a supply of clean water and soap available, and if possible, do not work alone.

Do not tear paper containers to open them; use a sharp knife or a scissors. When pouring from a container, keep the container at or below eye level and avoid splashing or spilling chemical on your face or protective clothing. Never use your mouth to siphon a pesticide from a container. always stand upwind so the wind does not blow the pesticide towards you. If an accident occurs, attend to it immediately. Remove any contaminated clothing and wash yourself thoroughly with soap and water. Spills should be attended to promptly. Note the section on spills in the chapter on "Pesticide Emergencies."

Follow label instructions and mix only the amount

you plan to immediately use. Measure accurately! The effectiveness and safety of an application is jeopardized if too much or too little chemical is used. Refer to the section "Conversions and Calculations" for unit conversion tables and sample pesticide calculations. Measuring devices such as "tip and pours" are a great help in handling small amounts of concentrate. All measuring devices (spoons, cups, scales) should be kept in the pesticide storage area and never used for other purposes. Label them accordingly to prevent their use for anything else. Measuring cups should be rinsed and the rinsate put into the spray tank. Pesticide containers should be triple rinsed as soon as they are emptied because residues can dry and become difficult to remove later. Pour the rinsate into the spray tank to avoid disposal problems and wasting product. Close containers tightly and return them to the pesticide storage area.

Equipment should be checked and calibrated prior to filling and use. The spray tank must also be clean; oil, grease, and chemical residues can cause incompatibility problems. The agitation system should be running and the spray tank should be approximately half filled with water before any pesticide is added.

Always keep your head above the fill hole. Do not spill or splash any chemical when putting it into the tank. If two or more pesticides are to be mixed, they must be compatible and mixed in the correct order. Small quantities of wettable powders often mix more easily if a slurry is made first. Compatibility is discussed further in the chapter on "Pesticide Formulations."

When adding water to the spray mixture, leave an air gap between the end of the waterpipe or hose and the top of the water level. This prevents contaminat-

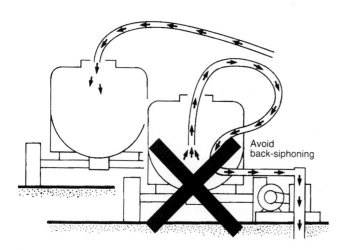

Avoid back-siphoning

ing the pipe or hose and avoids the possibility of back-siphoning the spray mixture into the water source. Never leave a spray unit unattended while it is being filled. Install check-valves or other anti-backflow device to prevent back-siphoning. Prevent water contamination from back-siphoning by filling the spray tank from a nurse tank that contains only water or by adding the pesticide in the field after the tank has been filled with water. Back-siphoning pesticide into a water system is a very costly mistake that can be easily avoided by good management practices.

Keep in mind that water characteristics influence the effectiveness of some pesticides. Alkaline spray water, for example, promotes chemical breakdown of many organophosphates and carbamates. The recommended pH of water for mixing most pesticides is between 5.0 and 7.0. Buffers and acidifying agents can be used to adjust the pH of the water. If water is high in suspended solids, such as silt or organic matter, certain pesticides can be rendered completely ineffective because they bind to the contaminants in the water.

Closed handling systems can reduce user exposure to pesticide concentrates. A closed handling system has interconnected equipment that allows the applicator to remove a pesticide concentrate from its original container, rinse the empty container, and transfer the pesticide and rinsate to the spray tank without the applicator being exposed to the chemical.

Apply Pesticides Safely and Effectively

The safety and effectiveness of a pesticide application hinge largely on using the correct amount of pesticide and an appropriate application method. This assumes, however, that the pest problem has already been correctly diagnosed and monitored, and the pesticide carefully selected to consider performance, worker safety, cost, compatibility with other chemicals, preharvest and re-entry intervals, carryover, and nontarget exposure.

Before application

Before making a pesticide application, be sure to read the product label. For safety precautions, never let an inexperienced person apply pesticides along.

Correct handling procedures require that clean clothing and proper protective equipment be worn. Respiratory protection may be essential if the applicatin is made indoors or if the applicator is in an enclosed cab without air filters.

Never eat, smoke, or drink while handling pesticides; do not even carry food or smoking items with you. Fresh water, soap, and paper towels should be carried in a protected container to allow for quick removal of pesticide contaminants from the body in the event of a spill or exposure to spray drift. A first aid kit and a plastic, flushing action, eyewash bottle are also good precautions, particularly in service vehicles. Applicators should plan to work in pairs when applying highly toxic pesticides.

Livestock, pets, and farm equipment should be removed from the area to be treated. Any persons not involved in the application should leave the area to be treated. Posting of placards may be required to keep unauthorized or unprotected persons from entering the area.

Check application equipment carefully, particularly for leaking hoses and connections and plugged or worn nozzles.

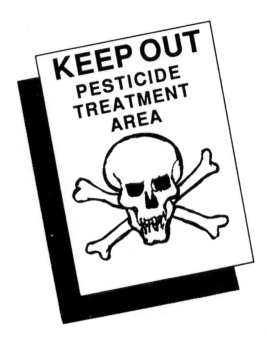

During application

During the pesticide application the weather should be carefully monitored. Pesiticides should be applied only under favorable weather conditions. Do not apply pesticides during or just before expected high winds. As wind velocity increases the chance of drift and volatilization also increases. Do not apply pesticides just before an expected heavy rain. Rain can wash the chemicals off treated surfaces or cause pesticide runoff from a treatedarea. It is often preferable to apply pesticides in the early morning or early evening when wind speeds are usually lower and protective clothing and equipment can be worn with less discomfort.

Applications should be made in a manner that guards against pesticide drift onto nearby water bodies, crops, pastures, livestock, or residential areas. Drift is the movement of airborne pesticides (particles, spray droplets, or gases) beyond the intended contact area. Drift becomes more severe when wind speeds and air temperatures increase, when relative humidity is low, when nozzle height and pump pressure are high, and when spray droplets are small.

Significant drift can also occur when calm coditions exist with a temperature inversion. An inversion occurs when the air temperature at the ground is lower than that of the air above it. The warmer air does not allow the cooler air to rise, but instead causes it to move laterally. Small spray droplets from the application can remain suspended in this layer of cool air and move with it until deposited on a sensitive crop or area.

Certain application measures can help to reduce drift. Droplet size, which is a major factor in spray drift, can vary significantly with different nozzle types. Nozzle types vary in the percentage of fine droplets that they produce and the pressures at which they operate. Use of low-drift nozzles, reduced pump pressure, and the addition of a drift-control agent in the spray tank can help to increase droplet size.

Low humidity and high temperatures favor water evaporation from spray droplets. These smaller droplets remain airborne longer and are more prone to drift from the intended target site.

Be sure to also:
• Replace worn nozzles.
• Set the boom only as high as necessary for adequate coverage.
• Avoid spraying when conditions favor drift.
• Select nonvolatile or low volatile formulations.

Some problems that can result from pesticide drift can be avoided by leaving an untreated border around the field and by spraying downwind from sensitive areas such as residential properties and beehives. Position yourself and your equipment to prevent the pesticide from blowing in your face.

Further minimize your exposure to the chemical when working on equipment. If a nozzle becomes clogged while making an application, stop the sprayer and move to an untreated area before correcting the problem. Never touch your mouth to a spray nozzle or a clogged pump part.

After application

In order to increase the efficacy and safety of a pesticide application, be sure to follow any post-application procedures listed on the label, such as reentry periods and incorporation procedures if the pesticide was soil applied. Never leave equipment unattended at the application site.

Clean all equipment after the pesticide application. Follow any cleaning recommendations on the label. Cleaning should be done in a designated area away from water supplies. Wear the appropriate protective equipment and clothing, and keep in mind that the pesticide has contaminated all equipment parts (pumps, tanks, and hoses). Exercise extreme caution if a sprayer used for herbicides is to be used to apply

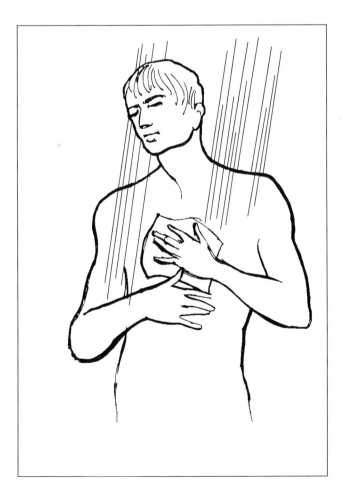

another type of agricultural chemical. The chapter "Pesticide Application Equipment" outlines some procedures for cleaning spray equipment.

After cleaning application equipment, clean your protective equipment. Personal clean up is next. In particular, wash your hands and face thoroughly with soap and water before eating, drinking, or smoking. Shower and change clothing as soon as possible. Be sure to scrub your scalp, neck, behind your ears, and under your nails.

Dispose of Pesticides Safely

It is the responsibility of the pesticide user to see that pesticide wastes such as unused chemicals and empty pesticide containers are disposed of properly. Improperly disposed, pesticide wastes can create serious hazards for both humans and the environment.

It makes good business sense to deal with pesticide wastes properly and safely. Plan carefully and observe the following guidelines.

- Avoid disposal problems associated with excess pesticide by purchasing only the amount you will need for one growing season. Product registrations may change and new chemicals may be better than old ones. A long storage period may also exceed the effective shelf life of the product.
- Always read the label as your first source of disposal information. Recognize, however, that the label may not always give you clear, practical guidance. And, if the product is old, the label recommendations may be out-dated and no longer appropriate.
- During disposal of unwanted pesticides or containers, wear appropriate protective clothing and equipment.
- Clothing and protective equipment to be discarded, contaminated soil, and materials used to clean up spills should be considered pesticide waste and handled as such.
- Federal and state laws regulate the disposal of containers and other pesticide wastes. If you have a question or problem relating to pesticide disposal, contact a regional office of the Pennsylvania Department of Agriculture (PDA), the Regional Chemist in one of the regional offices of the Pennsylvania Department of Environmental Resources (DER), or the regional office of the U.S. Environmental Protection Agency (EPA) in Philadelphia.

An important part of managing pesticide waste is waste reduction. Any reduction in the amount of waste generated can reduce disposal problems and costs. Reducing pesticide waste requires careful planning of purchases as well as careful handling and application of pesticides.

Pesticide concentrates

Carefully read the label instructions for storage requirements. Some pesticides are destroyed by freezing temperatures. Once frozen, they often cannot be used and become a disposal problem. Similarly, pesticide containers can corrode, and some pesticides are destroyed if they become wet. If a pesticide container does not have a legible label, it cannot be identified and, therefore, cannot be used. The container now becomes a disposal problem for the applicator.

The safest means of disposal for pesticide concentrates is to use the product in a manner consistent with its label. If this is not possible, return it to the dealer or manufacturer or offer it to another qualified applicator. If no disposal option is available, then check with a regional office of the PDA or the Regional Chemist in a regional DER office.

Certain pesticides may be disposed of through a municipal refuse collection service; others may require more stringent and costly disposal procedures such as the need to hire a licensed hazardous waste transporter.

Commercial and public applicators should be aware of the current hazardous waste guidelines established under the Resource Conservation and Recovery Act (RCRA) as well as all comparable state hazardous waste statutes and regulations. They should be thoroughly familiar with the guidelines prior to disposing of pesticide wastes. For instance, pesticide wastes classified as hazardous require special disposal and recordkeeping practices. The Pennsylvania DER can provide more information on RCRA and your specific disposal responsibilities under the law.

Spray mixes

To minimize problems with excess spray mix, estimate job needs carefully so you will mix only as much pesticide as needed for a particular application. To do this, you must know the size of the area to be treated. The capacity of the spray equipment and its output must also be known to determine the quantity of water and the amount of pesticide product to place in the spray tank. Monitor weather conditions before mixing pesticides to ensure that you will actually be able to spray at the predetermined time. Check spray equipment to see that it is in good working order before the spray tank is filled. Equipment must be calibrated to apply the pesticide at the correct rate and minimize leftover spray mix. If you do mix too much, apply the material in the recommended manner to another crop or site listed on the label.

Equipment rinsates

Equipment rinsate is generated when spray application equipment is washed and rinsed after use. Rinsates must be handled carefully to avoid water contamination or injury to nontarget plants and animals.

When possible, rinse your equipment at the application site and spray the rinsate on the treated area. This is feasible only if a water source is available at the application site. A more practical option for most pesticide users is to rinse equipment at the mixing site and then apply the rinsate to a crop or site listed on the product label.

Another option is to collect and store the rinsate for future use. Collection and storage systems usually consist of a concrete pad or platform on which equipement is washed, a drainage system that connects to a holding tank, and a pump to dispense the liquid from the holding tank into the sprayer. Above ground holding tanks are usually preferred over buried tanks because they can be more easily monitored for leaks. These systems can be very useful in managing pesticide wastes, but must be used responsibly. Careful records must be kept of all pesticide rinsates put into the holding tanks to avoid subsequent plant injury or illegal residues on a food or feed crop when the rinsates are used.

Do not allow equipment rinsate to enter a sewer or a drain that leads to a water/sewage treatment system. Also, remember that repeated cleaning of application equipment on bare ground in the same location can lead to pesticide levels in the soil that exceed the soil's capacity to bind or degrade the chemical.

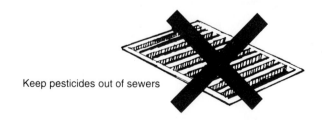

Keep pesticides out of sewers

Pesticide leaching from such areas can lead to groundwater contamination.

Pesticide containers

Properly rinsing glass, metal, plastic, and even some heavy paper containers effectively removes most pesticide remaining in the container. Rinsing not only saves the applicator money by using the rinsate in the spray tank, but also allows disposal of the containers as nonhazardous waste. Rinse containers as soon as they are empty. Some pesticide residues become very difficult, if not impossible, to remove after they dry. Rinse containers using either the triple rinse method or an equivalent procedure such as pressure rinsing. To triple rinse:

1. Drain the concentrate from the pesticide container into the spray tank for at least 30 seconds after the flow begins to drip.
2. Fill approximately one-fourth of the container volume with water or an appropriate solvent, replace the cap, and rotate the container so all of the interior surfaces are rinsed.
3. Pour the rinsate into the spray tank, allowing it to drain for at least 30 seconds after the flow begins to drip.
4. Repeat this procedure two more times.

Triple-rinsed or pressure-rinsed containers that are being held for disposal at a later date should be marked to indicate that rinsing has been done and the date. Containers that cannot be recycled through a recycling facility or the dealer should be rendered unusable by being pierced or crushed. Never reuse pesticide containers for any prupose. All containers should be kept in a locked storage facility until disposal, and away from all possible contact with children and animals.

Few disposal options exist for empty pesticide containers. Municipal sanitary landfills are not required to accept pesticide containers, but at this time, rinsed containers are still being accepted at many licensed municipal landfills. It is a good policy to check with your local solid waste authority prior to discarding pesticide containers this way.

Triple-rinsed or pressure-rinsed containers should be recycled whenever feasible. For information on recycling facilities, consult your local solid waste disposal authorities, or the Regional Resource Recovery and Planning Coordinator at a regional DER office.

Never leave pesticide containers in fields, even if they have been rinsed. Properly rinsed containers can be buried on your own property, but the site should

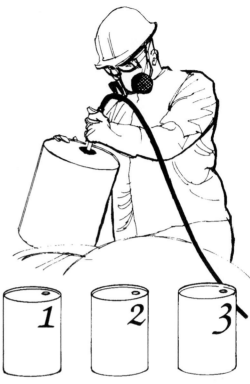

Triple rinse containers

be located away from houses, crop growing areas, livestock areas, farm ponds, irrigation channels, wells, and streams.

Combustible containers can be burned only if permitted by the instructions on the label and by local and state ordinances and policies. Those planning to burn combustible containers should contact the Bureau of Air Quality at a regional DER office. Remove as much residue from combustible containers as possible; triple rinse containers if feasible. Burn pesticide containers in an approved site, away from residential areas or where persons can come in contact with the smoke. Always stand upwind when burning pesticide containers; the smoke may be toxic. Herbicide vapors, particularly those from growth-regulating herbicides such as 2,4-D and dicamba, can cause injury to nearby plants.

Follow disposal instructions on the label; seek assistance with disposal problems.

Transport Pesticides Safely

Once a pesticide is in your possession, you are responsible for its safe transportation. Accidents can and do occur even when transporting pesticides a short distance. Know how to prevent transportation problems and be prepared in case of an emergency.

Transport vehicle

The safest way to carry pesticides is usually in the back of a truck. Steel beds are preferable since they are more easily cleaned if a spill should occur. Flatbed trucks should have side and tail racks. Any vehicle used to transport pesticides should be in safe driving condition; in particular, check the tires, brakes, and steering.

Pesticides should never be carried in the passenger compartment of a vehicle because spilled chemical and hazardous fumes can cause serious injury to the occupants. Spilled pesticides can also be very difficult if not impossible to remove from upholstery. If pesticides must be transported in a station wagon, windows should remain open and no one should be permitted to ride near the containers.

Food, livestock feed, fertilizers, seed, veterinary supplies, and plant materials should always be kept separate from pesticides because danger of contamination is too great. If at all possible, herbicides should be transported separately from other pesticides because a herbicide spill could lead to contamination of the other pesticides.

Containers should be inspected prior to loading to be certain legible labels are attached, all caps and plugs are tightly closed, and the outsides of the containers are not contaminated with pesticide. Obtain a current Material Safety Data Sheet (MSDS) for each pesticide at the time of purchase; it provides information on the toxicity and chemical and physical characteristics of the product. Such information is essential in a pesticide emergency.

Handle containers carefully when loading to avoid rips and punctures. Inspect the truck bed for nails, stones, and sharp edges that could damage containers. Secure anything in the vehicle that could move during transport and potentially puncture a container. Use a brace bar, rope, or other device to prevent containers from sliding or rolling in the truck bed. Packing or shipping containers can be used to provide extra protection.

Pesticides should be protected from temperature extremes and moisture during transport. In hot weather the temperature inside a closed vehicle is always considerably higher than outside. Extremely high or low temperatures can alter the effectiveness of certain chemicals. Rain can destroy paper and cardboard pesticide containers and promote rusting of metal containers. A tarp or a sheet of water repellent material should be placed over the containers to protect them from moisture.

A vehicle should always carry the basic equipment and material necessary for emergency spill containment and cleanup.

Safety precautions

Never leave your vehicle unattended when transporting pesticides in an open vehicle. You are legally responsible if curious children or careless adults are accidentally poisoned from pesticides left unattended. Theft and vandalism are also potential problems. Whenever possible, transport pesticides in a locked compartment.

Transporting diluted pesticides in either trailer- or truck-mounted spray tanks over public highways requires the same precautions as transporting concentrates. Perform a detailed safety check before leaving the mixing area. Check the tank for leaks. Make sure that all clamps, connections, and fittings are secure. Spray tanks should be securely fastened with a chain tightener. Spray tank covers must fit tightly to prevent the pesticide mix from splashing out during transportation and operation.

Finally, be familiar with the transportation route when carrying pesticides. Anticipating potential hazards can help drivers complete their journey safely.

Regulations

Federal and state laws regulate the transportation of hazardous chemicals, including many pesticides, over public roads. The most common requirements for the transportation of pesticides are placarding and the possession of shipping papers. Placards are placed on vehicles to warn of the potential danger of the materials being carried. The type of placard(s) required depends on the hazard class (i.e., poison, flammable, corrosive, oxidizer) of the chemical, and in most cases the amounts of chemical present.

Placarding is always required when transporting materials with a Poison A classification. These materials (such as phosphine or chloropicrin compressed gas) would be dangerous to life if a very small amount of gas or vapor from the liquid were to be mixed with ambient air.

Poison B substances are those that are known to present a potential health hazard to humans during transportation, or in the absence of human health information are known to meet one of the following acute toxicity criteria: acute oral $LD_{50} \leq 50$ mg/kg; acute inhalation $LC_{50} \leq 2$ mg/l; or dermal $LD_{50} \leq 200$ mg/kg. Poison B substances include such pesticides as azinphos-methyl, carbofuran, DDVP, disulfoton, and paraquat.

Placarding is required when transporting 1,000 pounds or more gross weight of a Poison B substance. Placarding is also required when transporting a Poison B substance in a portable or cargo tank. A portable tank includes bulk containers, usually equipped with skids or racks and designed primarily to be loaded onto a vehicle. A portable tank, by definition, includes minibulk or bulk containers, but not drums and other types of common packaging. A cargo tank is any tank that is permanently attached to a vehicle or is mounted onto a frame with wheels that is part of a motor vehicle. When placarding is used, it must always remain on a tank until the unit has been cleaned.

Placarding is not usually needed when carrying dilute spray mixes (i.e., when mixing 10 pounds of a Poison B insecticide with 1000 gallons of water). When this occurs the mixture is usually so dilute that it no longer meets the toxicity criteria for a Poison B chemical.

A shipping paper, which can be a bill of lading, manifest, or other shipping document, is required when transporting certain quantities of some pesticides. The purpose of a shipping paper is to provide relevant information about the chemicals being transported should there be an accident and the driver of the vehicle becomes incapacitated. The shipping paper must state the total quantity of chemicals present and identify all hazardous chemicals with their proper shipping names, hazard classes, and identification numbers. The type of packaging, number of pieces, and information about placarding may also appear on the shipping paper, but are not required. The shipping paper should be within the driver's reach and kept either in a pouch attached to the inside of the driver's door or in some other readily visible place.

A shipper of hazardous chemicals is also responsible for proper packaging. If repackaging is done, it must be done in compliance with all regulations.

The Motor Carrier Safety Division, Pennsylvania Department of Transportation (PennDOT), is responsible for the enforcement of the Hazardous Materials Regulations in the Commnwealth of Pennsylvaia.

Keeping Records

Certified applicators who use pesticides are required to keep records. Commercial and public applicators must keep records of all pesticide applications. Private applicators must keep records of all restricted use pesticide applications. All records must be kept for a minimum of three years and made available to the PDA upon request. The new federal farm bill also requires private applicators to keep records of restricted use pesticide applications. Useful information includes:

- Date and time of application
- What pesticide was used
- The formulation of the pesticide
- The way the pesticide was mixed (for example, pounds per 100 gallons of water)
- The rate of application (for example, gallons per acre and the total area treated)
- Type of equipment used
- What crop or site was treated (for example, corn, house foundation, turf)
- The target pest(s)
- Wheather conditions at the time of application
- Name of the applicator
- Results of the application

All pesticide users are strongly advised to keep thorough records for their protection should a problem arise from an application. Personal protection, however, is not the only reason for keeping pesticide records. Information on previous applications can prevent damage to sensitive crops and prevent the presence of illegal residues. Recordkeeping can save money. Records from year to year help the applicator to compare the results of pest control programs and practices, and can serve as a guide when making future purchases.

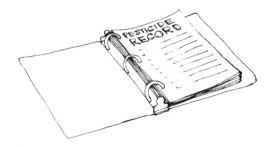

Bibliography

See end of Chapter 24.

24

PESTICIDE EMERGENCIES

Although accidents and emergencies involving pesticides are rare, they do, unfortunately, occur. Manufacturers, transporters, dealers, and users of pesticides must be prepared to respond to emergencies promptly and correctly. Do all you can to prevent an accident, but be prepared in case an emergency should arise.

Fires

Pesticide products vary significantly in their flammability and storage hazard. Those requiring extra precautions usually include the label statement "Do not use or store near heat or open flame." Pesticides containing oils or petroleum solvents are the ones most likely to have these warnings, although certain dry formulations also present fire and explosion hazards.

Potential problems associated with pesticide fires include:

- The pesticides may be highly flammable or explosive, for example, aerosols, solvents, dusts or powders, and chlorates in some herbicides and desiccants.

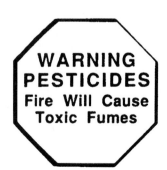

WARNING PESTICIDES Fire Will Cause Toxic Fumes

From Hock WK, Brown CL (editors): *Pesticide education manual*, ed 2, University Park, Penn, Penn State University.

- The pesticides may give off vapors or smoke which are highly toxic to fire fighters, nearby residents, and animals, for example, organophosphate, carbamate, and organochlorine pesticides and certain solvents.
- Some products may give off vapors or smoke which are toxic to plants (phytotoxic), for example, vapors from some herbicides.
- Pesticides may be present in the debris and soil.
- Run-off from the fire site is likely to contain highly toxic chemicals.

Precautions to Reduce Fire Hazards

By observing certain fundamental safety precautions, the threat of a serious pesticide fire can be reduced, or eliminated in some instances. Whenever possible, observe the following precautions:

- Locate storage facilities as far as possible from where people and animals live.
- Keep storage facility locked at all times.
- Post signs that indicate combustible materials are stored in the facility.
- Store combustible materials away from steam lines and other heating systems.
- Do not store glass or pressurized containers in sunlight where they can concentrate heat rays and possibly explode or ignite.
- Install fire detection systems in large storage areas.
- Keep foam-type fire extinguishers that are approved for chemical fires in all storage areas.
- Notify the servicing fire company as to the location and contents of the storage facility. It may save their lives and the lives of others should there be fire.
- Develop an emergency plan and train all workers in its execution.
- Keep a written inventory of the pesticides held in storage and file the list away from the main

office. If a fire occurs during nonbusiness hours, emergency personnel will need to know what chemicals are present.

Action in the Event of a Fire

Prompt and responsible action is essential in the event of a toxic chemical fire. Emergency (or contingency) planning prior to the occurrence of a fire or other catastrophe is the cornerstone of a responsible action plan. All details on how to respond to a fire should be coordinated with local emergency response officials and reviewed at least annually. Then the following actions can be taken promptly with a minimum of confusion should a toxic chemical fire occur:

- Evacuate the premises.
- Notify the fire department and inform the fire fighters of the nature of the pesticides involved. Warn all firefighters of the dangers from exploding containers, chemical vapors, smoke, run-off, and debris. MSDSs provide technical and emergency information.
- Keep people away.
- If significant smoke is generated, evacuate all people and animals in the vicinity, especially those downwind.
- Have a doctor and/or ambulance standing by at the site.
- Notify all fire fighter that they must wear protective clothing and use a self-contained breathing apparatus.

Other respirators will not provide adequate protection.

- Avoid eating, drinking, or smoking during fire-fighting operations—they increase the danger of exposure to hazardous chemicals.
- Fight fire with fog, foam, or dry powder. If only water is available, use it as a fine spray of fog. Do not use water jets because they can break bags and glass containers.
- Check that water and spilled chemicals are being contained. Use only as much water as absolutely necessary.
- If run-off occurs or dangers arise from exploding containers, consider withdrawing and allowing the fire to burn out. Dikes should be built to contain the run-off.
- Relieve from duty and place under medical care any person exposed to pesticide vapors or smoke or to splashing chemical, and any person showing signs of illness, dizziness or unusual behavior. Poisoning by pesticides can be mistaken for heat exhaustion, smoke inhalation, or physical stress. Remove contaminated clothing immediately.
- On completion of activities, equipment and all clothing should be cleaned and all personnel involved should take showers.

After the fire, clean-up and salvage operations should not be attempted until the area has cooled, and then, under expert supervision only.

Pesticide Spills

As careful as most people try to be, pesticide spills do occur. The spill may be a minor one involving only a few leaking containers; or it may be a major accident where a piece of equipment malfunctions and releases its contents, or a tank truck or rail car overturns and spills its cargo. It is very important that all users of hazardous chemicals be thoroughly familiar with the laws and guidelines governing chemical spills. Their inability to respond properly to such an emergency, no matter how minor the problem, could seriously endanger public health and environmental quality.

The suggested guidelines in the event of a hazardous chemical spill are included under the "Three C" program: control the spill, contain it, and clean it up.

Control the Spill

Immediate steps should be taken to control the flow of the liquid being spilled. If a sprayer has tipped

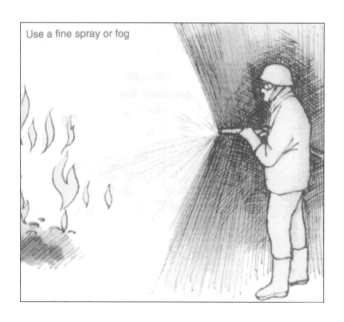

Use a fine spray or fog

over, or if a hazardous chemical is leaking from a damaged tank truck, or if a one-gallon can on a storage shelf has rusted through and is leaking, do whatever you can safely do to stop the leak or spill at once. For instance, smaller containers can be put into larger containers to prevent further release of the chemical. Stopping larger leaks or spills often isn't so simple.

Don't expose yourself unnecessarily to the leaking chemical; wear protective equipment when attempting to control the leak. Also, don't charge in blindly if someone is injured; again, make sure you are properly protected.

Get help. Have someone alert the state and local police if the spill occurs on a public highway. Contact the regional office of the Pennsylvania Department of Agriculture if the chemical is a pesticide or other agricultural chemical. Be sure to have the product label available! In certain cases, it may be necessary to alert the fire department, but be sure to caution them not be wash down the spill until advised to do so. At times it may also be necessary to contact public health officials and the nearest hospital emergency room.

If you encounter an accident that you can't handle or if problems occur during the clean-up phase, you should contact the Chemical Transportation Emergency Center (CHEMTREC) in Washington, D.C. at 1-800-424-9300. The CHEMTREC office is staffed 24 hours a day by trained personnel who are competent and knowledgeable in handling emergencies involving pesticide chemical, including spills and accidents.

Isolate the area. Rope off the contaminated area; keep people at least 30 feet away from the spill. Avoid contact with any drift or fumes that may be released. Do not use road flares if you suspect the leaking material is flammable. At times it may be necessary to evacuate people down-wind from the spill.

Do not leave the spill site until someone relieves you. Someone should be present at the spill site continuously until the chemical is cleaned up and the danger removed.

Contain the Spill or Leak

At the same time the leak is being controlled, contain the spilled material in as small an area as possible. Do everything possible to keep it from spreading or getting worse. In some situations you may need to use a shovel or power equipment to construct a dam. The important thing to remember is don't let the spilled material get into any body of water, including storm sewers, no mater how small the spill.

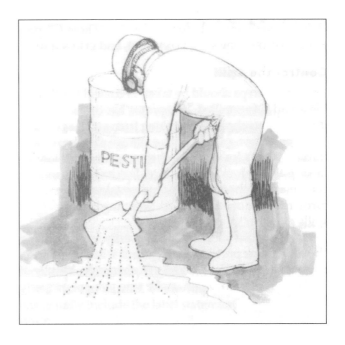

If the chemical does contaminate a stream, pond, or any other waterway, contact the Pennsylvania Department of Environmental Resources (DER), the Pennsylvania Fish Commission, and the Pennsylvania Department of Agriculture immediately. Discharge of chemical substances into waterways must also be reported to the U.S. Environmental Protection Agency under the authority of the Clean Water Act (National Response Center, 1-800-424-8802). Have the authorities notify downstream users as soon as possible to prevent accidental poisoning of livestock and to avoid contamination of irrigated crops and soil.

Liquid spills can be further contained by spreading absorbent materials such as fine sand, vermiculite, clay, or pet litter over the entire spill. However, a word of caution. Avoid using sawdust or sweeping compounds if the material is a strong oxidizer, because such a combination presents a possible fire hazard. Several manufacturers now have nonselective, universal sorbents packed in porous fabric pillows. These pillows or "tubes" can be placed directly on the spill or used to dike around the spill area. Waste disposal is also simplified since the contaminated pillows can be placed into heavy-duty disposal bags without dust or spillage.

In the case of dust, wettable powder, or granular material, you can reduce further spreading by lightly misting the material with water, or covering the spill with some type of plastic cover. Remember, however, that this cover is now contaminated and should be discarded after use.

Disposal of all hazardous wastes must be done in strict accordance with state and federal (RCRA) laws. This applies to any pesticide spill—insecticide, fungicide, or herbicide.

Clean Up the Spill

Keep adding absorbent material to the contaminated area until all the liquid is soaked up, sweep it up, and place it in a steel or fiber drum lined with a heavy-duty plastic bag. Once the spill has been cleaned up, it may be necessary to decontaminate or neutralize the area, especially if a carbamate or organophosphate insecticide was involved.

Use ordinary household bleach in water (approximately 30 percent) or hydrated lime. Remember to wear protective equipment if needed. Do not use bleach and lime together. Work this cleaning material into the spill area with a coarse broom. Then add fresh absorbent material to soak up the now contaminated cleaning solution. This material should then be swept up and placed in a plastic bag or drum for disposal. It will be necessary to repeat this procedure several times to ensure that the area has been thoroughly decontaminated.

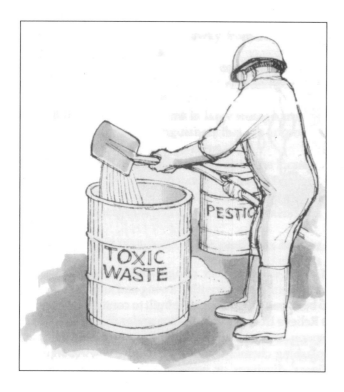

Soil contamination

The only effective way to decontaminate soil saturated with a hazardous chemical is to remove the top 2 to 3 inches of soil. Be sure to dispose of this contaminated soil at a proper disposal site. Then cover the area with at least 2 inches of lime, and finally, cover the lime with fresh topsoil.

Soils contaminated as the result of application errors or minor spills can sometimes be cleaned up by applying activated charcoal to the contaminated surface immediately after the spill or misapplication. The charcoal may absorb or tie up enough chemical to avoid significant plant injury and long-term contamination. However, application of activated charcoal to areas where large spills have occurred will do little to reduce soil contamination and subsequent plant damage.

Clean the equipment and vehicles

Clean any vehicles and equipment that were contaminated either as a result of the original accident or during the clean-up and disposal procedures. Before you begin, however, be sure you are properly clothed and protected to avoid contact with the chemical. Use ordinary household bleach in water (approximately 30 percent bleach) or an alkaline detergent (dishwasher soap) solution to clean your equipment. Do not mix bleach and alkaline detergent together.

Porous material and equipment such as brooms, leather shoes, and cloth hats cannot be effectively decontaminated and must be discarded or destroyed. Also, don't save disposable garments and gloves or badly contaminated clothing. You should dispose of them properly and immediately after completing the clean up.

Serious accidents

Serious accidents involving chemicals present unusually hazardous conditions—perhaps a major spill has occurred or the chemical is particularly dangerous to handle.

To protect the public and to assist public agencies in handling such mishaps, the chemical industry has in place an emergency response system. Here is how this response system works.

1) Caller reports an incident to CHEMTREC in Washington, D.C., using the telephone number 1-800-424-9300. The individual answering the CHEMTREC will ask the caller for information about the incident being reported and to identify the chemical(s) involved.

2) CHEMTREC will then provide basic emergency information on the chemical(s) reported.

3) CHEMTREC will then contact the manufacturer(s) of the chemical(s) involved so that the company can initiate its own technical assistance and response procedures. Pesticide manufacturers have technical staff skilled in dealing with emergencies involving their products.

Emergency telephone number on pesticide labels

An additional and very important number to remember is the emergency telephone number found on many product labels and on transportation shipping papers. The lines are answered 24 hours per day by people who are prepared to handle pesticide emergencies involving their products.

Follow up

For legal protection, it is advisable to keep records of your activities and conversations with regulatory authorities, emergency response personnel, and the general public when dealing with a pesticide spill. Photographs help to document any damage as well as the clean-up process. Be sure the spill has been reported to the appropriate regulatory agencies (Pennsylvania Departments of Agriculture and Environmental Resources).

SARA Title III also requires the reporting of certain pesticide spills if the amount spilled is greater than the "reportable quantity" for that chemical.

Discharge of chemical substances into waterways must also be reported to the U.S. Environmental Protection Agency under the authority of the Clean Water Act.

Spill Prevention and Preparation

A key to preventing pesticide spills is to properly maintain all vehicles and application equipment. Leaks and drips from cracks or loose fittings in equipment are indications of potential trouble. An under-standing of how spray equipment works, especially a pumping system, is often essential to controlling the flow of a product and minimizing equipment damage should a problem occur. Safe driving and other good operating habits further reduce the likelihood of a spill.

Knowing how to safely handle pesticide spills and leaks is as important as knowing how to correctly apply the material. All facilities in which pesticides are handled should have a complete listing of emergency telephone numbers readily available. Always have the product label with you! A Material Safety Data Sheet (MSDS) for every pesticide on the premises is a must. Proper equipment and supplies for cleaning up spills are essential in every storage establishment.

All persons using or transporting pesticides and other hazardous chemicals have a responsibility to protect the public and the environment. Doing everything possible to avoid spills, and adhering to a few basic guidelines when handling spills and leaks, can go a long way toward meeting that responsibility.

Bibliography (Chapters 20-24)

Bohmont BL: *The standard pesticide user's guide*, Englewood Cliffs, NI, 1990, Prentice Hall.

Farm chemicals handbook: Willoughby, Ohio, 1993, Meister Publishing.

Herbicide handbook of the weed science society of America: ed 6, Champaign, Ill 1989, The Society.

Marer PJ, Flint ML, Stimmann MW: *The safe and effective use of pesticides*, Pesticide Application Compendium 1, Publ. 3324, 1988, UCD.

Morgan DP: *Recognition and management of pesticide poisoning*, ed 4, 1989, US Environmental Protection Agency.

Thomson WT: *Agricultural chemicals, book 1: insecticides (1989); book II: herbicides (1989-90); book III: miscellaneous agricultural chemicals (1991-92); book IV: Fungicides (1991)*, Thomson Publications, Fresno, Calif.

Ware GW: *The pesticide book*, 1989, Fresno, Calif. Thomson Publication.

GLOSSARY (CHAPTERS 20-24)

absorption The movement of a chemical into plants, animals (including humans), microorganisms, or soil.

acaricide A pesticide used to control mites and ticks. A miticide is a type of acaricide.

activated charcoal Finely gorund charcoal which adsorbs chemicals.

activator An adjuvant added to a pesticide to increase its toxicity.

active ingredient The chemical or chemicals in a product responsible for pesticidal activity.

acute toxicity Injury produced from a single exposure. LD50 and LC50 are common indicators of the degree of acute toxicity (see chronic toxicity).

adjuvant A substance added to a pesticide to improve its effectiveness or safety. Same as additive. Examples: Penetrants, spreader-stickers, and wetting agents.

adsorption The process where chemicals are held or bound to a surface by physical or chemical attraction. Clay and high organic soils tend to adsorb pesticides.

adulterated pesticide A pesticide that does not conform to the professed standard or quality as documented on its label or labeling.

aerosol A chemical stored in a container under pressure. An extremely fine mist is produced when the material, dissolved in a liquid, is released into the air.

agitation Process of stirring or mixing in a sprayer.

algae Relatively simple plants that are photosynthetic and contain chlorophyll.

algaecide (algicide) A pesticide used to kill or inhibit algae.

annual A plant that completes its life cycle in one year.

antagonism The reduction of pesticide activity when two or more different pesticides are mixed together.

antibiotic Chemical produced by a microorganism which is toxic to other microorganisms. Examples: Streptomycin and penicillin.

anticoagulant A chemical which prevents normal bloodclotting. The active ingredient in some rodenticides.

antidote A practical treatment used to counteract the effects of pesticide poisoning or some other poison in the body.

anti-siphoning device
A hose attachment designed to prevent backflow of a pesticide mix from the spray tank into a water source.

anti-transpirant A chemical applied to a plant to reduce the rate of transpiration or water loss.

arachnid A wingless arthropod with two body regions and four pairs of jointed legs. Spiders, ticks, and mites are arachnids.

arthropod An invertebrate animal characterized by a jointed body and limbs and usually a hard body covering that is molted at intervals. Insects, mites, and crayfish are arthropods.

atropine (atropinesulfate) An antidote used to treat organophosphate and carbamate poisoning.

attractant A substance or device to lure insects or other pests to a trap or poison bait.

avicide A chemical used to kill or repel birds.

bacteria
Microscopic organisms, some of which are capable of producing diseases in plants and animals.

bactericide Chemical used to control bacteria.

bait A food or other substance used to attract a pest to a pesticide or to a trap.

band application Application of a pesticide or other material in or beside a crop row rather than over the entire field. (See Broadcast Application)

basal application Application to plant stems or trunks at or just above the ground line.

beneficial insect Insect that is useful or helpful to humans. Examples are pollinators and parasites and predators of pests.

biennial A plant that completes its life cycle in two years.

bioaccumulation The ability of organisms to accumulate or store chemicals in their tissues.

biological control Control of pests using predators, parasites, and disease-causing organisms. May be naturally occurring or introduced.

biomagnification The process where some organisms accumulate chemical residues in higher concentrations than those found in the organisms they consume.

botanical pesticide A pesticide produced from naturally occurring chemicals in plants, Examples are nicotine, pyrethrum, and rotenone.

brand name The name, number, or designation of a specific pesticide product or device made by a manufacturer or formulator.

broadcast application The uniform application of a pesticide or other material over an entire field or area.

broadleaf plants Plants with broad, rounded, or flattened leaves with netted veins (examples: dandelion and rose). Different from the narrow blade-like leaves with parallel veins of grasses sedges, rushes, and onions.

broad-spectrum pesticide A pesticide that is effective against a wide range of pests.

buffers Adjuvants used to retard chemical degradation of some pesticides by lowering the pH of alkaline water.

calibrate-calibration To properly adjust equipment; to determine the correct amount of material to be applied to the target area.

carbamates A group of pesticides containing nitrogen, formulated as insecticides (Sevin, Furadan, Lannate), fungicides (Mancozeb, Maneb), and herbicides (IPC, CIPC).

carcinogen A substance or agent able to induce malignant tumors (cancer).

carrier An inert liquid, solid, or gas added to an active ingredient to make a pesticide formulation. A carrier is also the material, usually water or oil, used to dilute the formulated product for application.

causal organisms The organism (pathogen) that produces a given disease.

chemical name The technical name of the active ingredient(s) found in the formulated product. This complex name is derived from the chemical structure of the active ingredient.

chemigation The application of fertilizers or pesticides to soil or plants by inclusion in irrigation water.

chemosterilant A chemical compound capable of inhibiting reproduction.

chemtrec The Chemical Transportation Emergency Center has a toll-free number that provides 24-hour information for chemical emergencies such as a spill, leak, fire, or accident. 1-800-424-9300.

chlorinated hydrocarbon A pesticide containing chlorine, carbon, and hydrogen. Many are persistent in the environment. Examples: Chlordane, DDT, methoxychlor. Also called ORGANOCHLORINES

chlorosis The yellowing of a plant's normally green tissue.

cholinesterase A chemical catalyst (enzyme) found in humans and many other animals that regulates the activity of nerve impulses.

chronic toxicity The ability of a material to cause injury from repeated, prolonged exposure to small amounts. (See Acute Toxicity)

common name A name given to a pesticide active ingredient by a recognized committee on pesticide nomenclature. Many pesticides are known by a number of trade or brand names but the active ingredient(s) has only one recognized common name. Example: The common name for Sevin insecticide is carbaryl.

compatibility agents Adjuvants used to enhance the mixing of two or more different pesticide products and/or fertilizers.

compatible Chemicals are said to be compatible if they can be mixed together without reducing the effectiveness of any individual chemical.

concentration Refers to the amount of active ingredient in a given volume or weight of formulated product.

contract herbicide A chemical that kills primarily by contact with plant tissue, with little or no translocation.

contact insecticide A compound that causes death or injury to insects upon contact. It does not need to be ingested to be toxic to the insect.

contamination The presence of an unwanted substance in or on a plant, animal, soil, water, air, or structure. (See Residue)

corrosive poison A poison containing a strong acid or base which will severely burn the skin, mouth, stomach, etc.

curative pesticide A pesticide which can inhibit or kill a disease-causing organism after it is established in the plant or animal. Also known as CHEMOTHERAPY.

days to harvest The minimum number of days permitted by law between the last pesticide application and the harvest date. (Same as Preharvest Interval.)

days to slaughter The minimum number of days permitted by law between the last pesticide application and the date the animal is slaughtered.

decontaminate To remove or degrade a chemical residue from a surface or substance.

defoliant A chemical which initiates the premature drop of leaves.

degradation The process by which a chemical compound is broken down to a simpler compound by the action of microorganisms, water, air, sunlight, or other agents. Degradation products are usually, but not always, less toxic than the original compound.

deposit The occurrence of pesticide on a treated surface after application.

dermal toxicity The ability of a pesticide to cause injury to a human or animal when absorbed through the skin.

desiccant A chemical that promotes drying or loss of moisture from leaves or other plant parts.

detoxify To render a pesticide active ingredient or other poisonous chemical harmless.

diagnosis The positive identification of a problem and its cause.

diluent Any liquid, solid, or gaseous material used to dilute or carry an active ingredient.

dip Complete or partial immersion of a plant, animal, or object in a pesticide mixture.

disinfectant A chemical or other agent that kills or inactivates disease-producing microorganisms in animals, seeds, or other plant parts. Also, commonly refers to chemicals used to clean or surface-sterilize inanimate objects.

dispersing agent An adjuvant that facilitates mixing and suspension of a pesticide formulation in water.

dormant spray A pesticide application made in late winter or early spring prior to the resumption of active growth by plants.

dose, dosage Quantity of pesticide applied to a given site or target.

drift The airborne movement of a pesticide spray or dust beyond the intended contact area.

drift retardant An adjuvant added to a spray mixture to reduce drift.

dry flowable A dry, granular pesticide formulation that forms a suspension when added to water. Same as WATER DISPERSIBLE GRANULE.

dust A finely ground, dry pesticide formulation containing a small amount of active ingredient and a large amount of inert carrier or diluent such as clay or talc.

emulsifiable concentrate A pesticide formulation produced by mixing an active ingredient and an emulsifying agent in a suitable petroleum solvent. When added to water, a milky emulsion is formed.

emulsifying agent (emulsifier) A chemical which aids in the suspension of one liquid in another which normally would not mix together.

emulsion A mixture of two liquids which are not soluble in one another. One is suspended as very small droplets in the other with the aid of an emulsifying agent. Example: Emulsifiable concentrate in water.

encapsulated pesticide A pesticide formulation with the active ingredient enclosed in capsules of polyvinyl or other synthetic materials; principally used for slow release. May also refer to a method of disposal of pesticides and pesticide containers by sealing them in a sturdy, water-proof container to prevent leakage of contents.

endangered species Individual plants or animals with a population that has been reduced to near extinction.

environmental protection agency (EPA) The federal agency responsible for implementing pesticide rules and regulations, and registering pesticides.

environment All the features that surround and affect an organism or group of organisms.

EPA establishment number A number assigned to each pesticide production facility by EPA. The number indicates the plant at which the pesticide product was produced and must appear on all labels of that product.

EPA registration number A number assigned to a pesticide product by EPA when the product is registered by the manufacturer or the designated agent. The number must appear on all labels for a particular product.

eradicant A chemical or other agent (steam, heat) used to eliminate an established pest from a plant, animal, or specific site (soil, water, buildings).

fetotoxin A substance able to cause harm to a developing fetus but not necessarily cause deformities. (See Teratogen)

field scout A person who samples fields for pests infestations.

FIFRA The Federal Insecticide, Fungicide, and Rodenticide Act; a federal law dealing with pesticide regulations and use.

flowable A pesticide formulation in which a very finely ground solid particle is suspended (not dissolved) in a liquid carrier.

foam retardant An adjuvant used to reduce the foaming of a spray mixture due to agitation.

foaming agent An adjuvant designed to reduce pesticide drift by producing a thick foam.

fog treatment The application of a pesticide as a fine mist or fog.

food chain Sequence of species within a community, each member of which serves as a food source for the species next higher in the chain.

forecasting The prediction of pest incidence using weather, host, and pest characteristics.

formulation The pesticide product as purchased, containing a mixture of one or more active ingredients, carriers (inert ingredients), and other additives diluted for safety and ease of application.

fumigant A pesticide that forms gases that are toxic to plants, animals, and microorganisms.

fungi (singularfungus) Non-chlorophyll-bearing plants, living as saprophytes or parasites. Some infect and cause diseases in plants, animals, and humans or destroy wood and fiber products. Others are beneficial, for instance, decomposers and human food sources. (Examples: rusts, mildews, smuts.)

fungicide A chemical used to control fungi.

fungistatic agent A chemical that inhibits the germination of fungal spores or the growth of mycelium, but does not kill the fungus.

general use pesticide A pesticide which can be purchased and used by the general public. (See Restricted Use Pesticide)

germination The sprouting of a seed or the production of a germ tube (mycelium) from a fungus spore.

GPA Gallons per acre.

GPM Gallons per minute.

granule A dry pesticide formulation. The active ingredient is either mixed with or coated onto an inert carrier to form a small, ready to use, low-concentrate particle which does not normally present a drift hazard. Pellets differ from granules only in their precise uniformity, large size, and shape.

groundwater Water located beneath the soil surface from which well water is obtained or surface springs are formed.

growth regulator A chemical which alters the growth processes of a plant or animal.

harvest aid chemical Material applied to a plant prior to harvest to reduce the amount of plant foliage. (See Defoliant.)

hemotoxin A substance or agent able to cause blood disorders.

herbaceous plants Plants that do not develop woody tissues.

herbicide A pesticide used to kill or inhibit plant growth.

host A plant or animal on or in which a pest lives.

hydrolysis Breakdown of a chemical in the presence of water.

illegal residue A quantity of pesticide remaining on or in the crop/animal at harvest/slaughter which is either above the set tolerance or which is not allowed to be used on the crop/animal.

incompatible Two or more materials which cannot be mixed or used together.

inert ingredient An inactive material in a pesticide formulation which does not have pesticidal activity.

ingredient statement The portion of the label on a pesticide container which gives the name and amount of each active ingredient and the total amount of inert ingredients in the formulation.

inhalation toxicity The property of a pesticide to be poisonous to humans or animals when breathed in through the lungs.

inoculum That portion of the pathogen that can cause disease in a host.

insecticide A pesticide used to control or prevent damage caused by insects.

insects Arthropods characterized by a body composed of three segments and three pairs of legs.

integrated pest management The use of all suitable pest control methods to keep pest populations below the economic injury level. Methods include cultural practices, use of biological, physical, and genetic control agents, and the selective use of pesticides.

labeling Supplemental pesticide information which complements the information on the label, but which is not necessarily attached to or part of the container.

label All printed material attached to or part of a pesticide container.

larvae (singular larva) The immature form of an insect or other animal that hatches from the egg.

LC50 The concentration of a pesticide, usually in air or water, which can kill 50 percent of a test population of animals. LC50 is usually expressed in parts per million (ppm). The lower the LC50 value, the more acutely toxic the chemical.

LD50 The dose or amount of a pesticide which can kill 50 percent of the test animals when eaten or absorbed through the skin. LD50 is expressed in milligrams of chemical per kilogram of body weight of the test animal (mg/kg). The lower the LD50 the more acutely toxic the chemical.

leaching The movement of a substance through soil with water.

metabolite In the case of pesticides, a compound derived from changes in the active ingredient through chemical, biological, or physical reactions. The metabolite may be simpler or more complex and may or may not be more poisonous than the original chemical.

metamorphosis A change in the shape, size, and/or form of an animal.

microbial degradation Breakdown of a chemical by microorganisms.

microbial pesticide Bacteria, viruses, fungi, and other microorganisms used to control pests. Also called BIORATIONALS.

microorganism An organism that is so small it cannot be seen without the aid of a microscope.

miscible liquids Two or more liquids which can be mixed and will remain mixed under most conditions. Water and ethyl alcohol are miscible; water and oil ar not.

mite A small arthropod similar to an insect but with eight legs. Its body is divided into two parts and has no antennae.

miticide A pesticide used to control mites; synonymous with acaricide.

mode of action The way in which a pesticide exerts a toxic effect on the target plant, animal, or microorganism.

molluscicide A chemical used to control snails and slugs.

mutagen A substance or agent able to cause genetic changes in living cells.

mycelium The mass of filaments that forms the body of a fungus.

mycoplasma A microorganism possessing many virus-like properties. Some cause plant diseases.

necrosis Death of plant or animal tissues which results in the formation of discolored, sunken, or necrotic (dead) areas.

nematicide A pesticide used to control nematodes.

nematodes Microscopic, colorless, worm-like animals that live as saprophytes or parasites. Many cause diseases of plants or animals.

neurotoxin A substance or agent able to cause disorders of the nervous system.

nonpersistent pesticide A pesticide that does not remain active in the environment more than one growing season.

nonselective pesticide A pesticide that is toxic to a wide range of plants or animals without regard to species. For example, a nonselective herbicide can kill or damage all plants it contacts.

nontarget organism A plant or animal other than the intended target(s) of a pesticide application.

noxious weed A plant defined by law as being particularly troublesome, undesirable, and difficult to control.

oncogen A substance or agent able to induce tumors (not necessarily cancerous) in living tissues. (See Carcinogen.)

oral toxicity The occurrence of injury when a pesticide is taken by mouth.

organophosphates A large group of pesticides which contain the element phosphorus. Most are nonpersistent insecticides, miticides, and nematicides. Many are highly toxic. Examples: Malathion, parathion, diazinon, chlorpyrifos.

ovicide A material that destroys eggs.

parasite A plant, animal, or microorganism living in, on, or with another living organism for the purpose of obtaining all or part of its food.

pathogen A disease causing organism.

penetrant An adjuvant added to a spray mixture to enhance the absorption of a pesticide.

perennial A plant that lives for more than two years.

persistent pesticide A pesticide chemical (or its metabolites) that remains active in the environment more than one growing season. Some compounds can accumulate in animal and plant tissues or remain in soil for years.

pesticide A chemical or other agent used to kill or otherwise control pests, or to protect from a pest.

pest An undesirable organism (insect, bacterium, fungus, nematode, weed, virus, rodent) which is injurious to humans, desirable plants and animals, manufactured products, or natural products.

pheromone A substance emitted by an animal to influence the behavior of other animals of the same species. Some are synthetically produced for use in insect traps.

photodegradation Breakdown of chemicals by the action of sunlight.

phytotoxicity Injury to plants. pH A measure of acidity/alkalinity; acid below pH7, basic or alkaline above pH7.

piscicide A chemical used to control pest fish.

point of runoff When a spray starts to run or drip from the leaves and stems of plants or the hair or feathers of animals.

poison control center An agency, generally a hospital, which has current information on proper first aid techniques and antidotes for poisoning emergencies.

postemergence After the weed or crop plants have appeared through the soil. Usually used to specify the timing of herbicide applications.

PPM Parts per million. A means to express amounts of chemicals in or on food, plants, animals, water, soil, or air. One part per million equals 1 pound in 500 tons. PPB is part per billion.

precipitate A solid substance that forms in a liquid and settles to the bottom of a container. A material that no longer remains in suspension.

predator An animal that attacks, feeds on, and kills other animals. Examples of predaceous animals are hawks, owls, snakes, fish, spiders and many insects and mites.

preemergence Before the weed or crop plants have appeared through the soil. Usually used to specify the timing of herbicide applications.

preharvest interval Same as days to harvest.

premix A pesticide product formulated with more than one active ingredient.

preplant pesticide A pesticide applied prior to planting a crop.

propellant The inert ingredient in self-pressurized products that forces the active ingredient from the container. (See Aerosol)

protectant A pesticide applied to a plant or animal prior to infection or attack by the pest in order to prevent infection or injury by the pest.

protective equipment Equipment intended to protect a person from exposure during the handling and application of pesticides. Includes long-sleeved shirts and long trousers, coveralls, suitable hats, gloves, shoes, respirators, and other safety items as needed.

pupa The developmental stage of some insects between larva and adult.

quarantine Regulatory method to control the introduction and dissemination of plant and animal pests (animals, insects, weeds, and disease-causing organisms) into new areas. Involves inspections, treatments, and destruction of contaminated plants/animals or their parts.

rate of application The amount of pesticide applied to a plant, animal, unit area, or surface; usually measured as per acre, per 1,000 square feet, per linear feet, or per cubic feet.

RCRA The Resource Conservation and Recovery Act; the federal law regulating the transport, storage, treatment, and disposal of hazardous wastes.

reentry interval The period between treatment of the crop and the time when the crop can be reentered and handled without a person wearing protective clothing and equipment in the treated field.

Registered pesticides Pesticide products which have been registered by the Environmental Protection Agency for the uses listed on the label.

repellent A compound that keeps insects, rodents, birds, or other pests away from plants, domestic animals, buildings, or other treated areas.

residual pesticide A pesticide that continues to remain effective on a treated surface or area for an extended period following application.

residue The pesticide active ingredient or its breakdown product(s) which remains in or on the target after treatment.

resistant A population of organisms that are uninjured or unaffected by a certain dosage of pesticide chemical used to control other populations of the same organism successfully. Also, plants and animals that are unaffected by a pest species. (See Tolerant)

restricted use pesticide A pesticide which can be purchased only by certified pesticide applicators and used only by certified applicators or persons directly under their supervision. Not available for use by the general public because of the high toxicities and/or environmental hazards.

rodenticide A chemical used to control rodents.

runoff The movement of water and associated materials on the soil surface.

safener An adjuvant used to reduce the phytotoxic effects of a pesticide.

saprophyte An organism which obtains its food from dead or decaying organic matter.

seed protectant A pesticide applied to seeds prior to planting to protect them from insects, fungi, and other soil pests.

selective pesticide A pesticide that is toxic to some pests, but has little or no effect on other similar species. Example: Some fungicides are so selective that they control only powdery mildews and no other fungi.

serial application The application of one pesticide immediately or shortly after the application of another.

signal words Required word(s) which appear on every pesticide label to denote the relative acute toxicity of the product. The signal words are either DANGER-POISON used with a skull and crossbones symbol for highly toxic compounds, DANGER for skin and eye irritants, WARNING for moderately toxic, or CAUTION for slightly toxic compounds.

silvicide A herbicide used to destroy brush and trees such as in wooded areas.

slurry A thick suspension of a pesticide made from a wettable powder and water.

soil drench To soak or wet the ground surface with a pesticide. Large volumes of the pesticide mixture are usually needed to saturate the soil to any depth.

soil incorporation The mechanical mixing of a pesticide product with soil.

soil injection The placement of a pesticide below the surface of the soil. Common application method for fumigants and termiticides.

soil sterilant A chemical or agent that prevents the growth of all organisms present in the soil; a nonselective pesticide. Soil sterilization may be temporary or permanent depending on the chemical.

soluble powder A finely ground dry pesticide formulation which will dissolve in water or some other liquid carrier.

solution Mixture of one or more substances in another substance (usually a liquid) in which all the ingredients are completely dissolved. Example: Sugar in water.

solvent A liquid such as water, oil, or alcohol which will dissolve another

substance (solid, liquid, or gas) to form a solution.

space spray A pesticide which is applied as a fine spray or mist to a confined area.

spore The reproductive unit of a fungus. A spore is analagous to a plant seed.

spot treatment Application to small areas.

spray deposit The amount of pesticide chemical that remains on a sprayed surface after the droplets have dried.

spreader An adjuvant used to enhance the spread of a pesticide over a treated surface, thus improving the coverage.

sticker An adjuvant used to improve the adherence of spray droplets to a plant, animal, or other treated surface.

stomach poison A pesticide that must be eaten by an animal in order to be effective; it will not kill on contact.

structural pests Pests that attack and destroy buildings and other structures, clothing, stored food, and manufactured/processed goods. Examples: Termites, cockroaches, clothes moths, rats, dry-rot fungi.

summer annual Plants that germinate in the spring or summer and complete their life cycle within one year.

surfactant An inert ingredient which improves the spreading, dispersing, and/or wetting properties of a pesticide mixture.

susceptible A plant, animal, or site that is affected by a pest. Also refers to pest populations that can be controlled by pesticides.

suspension A pesticide mixture consisting of fine particles dispersed or floating in a liquid, usually water or oil. Example: Wettable powders in water.

swath The width of the area covered by one sweep of an airplane, ground sprayer, spreader, or duster.

synergism The effect of two or more pesticides applied together which is greater than the sum of the individual pesticides applied separately. Example: Pesticide X kills 40 per-

cent of an insect population. Pesticide Y kills 20 percents. When applied together, X and Y kill 95 percent.

systemic A chemical that is absorbed and translocated within a plant or animal.

tank mix A mixture of products in a spray tank.

target The plants, animals, structures, areas, or pests at which the control method is directed.

technical material The pesticide active ingredient in pure form, as it is manufactured by a chemical company. It is usually combined with inert ingredients or additives in formulations such as wettable powders, dusts, emulsifiable concentrates, or granules.

teratogen A substance or agent able to produce abnormalities or defects in living human or animal embryos and fetuses. These defects are not usually inheritable.

termiticide An insecticide used to control termites.

thickener A drift control adjuvant such as cellulose or gel used to promote the formation of a greater proportion of large droplets in a spray mixture.

tolerance A regulation that establishes the maximum amount of pesticide residue (active ingredient or certain metabolites) that may legally remain in or on a raw agricultural commodity (food or feed product) at harvest or slaughter.

tolerant The property of organisms, including pests, to withstand a certain degree of stress, such as pest attack, weather, or pesticides.

toxicant A poisonous substance such as the active ingredient in a pesticide formulation.

toxicity The degree or extent that a chemical or substance is poisonous.

toxic Poisonous to living organisms.

toxin A naturally occurring poison produced by plants, animals, or microorganisms. Examples: The poison produced by the black widow spider, the venom produced by snakes, the botulism toxin.

translocation The movement of material within a plant or animal from the site of entry. A systemic pesticide is translocated.

ultra low volume (ULV) Sprays that are applied at 0.5 gallon or less per acre, often as the undiluted formulation.

vapor pressure The property which causes a chemical to evaporate. The higher the vapor pressure, the more volatile the chemical or the easier it will evaporate.

vector An animal (insect, nematode, mite) or plant (dodder) that can carry and transmit a pathogen from one host to another.

vertebrate Animal characterized by a segmented backbone or spinal column.

virus Ultramicroscopic parasites. Viruses can only multiply in living tissues and cause many animal and plant diseases.

volatility The degree to which a substance changes from a liquid or solid state to a gas at ordinary temperatures when exposed to air.

water table The upper level of the water saturated zone in the ground.

weed An unwanted plant.

wettable powder A dry pesticide formulation in powder form which forms a suspension when added to water.

wetting agent An adjuvant used to reduce the surface tension between a liquid and the contact surface for more thorough coverage.

winter annual Plants that germinate in the fall and complete their life cycle within one year.

ANSWERS TO REVIEW QUESTIONS

Chapter 1

1. A public pool is typically larger than 1800 sq ft of surface area, is owned by some legal entity, and is available to anyone paying a small entry fee. Semipublic pools have a specific entry requirements and restrictions like a fitness club or a country club would have. Most semipublic pools are considered as public pools by health departments.

2. Hotel/motel/resort pools, country club pools, fitness center, and agency (YM/WCA, Boys Club, etc.) pools can all be classified as semipublic pools. NSPI states that semipublic pools must involve lodging.

3. Residential pools are private pools.

4. Residential pools are basically unregulated. Although there may be some exceptions, typically there are no agencies that regulate residential pools.

5. The pool itself, inlets and outlets, the surge (balancing tank), pump, hair/lint strainer, filter(s), heater, disinfectant system, are all part of circulation system.

6. Most headfirst entries causing serious neck injuries occur in a depth of water that is less than five (5) feet deep.

7. A good pool deck is nonslip, has good sloping and drains well, has adequate space for activities, is free of obstructions, does not have cracks or dimpled, and does not promote algae, fungal, or bacterial growth.

8. Sanitation refers to killing bacteria in the water while oxidation is the "burning-up" of organic debris.

9. Divers can hit their heads on the slope. Nonswimmers may also slip down the slope into keep water.

10. No. Chlorine readings are not used to determine water balance in swimming pools.

Chapter 2

1. Sixty percent of all new pools constructed are residential pools.

2. An above-ground pools is both portable and temporary and has a water depth between 36-48 inches. An in-ground pool is permanent. The sides of the in-ground pool are in partial of full contact with the earth.

3. A toddler between the ages of 1 to 3 should be of special concern around a residential pool.

4. Safety layers include supervision, fencing, pool alarms, and pool covers.

5. Pool fencing should between 4 and 6 feet high, have vertical slats no more than 4 inches apart, be free of footholds and handholds, and have a self-closing and self-latching gate with the latch at least 48 inches high.

6. The pool cover must be completely removed before swimming.

7. A separate phone is a must for pools to save time in case of emergencies.

8. NO—Headfirst entries must never be allowed in aboveground pools.

9. YES—Above-ground pools are usually removable.

10. Vinyllined pools have lowered the cost of residential pools.

11. Electrical outlets should be protected with GFIs.

12. Never mix chemicals, wear eye and face protection, do not add chemicals directly to the pool with swimmers present, store different chemicals separately, keep lids tightly sealed.

13. NO—A pool does not usually affect the cost of homeowners insurance.

Chapter 3

1. Competitive starting blocks should always be located at the DEEP end to the pool.

2. Headfirst entries should never be allowed in water that is less than 5 but preferably 9 feet deep.

3. A dry niche light can be accessed from out of the

water; both the light and the pool operator stay dry. The wet niche must be accessed from inside the pool.

4. Major pool finishing types include plaster, tile, and vinyllined.

5. Safety markings should be in contrasting colors with letters and numbers at least 4 inches high and conspicuously placed.

6. Outdoor pools lose chlorine to the UV rays of the sun, promote algae growth, receive airborne debris like grass, leaves, pollen, etc., tend to have more trespassers and vandals at night, and need to pride shade.

7. Trespasser swimming late at night, vandals destroying property, thieves stealing equipment.

8. The American disabilities Act (ADA) is designed to make public facilities more accessible to individuals with disabilities.

9. Special concerns that many hotel/motel/resort pools have include very young and very old guests, a transient clientele, patrons unfamiliar with the facility, alcohol, and frequent parties.

Chapter 4

1. A "turnover" is the number of times a quantity of water equal to the pool volume passes through the filtration system in 24 hours.

2. A gutter is an overflow trough taking water from the surface of the water and is located continuously around the perimeter. A skimmer is an overflow box or outlet located intermittently around the perimeter of the pool. Gutters are usually much more effective than skimmers.

3. A weir is a moving door or flap controlling the flow of water into the skimmer box.

4. A surge tank collects and saves large volumes of water displaced by large bather loads. The surge tank also protects the pool pump by keeping the water level in the tank above the suction port of the pump.

5. The hair and lint strainer protects the recirculating pump.

6. Three major filter types include Sand, DE, and Cartridge.

7. 84° to 86° F is the recommended temperature for special populations.

8. A heat exchanger is a device composed of coils, tubes, or plates that transfers heat from a source to the pool water without mixing.

9. An erosion feeder is an canister attached to a circulation line that permits solid disinfectants to dissolve slowly.

10. Centrifugal pumps are most often used for swimming pool circulation.

11. The impeller is the working part in the centrifugal pool pump.

Chapter 5

1. Filter Media

Sand: Advantage—permanent media does not require frequent changing
Disadvantage—cannot trap finer particles

DE: Advantage—superior filtration and water clarity
Disadvantage—temporary media that must be placed often

Cartridge: Advantage—saves water because it is not backwashed
Disadvantage—difficult to clean

2. Pressure filters are in an enclosed tank. Vacuum filters are in an open tank or vat.

3. Regenerative DE filters can be "bumped" to readjust the DE to extend the filter cycle, avoid backwashing, and thus save DE and water.

4. Slurry feeding provides the slow, continuous addition of DE which extends the filter cycle.

5. "Channeling" is a filtration problem allowing water to pass through holes or channels in the filter bed, thereby missing filtration.

6. Not all filters are backwashed during cleaning. Filters like vacuum DE and cartridge filters are cleaned without reversing the flow of water through the filter bed.

7. Conventional pressure sand and gravel filters are typically much larger and slower than high rate filters.

Chapter 6

1. Disinfectant

Iodine: Advantage—decreased pH dependence, no residual, increased killing poser, long residual
Disadvantage—expensive, not an oxidizer, discolors jewelry

Ozone: Advantage—no smell or chloramines, increased killing power
          Disadvantage—unstable in pool water, no residual

Ionization: Advantage—no effect on pH, reduced chemical usage
             Disadvantage—no oxidation, green/black staining possible

Chlorine
Generative: Advantage—do not purchase chemicals, regenerates itself
             Disadvantage—expensive to install, water tastes salty

U/V
Hydrogen
Peroxide: Advantage—less chemical consumption
           Disadvantage—weak disinfectant, no residual

Polymeric
Biquanide: Advantage—very little use of chemicals
            Disadvantage—incompatible with many pool chemicals

Chapter 7

1. Chlorine type

Gas chlorine: 100% available
                     Lowers pH

Calcium
hypochlorite: 65% available
                     Raises pH

Sodium
hypochlorite: 12%-15% available
                     Raises pH

Lithium
hypochlorite: 35% available
                     Raises pH

Dichlor: 56% or 62% available
                     Neutral pH

Trichlor: 90% available
                     Lowers pH

2. Dichlor and Trichlor are stabilized chlorines.

3. Disinfection is the process of killing germs, bacteria, algae, fungus and prevents the transmission of disease. Oxidation helps filtration by "burning-up" organic impurities and particulate matter.

4. Gas chlorine requires a separate room, SCBA for emergencies, an exhaust fan near the floor, secured tank, emergency action plan leaks.

5. No—sodium hypochlorite has a SHORT shelf life.

6. No—calcium hypochlorite is combustible.

7. Lithium hypochlorite is very soluble, making it suitable for superchlorination.

8. Cyanuric acid stabilizes chlorine to protect it from the damaging U/V rays of the sun, thereby making it last longer.

9. Organic chlorines are stabilized (Dichlor, Trichlor). Inorganic chlorines are unstabilized, therefore lost in sunlight.

10. Yes—Bromine requires the addition of an oxidizer.

11. NO—Bromamines are more effective than chloramines.

Chapter 8

1. "Chlorine odor" is caused by combined available chlorine (CAC), or chloramines.

2. Add FAC 10 X's greater than the CAC level.

3. Potassium Peroxymonosulfate is a nonchlorine shocking agent.

4. $6.0 \text{ ppm} \quad \times \quad \dfrac{75{,}000}{120{,}000} \quad \times \quad 1 \text{ gal} \quad = \quad 3.75 \text{ gals}$

5. $4.0 \text{ ppm} \quad \times \quad \dfrac{200{,}000}{120{,}000} \quad \times \quad 1.6 \text{ lbs} \quad = \quad 6.66 \text{ lbs}$

6. $10 \text{ ppm} \quad \times \quad \dfrac{120{,}000}{120{,}000} \quad \times \quad 1 \text{ lb} \quad = \quad 10 \text{ lbs}$

NOTE: The answer to no. 4 should be rounded up to 4 gallons and no. 5 should be rounded up to 7 pounds if you were actually going to superchlorinate these pools.

Chapter 9

1. Unbalanced water can be either acidic, aggressive, corrosive, or basic, scaling.

2. To raise pH add soda ash or sodium hydroxide.

3. To lower pH add muriatic acid or sodium bisulfate.

4. Total Alkalinity (TA) should be generally be maintained between 100 and 150 ppm.

5. To raise TA, add sodium bicarbonate.

6. To lower TA, add muriatic acid or sodium bisulfate.

7. Low calcium hardness (CH) will pull calcium (leaching) from pool finishes like plaster, tile, and grout.

8. To raise CH, add calcium chloride.

9. High TDS can only be lowered by removing water from the pool and replacing it with fresh water.

10. Langelier Saturation Index requires pH, Temperature, TA, CH, TDS.

Chapter 10

1. Phenol red is used to test for pH.

2. DPD is the preferred method of testing for chlorine.

3. ORP is now the preferred method of testing.

4. ORP sensors are the most accurate, they monitor the water continuously, and they can be adapted to make chemical adjustments automatically.

5. TA should be checked every 2 weeks.

6. The TA test is titrimetric test.

7. CYA should not exceed 100 ppm.

8. Bacteriological tests in most states are usually required weekly.

Chapter 11

1. 5.0 ppm FAC is required to rid a pool with 0.5 ppm CAC.

2. One pound of gas chlorine in a 120,000 gallon pool will raise the FAC by 1 ppm.

3. Sodium thiosulfate or sodium sulfite would be added to reduce high levels of FAC.

4. 75 lbs of sodium bicarbonate will increase the TA by 50 ppm in a 100,000 gallon pool.

5. To lower TA, muriatic acid must be added full strength at one end of the pool in one spot so as to make a "hole" in water as the acid is being added.

6. Oval pool Volume = maximum length X maximum width X Average depth X 5.9 gallons.

7. One pound of sodium thiosulfate added to 100,000 gallons of pool water will reduce the chlorine by 1 ppm.

Chapter 12

1. An algicide kills algae, whereas an algistat prevents algae growth.

2. There are numerous species of algae that create pool problems.

3. "QUATS" are algicides that tend to foam.

4. No—once algae begins to grow, it is extremely difficult to remove from a pool.

5. Cloudy, milky water can be caused by inadequate filtration, no disinfectant, DE in the pool, unbalanced water, high TDS, and others.

6. WATER COLOR   PROBLEM
    A. blue/green   C. Manganese
    B. red or brown   A. Copper
    C. blue or black   B. Iron

7. Rough finishes, clogged pipes, and filter calcification are caused by excessively high calcium hardness, or a very basic saturation index.

8. The main drain box is often the location for most large pool leaks.

Chapter 13

1. A hot tub is made of wood. A spa is made of fiberglass, acrylic, or some similar material.

2. Yes—hot water pools require more attention to chemicals than public pools.

3. Soaker load for spas = area of the spa ÷ 10 (in a circular spa this would be 3.14 x radius² ÷ 10)

4. The heater is most susceptible to unbalanced water.

5. Spa/hot tub rules should include: No children under 12 years permitted, no diving, no handstands or underwater swimming, do not soak for more than 15 minutes, water must not be hotter than 104° F, no electrical appliances allowed, no medical contraindication.

6. An antivortex plate prevents hair and suit entanglement in return lines and drains.

7. A timer switch is intended to force soakers to leave the hot tub/spa every 15 minutes.

8. 104° F

Chapter 15

1. Winterizing a pool while full is preferred.

2. The hydrostatic pressure relief valve protects an empty pool from excessive ground water.

3. Propylene glycol is the antifreeze recommended for pools.

4. Empty pools can stretch the liners. Shocking can bleach the liner.

5. A winter cover simply prevent debris from entering the pool. A safety cover prevents people from entering the pool.

6. Pool lights must be turned off at the circuit breaker and either boxed on the pool deck or sunk to the bottom. Care must be taken not to damage the lens.

Chapter 16

1. Nearly 70% of all sport-related injuries are the result of entering shallow water headfirst.

2. Ninety-five percent of all headfirst injuries occur in less than 5 feet of water.

3. Paralysis results to trauma to the spine or spinal column.

4. A young athletic male between the ages of 18 to 31 years old is most likely to suffer from headfirst injuries.

5. The safe diving envelope is an underwater area that guarantees that any diver is unable to become injured by the side, slope, or bottom.

6. Above-ground pools must completely prohibit headfirst entries.

7. Starting blocks should be located in the deep end of the pool.

Chapter 17

1. Lifesaving involves rescue skills intended to save lives in the water. Lifeguarding involves skills for predicting and preventing accidents.

2. Systematic scanning techniques include circular scanning, monitoring hazardous areas, high risk watching, etc.

3. Recognition
   Intrusion
   Distraction

4. The 10/20 rule means 10 seconds to spot a victim and 20 seconds to make the rescue.

5. High risks guests vary from pool to pool but most often include young children, older people, minority groups, those visiting the pool for the first time, those consuming alcohol.

6. Commodore Wilbert E. Longfellow started the American Red Cross Lifesaving.

7. Typical types of pool accidents include:
   • Running—cuts and scrapes
   • Collisions with equipment and others
   • Headfirst entries into shallow water
   • Heart exhaustion/stroke
   • Heart attacks

8. Lifeguard communications include:
   Whistles
   Flags
   Hand signals
   Bullhorns
   Walkie-talkies
   Electric devices

Chapter 19

1. Priority items to check before opening include:
   Water clarity
   Water quality
   Water level
   Drain covers
   Bottom conditions
   Filtration
   Pool deck
   Flow rate

2. Priority areas to check before closing include:
   Securing all building and structures
   Water chemistry
   Backwashing and chemical adjustments
   Pool decks

3. The saturation index should be conducted at least once a week.

4. Chemical feeders must be cleaned regularly because they become clogged easily.

APPENDIX A
GENERAL INFORMATION

APPENDIX **A1**

In-Ground Pools by Construction

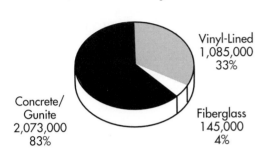

Vinyl-Lined
1,085,000
33%

Concrete/
Gunite
2,073,000
83%

Fiberglass
145,000
4%

Total Pools • 3,303,000

In-Ground Pool Equipment

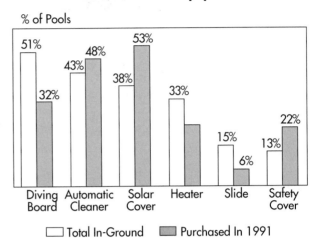

% of Pools

51% 32% | 43% 48% | 38% 53% | 33% | 15% 6% | 13% 22%

Diving Board | Automatic Cleaner | Solar Cover | Heater | Slide | Safety Cover

☐ Total In-Ground ☐ Purchased In 1991

Type of Pool Filter

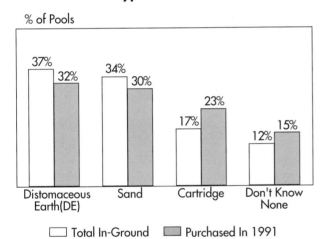

% of Pools

37% 32% | 34% 30% | 17% 23% | 12% 15%

Distomaceous Earth(DE) | Sand | Cartridge | Don't Know None

☐ Total In-Ground ☐ Purchased In 1991

In- Ground Pools by Construction

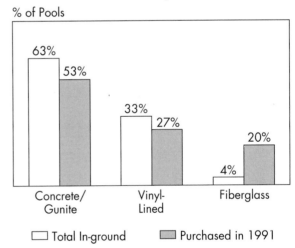

% of Pools

63% 53% | 33% 27% | 4% 20%

Concrete/ Gunite | Vinyl- Lined | Fiberglass

☐ Total In-ground ☐ Purchased in 1991

Above-Ground Pool Equipment

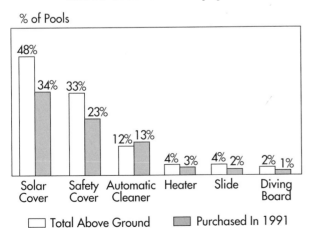

% of Pools

48% 34% | 33% 23% | 12% 13% | 4% 3% | 4% 2% | 2% 1%

Solar Cover | Safety Cover | Automatic Cleaner | Heater | Slide | Diving Board

☐ Total Above Ground ☐ Purchased In 1991

Type of Pool Filter

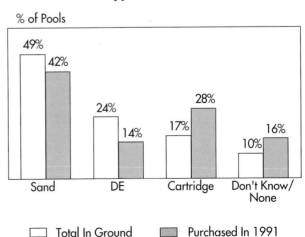

% of Pools

49% 42% | 24% 14% | 17% 28% | 10% 16%

Sand | DE | Cartridge | Don't Know/ None

☐ Total In Ground ☐ Purchased In 1991

From NSPI: *Pool and spa market study for the year 1991, 1992,* The Institute.

APPENDIX A2: ASSOCIATIONS

American Camping Assn.
5000 St. Rd. 67 N.
Martinsville, IN 46151-7902
317 342-8456; Fax 317 342-2065
Gary Abell, Public Relations Mgr.

American Red Cross, Nat'l
    Headquarters
431 18th St. N.W.
Washington DC 20006
Health & Safety - Development

American Swimming Coaches
    Assoc./Swim America
304 S.E. 20th St.
Ft. Lauderdale, FL 33316
305 462-6267, 800 356-ASCA; Fax:
    305 462-6280
John Leonard

Aquatic Exercise Assn.
1032 S. Spring, P.O. Box 497
Port Washington, WI 53074 414
    284-3416; Fax 414 284-1944
Gina Taucher, Editor

Commodore Longfellow Society
2531 Stonington Rd.
Atlanta, GA 30338
404 451-7175
Don Stephens, Nat'l Membership
    Chmn.

Council for National Cooperation
    in Aquatics (CNCA)
P.O. Box 351743
Toledo, OH 43635
419 867-3326
Louise Priest, Exec. Dir.

IDEA: The Assn. for Fitness
    Professionals
6190 Cornerstone Ct. E., Ste. 204
San Diego, CA 92121-3773
619 535-8979; Fax: 619 535-8234
Tracy R. Schauer, Resource Ctr.
    Coord.

International Racquet Sports
    Association (IRSA)
253 Summer St.
Boston, MA 02210
800 232-4772
Pam O'Donnell

International Swimming Hall of
    Fame
1 Hall of Fame Dr.
Ft. Lauderdale, FL 33316
305 462-6536; Fax 305 525-4031

NSF International
3475 Plymouth Rd.
Ann Arbor, MI 48105
313 769-8010; Fax: 313 769-0109
Jim Paschal, Program Mgr.

National Intramural-Recreational
    Sports Assoc. (NIRSA)
850 S.W. 15th St.
Corvallis, OR 97333-4145
503 737-2088
Will Holsberry

National Recreation & Park Assn.
650 W. Higgins Rd.
Hoffman Estates, IL 60195
708 843-7529; Fax: 708 843-3058
Walter C. Johnson, C.A.E.

National Spa and Pool Institute
2111 Eisenhower Ave.
Alexandria, VA 22314
703 838-0083; Fax: 703 549-0493
Molly Finney, Dir. of Conventions

National Swim & Recreation
    Assn.
429 Ridge Pike
Lafayette Hill, PA 19444
215 828-8746
Paul Ryan, Pres.

National Swim School Association
1158 35th Ave. N.
St. Petersburg, FL 33704
813 528-9704
Steve Graves

National Swimming Pool
    Foundation
10803 Gulfdale, Ste. 300
San Antonio, TX 78126
512 525-1227; Fax 512 344-3713
Les Kowalsky, Exec. Dir.

National Water Features
    Association (NWFA)
2010 N.W. 1st. Ave.
Delray Beach, FL 33444
407 278-3320
Terrell K. Higgs, Pres.

Recreation Safety Institute
P.O. Box 392
Ronkonkoma, NY 11779
516 563-4806; Fax: 516 563-4807
Dr. Armur H. Mittelstaedt, Board
    Chmn.

Resort and Commercial
    Recreation Assn.
P.O. Box 1208
New Port Richey, FL 34656-1208
813 845-7373
Frank Oliveto, Exec. Dir.

Special Olympics Int'l
1350 New York Ave. N.W., Ste.
    500
Washington, DC 20005-4709
202 628-8298; Telex:
    6502841739MCI; Fax: 202 737-
    1937
Selden Fritschner, Aquatics Dir.

Swimming Teachers of America
1158 35th Ave. N.
St. Petersburg, FL 33704
813 528-9604
Steve Graves

From Aquatics International, November/December 1993.

Appendix A2—cont'd

U.S. Diving, Inc.
Pan American Plaza, 201 S.
   Capital Ave., Ste. 430
Indianapolis, IN 46225
317 237-5252; Fax: 317 237-5257

U.S. Lifesaving Association
P.O. Box 20737
Chicago, IL 60620
312 294-2333
Joe Pecoraro, Pres.

United States Masters Swimming,
   Inc.
2 Peter Ave.
Rutland, MA 01543
508 886-6631; Fax: 508 886-6265
Dorothy Donnelly, Exec. Sect'y

United States Swimming
1750 E. Boulder St.
Colorado Springs, CO 80909
719 578-4578; Fax: 719 578-4669
Ray B. Essick, Exec. Dir.
Jeff Dimond, Info. Svcs. Dir.

U.S. Water Fitness Assn.
P.O. Box 3279
Boynton Beach, FL 33424-3279
407 732-9908; Fax: 407 732-0950
John R. Spannuth, Exec. Dir.

World Swimming Coaches Ass'n
304 S.E. 20th St.
Ft. Lauderdale, FL 33316
305 462-6267
John Leonard, Vice Pres.

World Waterpark Assn.
10606 W. 87th St., P.O. Box 14826
Lenexa, KS 66285-4826
913 599-0300; Fax: 913 599-0520
Patti Miller

YMCA of the USA
101 N. Wacker Dr., 14th Fl.
Chicago, IL 60606
312 977-0031
Tom Massey, Dir. of Program
   Svcs.

YWCA of the USA
726 Broadway
New York, NY 10003
212 614-2700

Appendix A3: Sources of Materials

ANSI American National Standards
11 West 42nd Street
New York, NY 10036
(212) 642-4900

ASME American Society of Mechanical
Engineers
345 East 47th Street
New York, NY 10017-2392
(212) 705-7800

ASTM (formerly American Society of Testing &
Materials)
1916 Race Street
Philadelphia, PA 19103
(215) 299-5585

AWPA American Wood Preservative
Association
P.O. Box 286
Woodstock, MD 21163-0286
(301) 465-3169

NEC National Electrical Code see NFPA

NEMA National Electrical Manufactures
Association
2101 L St, NW
Washington, DC 20037
(202) 457-1963

NFPA National Fire Protection Association
Batterymarch Park
Quincy, MA 02269
(617) 770-0700

NSF National Sanitation Foundation
3475 Plymouth Road
P.O. Box 1468
Ann Arbor, MI 48106
(313) 769-8010

NSPF National Swimming Pool Foundation
10803 Gulfdale, Suite #300
San Antonio, TX 78216
(512) 344-3713

UL Underwriters Laboratories
333 Pfingsten Road
Northbrook, IL 60062-2096
(708) 272-8800

From ANSI/NSPI: *Standard for aboveground/onground residential swimming pools,* 1992, The Institute.

APPENDIX A4: POOL SIZING AND MATHEMATICAL CONVERSION CHARTS

Pool Sizing

Proper determination of pool capacity is critical to how well you run your pool. Pool capacity tells you how much water balance, shocking, and problem treatment chemicals are required for your pool.

Using the two step procedure below, one can quickly and easily determine pool capacity.

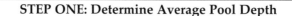

STEP ONE: Determine Average Pool Depth

Add _____ feet + _____ feet = _____ feet ÷ 2 = _____ feet
(Depth of Deep   (Depth of Shallow   (AverageDepth)
    End)   End)

STEP TWO: Determine Capacity for Your Pool

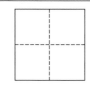 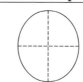 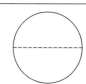

(Length)__feet X
(Width) __feet X
(Average Depth)__ feet X
7.5 = __gallons of water in
your pool.

(Long Diameter)__ feet X
(Short Diameter)__ feet X
(Average Depth)__ feet X
5.9 =__ gallons of water in
your pool.

(Diameter) __feet X
(Diameter) __feet X
(Average Depth __ feet X
5.9 = __ gallons of water in
your pool.

NOTE: Approximate capacity of free-form pool using one or more of formulas above.

Mathematical Conversion Chart

Pounds	X	0.454 =	Kilograms
Kilograms	X	2.205 =	Pounds
Ounces	X	28.35 =	Grams
Grams	X	0.0353 =	Ounces
Feet	X	0.305 =	Meters
Meters	X	3.729 =	Feet

U.S. Gallons	X	3.785	=	Liters
Liters	X	0.264	=	U.S. Gallons
U.S. Gallons	X	0.0038	=	Cubic Meters
Cubic Meters	X	264.2	=	U.S. Gallons
U.S. Gallons	X	0.833	=	Imperial Gallons
Imperial Gallons	X	1.201	=	U.S. Gallons

Useful Mathematical Equations

Circumference of a Circle	Area of Circle	Temperature Conversion
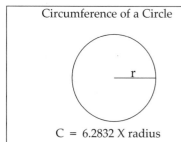 $C = 6.2832 \times radius$	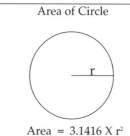 $Area = 3.1416 \times r^2$	I. Fahrenheit Degrees (°F)to Centigrade Degrees (°C) $$C = (F - 32) \times 0.555$$ II. Centigrade Degrees (°C) to Fahrenheit Degrees (°F) $$F = (C \times 1.8) + 32$$

Courtesy BioLab, Decatur, Ga.

APPENDIX A5: FILTRATION SYSTEM SIZES

Pool area (sq ft)	Capacity (gal X 1000)	High-rate sand filters			Pressure DE filters			Cartridge filters		
		Filter area (sq ft)	GPM	Pump HP	Filter area	GPM	Pump HP	Filter area	GPM	Pump HP
<375	<15	1.4	25-30	$^1/_2$	15	25-30	$^1/_2$	45	30	$^1/_3$-$^1/_2$
375-600	15-25	2.2	30-45	$^3/_4$	20-25	35-50	$^1/_2$-$^3/_4$	70	50	$^1/_2$-$^3/_4$
600-850	25-35	3.1	45-60	$^3/_4$-1	30-35	55-70	$^3/_4$-1	100	75	$^3/_4$-1
850	35-45	4.9	75-95	1-1$^1/_2$	35-40	70-80	1-1$^1/_2$	135	95	1-1$^1/_2$

[1]Average depth 5.5 feet, turnover rate 8 hours. May vary from manufacturer to manufacturer.

FILTER CHARACTERISTICS

Type Filter	Filter/Backwash Rates (GPM/sq ft filter area)		Filter additive	Notes
Slow rate/gravity (vacuum)	$^1/_2$-1	8-10	Alum (2 oz/sq. ft.)	Backwash one tank (or pit) at a time to achieve backwash rate.
Rapid rate sand	2-5	12-15	Alum (2 oz/sq. ft.)	(Same as preceding)
High rate sand	15-25[2]	15-25[2]	None	[2]20 GPM is recommended by most manufacturers. It is ineffective to run at a filter or backwash rate more or less than the recommended rate.
Pressure DE	1-2	1-2	DE (1$^1/_2$ oz-2$^1/_2$ oz/ 1 sq ft) or continuously feed 1-4 oz 1000 GPD	Backwash multiple tanks separately. Filtering at excessive flow shortens filter run.
Vacuum DE	2-3	External washing	Same as preceding	Above level tank requires 2 pumps. Filtering at excessive flow rate shortens filter run.
Cartridge surface	0.375-1	External	Small amounts of DE	The lower filter rate is required for public.

From NSPI: *Basic pool and spa technology*, ed 2, 1992, The Institute.

APPENDIX A6

Suggested Computations for Minimum Heights for Message Panel Wording Over Viewing Distances and Lighting Conditions		
Safe Viewing Distance	Minimum Letter Height for FAVORABLE Reading Conditions	Minimum Letter height for UNFAVORABLE Reading Conditions
Less than 24 inches	$Ht (in) = \dfrac{View\ Distance}{150}$	$Ht. (in.) = \dfrac{View\ Distance}{75}$
24 to 96	$Ht (in) = \dfrac{View\ Distance}{300}$	$Ht. (in.) = \dfrac{View\ Distance}{150}$
Greater than 96 inch	$Ht (in) = \dfrac{View\ Distance}{400}$	$Ht. (in.) = \dfrac{View\ Distance}{300}$

NOTE: (1) For purposes of computation, use of upper case letter height is acceptable. Final computation of letter height for viewing distances close to 24 inches and 96 inches can be based on either formula as long as readability can be demonstrated. (2) Letter height values derived from the above computations are not absolute due to variables that affect readability such as letter style, letter weight, contrast, and illumination. Final determination of letter height should be based on a visual examination of the composed word message in the reasonably expected environment of the use or one very similar to the expected environment of use. (3) Letter heights minimums indicated for favorable reading conditions may, in some instances, be reduced further for application to small products, products containers, or products having limited surface area on which to apply the message. However, a lower case letter height of .05 in (1.2 mm) or 6-pt. type is approaching the lower limits of legibility and should be considered as the minimum height for safety messages.

From McCormick EJ: *Alphanumeric and related displays*, Human Factors in Engineering and Design 88-97, McGraw Hill, Inc. 1976.

APPENDIX A7: BARRIERS FOR POOLS, SPAS, AND HOT TUBS

Application

The provisions of this document shall control the design of barriers for residential swimming pools, spas, and hot tubs. These design controls are intended to provide protection against potential drownings and near-drownings of children under the age of five by restricting access to swimming pools, spas, and tubs.

Requirements
Section I. outdoor swimming pool

An outdoor swimming pool, including an in-ground, or on-ground pool, hot tub, or spa shall be provided with a barrier which shall comply with the following:

1. The top of the barrier shall be at least 48 inches above grade measured on the side of the barrier which faces away from the swimming pool. The maximum vertical clearance between grade and the bottom of the barrier shall be 4 inches measured on the side of the barrier which faces away from the swimming pool. Where the top of the pool structure is above grade, such as an above-ground pool, the barrier may be at ground level, such as the pool structure, or mounted on top of the pool structure. Where the barrier is mounted on top of the pool structure, the maximum vertical clearance between

the top of the pool structure and the bottom of the barrier shall be 4 inches.

2. Openings in the barrier shall not allow passage of a 4 inch diameter sphere.

3. Solid barriers which do not have openings, such as a masonry or stone wall, shall not contain indentations or protrusions except for normal construction tolerances and tooled masonry joints.

4. Where the barrier is composed of horizontal and vertical members and the distance between the tips of the horizontal members is less than 45 inches, the horizontal members shall be located on the swimming pool side of the fence. Spacing between vertical members shall not exceed 1 3/4 inches in width. Where there are decorative cutouts within vertical members, spacing within the cutouts shall not exceed 1 3/4 inches in width. (This section is not intended to regulate fencing on top of aboveground/onground pools where the pool structure forms a barrier at least 48" above grade.)

5. Where the barrier is composed of horizontal and vertical members and the distance between the tops of the horizontal members is 45 inches or more, spacing between vertical members shall not exceed 4 inches. Where there are decorative cutouts within vertical members, spacing within the cutouts shall not exceed 1 3/4 inches in width. (This section is not intended to regulate fencing on top of aboveground/onground pools where the pool structure forms a barrier at least 48" above grade.

6. Maximum mesh size for chain link fences shall be a 1 1/4 inch square unless the fence is provided with slats fastened at the top or the bottom which reduce the openings to no more than 1 3/4 inches.

7. Where the barrier is composed of diagonal members, such as a lattice fence, the maximum opening formed by the diagonal members shall be no more than 1 3/4 inches.

8. Access gates shall comply with the requirements of Section I, Paragraphs 1 through 7, and shall be equipped to accommodate a locking device. Pedestrian access gates shall open outward away from the pool and shall be self-closing and have a self-latching device. Gates other than pedestrian access gates shall have a self-latching device. Where the release mechanism of the self-latching device is located less than 54 inches from the bottom of the gate, (a) the release mechanism shall be located on the pool side of the gate at least 3 inches below the top of the gate and (b) the gate and barrier shall have no opening greater than 1/2 inch within 18 inches of the release mechanism.

9. Where a wall of a dwelling serves as part of the barrier, one of the following shall apply: (a) All doors with direct access to the pool through that wall shall be equipped with an alarm which produces an audible warning when the door and its screen, if present, are opened. The alarm shall sound continuously for a minimum of 30 seconds immediately after the door is opened. The alarm shall have a minimum sound pressure rating of 85 dBA at 10 ft. and the sound of the alarm shall be distinctive from other household sounds such as smoke alarm, telephones and doorbells. The alarm shall automatically reset under all conditions. The alarm shall be equipped with manual rest means, such as touchpads or switches, to temporarily deactivate the alarm for a single opening from either direction. Such deactivation shall last for no more than 15 seconds. The deactivation touchpads or switches shall be located at least 45 inches above the threshold of the door. (b) The pool shall be equipped with a power safety cover which complies with ASTM F1346 listed below. (c) Other means of protection, such as self-closing doors with self-latching devices, which are approved by the governing body, shall be acceptable so long as the degree of protection afforded is not less than the protection afforded by (a) or (b) described above.

10. Where an aboveground/onground swimming pool structure is used as a barrier or where the barrier is mounted on top of the pool structure and the means of access is a ladder or steps that (a) the ladder or steps shall be capable of being secured, locked or removed to prevent access or (b) the ladder or steps shall be surrounded by barrier which meets the requirements of Section I, Paragraphs 1(a) through 1(h). When the ladder or steps are secured, locked, or removed, any opening created shall not allow the passage of a 4 inch diameter sphere.

Endorsed by US Consumer Products Safety Commission and NSPI: Approved by the NSPI Executive Committee: July, 1991. Issued by CPSC Staff: 4-5-91.

Section II. Indoor swimming pool.

All walls surrounding an indoor swimming pool shall comply with Section I, Paragraph 9.

Section III. Prohibited locations.

Barriers shall be located so as to prohibit permanent structures, equipment or similar objects from being used to climb the barriers.

Section IV. Exemptions

A spa with a safety cover which complies with ASTM F1346 listed below shall be exempt from the provision of this document.

ASTM F1346 New Standard Performance Specification for Safety Covers and Labeling Requirements for all Covers for Swimming Pools, Spas and Hot Tubs.

APPENDIX A8: ADDITIONAL SENSIBLE USE CONSIDERATIONS

The National Spa and Pool Institute (NSPI) suggests that builders of swimming pools advise the initial owner or operator of a public/commercial-type pool of the following:

1. A list of emergency telephone numbers should be kept at a telephone close to the pool. Numbers should include those for the nearest available police, fire, ambulance and/or rescue unit, and/or 911 if available, as well as the name and phone number of the nearest available physician and hospital. (Refer to Article 15.5.1.)

2. The availability of consumer awareness information from sources such as the following:

    (a) "The Sensible Way to Enjoy Your Pool" published by the NSPI, October 1983 (revised September 1986)*

    (b) "The Sensible Way to Enjoy Your Spa or Hot Tub" published by the NSPI, October 1983 (revised July 1986)*

    (c) The "Knowing How To Dive" published by the National Swimming Pool Foundation (NSPF), 1982 (revised 1985)†

3. For information regarding pool design requirements for competitive swimming and diving, obtain the "Official Swimming Pool Design Compendium, Updated 4th Edition," from the NSPF, or contact the appropriate national organization, such as the following:

    (a) Federation International de Natation Amateur (FINA)
    208-3340 West 41st Avenue
    Vancouver, British Columbia, Canada V6N 3E6

    (b) National Collegiate Athletic Association (NCCA)
    P.O. Box 1906
    Mission, KS 66201

    (c) National Federation of State High School Associations (NFSHSA)
    11724 Plaza Circle, Box 20626
    Kansas City, MO 64195

    (d) U.S. Swimming
    1750 East Boulder Street
    Colorado Springs, CO 80909

    (e) U.S. Diving
    901 West New York Street
    Indianapolis, IN 46202

---

* Contact: NSPI, 2111 Eisenhower Avenue, Alexandria, VA 22314, (703) 838-0083;
† Contact: NSPF, 10803 Gulfdale, Suite 300 San Antonio, TX 78216, (512) 525-1227
From ANSI/NSPI-1: *Standard for public swimming pools*, 1991, The Institute.

APPENDIX A9: COVER AND POOL DEFINITIONS

Covers: Something that covers, protects or shelters, or a combination thereof, a swimming pool, spa or hot tub.

Hard-top cover: A cover used on pools, spas or hot tubs that rests on the lip of the pool or spa deck (not a flotation cover) used as a barrier to users, for maintenance and thermal protection.

Winter cover: A cover that is secured around the perimeter of a pool or spa that provides a barrier to debris when the pool or spa is closed for the season.

Solar cover: A cover that, when placed on a pool or spa surface, increases the water temperature by solar activity and reduces evaporation.

Thermal cover: An insulating cover used to help prevent evaporation and heat loss from pools or spas.

Safety cover: As defined by ASTM F1346, Performance Specification for Safety Covers and Labeling Requirements for All Covers for Swimming Pools, Spas and Hot Tubs, a barrier (intended to be completely removed before entry of users), for swimming pools, spas, hot tubs or wading pools, attendant appurtenances and/or anchoring mechanisms which will—when properly labeled, installed, used and maintained in accordance with the manufacturers' published instructions—reduce the risk of drowning of children under five years of age by inhibiting their access to the contained body of water, and by providing for the removal of any substantially hazardous level of collected surface water. These covers may be power or manual.

Pools

Permanently installed swimming pool: A pool that is constructed in the ground or in a building in such a manner that it cannot be readily disassembled for storage (refer to NSPI-1 Standard for Public Swimming Pools or NSPI-5 Standard for Residential Swimming Pools as applicable).

Aboveground pool (Type 0): A removable pool of any shape that has a minimum water depth of 36 inches and a maximum water depth of 48 inches at the wall. The wall is located on the surrounding earth and may be readily disassembled or stored and reassembled to its original integrity. Diving and the use of a water slide are prohibited. (Refer to NSPI-4 Standard for Aboveground Residential Swimming Pools.)

On-ground residential swimming pool (Type 0): A removable pool package whose walls rest fully on the surrounding earth and has an excavated area below the ground level where diving and the use of a water slide are prohibited. (Refer to NSPI-4 Standard for Aboveground Swimming Pools.) The slope adjacent to the shallow area shall have a maximum slope of 3:1, and the slope adjacent to the shallow area shall have a maximum slope of 3:1, and the slope adjacent to the side walls shall have a maximum slope of 1:1.

Inground swimming pool: Any pool whose sides rest in partial or full contact with the earth. (Refer to NSPI-5 Standard for Residential Swimming Pools or NSPI-1 Standard for Public Swimming Pools, as applicable.)

Residential pool: A residential pool shall be defined as any constructed pool, permanent or non-portable, that is intended for noncommercial use as a swimming pool by not more than three (3) owner families and their guests and that is over 24 inches in depth, has a surface area exceeding 250 square feet and/or a volume over 3,250 gallons. (Refer to NSPI-5 Standard for Residential Swimming Pools.) Residential pools shall be further classified into types as an indication of the suitability of a pool for use with diving equipment.

Type 0: Any residential pool where the installation of diving equipment is prohibited.

Types I-V: Residential pools suitalbe for the installation of diving equipment by type. Diving equipment classifited at a higher type may not be used on a pool of lesser type (i.e., Type III equipment on a Type II pool).

Commercial/public pool: Any pool, other than a residential pool, which is intended to be used for swimming or bathing and is operated by an owner, lesse. operator, licensee or concessionaire, regardless of whether a fee is charged for use. References within the standard to various types of public pools (refer to NSPI-1 Standard for Public Swimming Pools) are defined by the following categories:

Class A (Competition pool): Any pool intended for use for accredited competitive aquatic events such as Federation Internationale De Natation Amateur

From ANSI/NPSI: *Standard for public swimming pools*, 1991, The Institute.

(FINA), U.S. Swimming, U.S. Diving, National Collegiate Athletic Association (NCAA), National Federation of State High School Associations (NFSH-SA), etc. The pool may also be used for recreation.

Class B (Public pool): Any pool intended for public recreational use.

Class C (Semi-public pool): Any pool operated solely for and in conjunction with lodgings such as hotels, motels, apartments, condominiums, etc.

Class D (Other pool): Any pool operated for medical treatment, therapy, exercise, lap swimming, recreational play and other special purposes, including, but not limited to, wave or surf action pools, activity pools, splash pools, kiddie pools and play areas. These pool are not intended to be covered within the scope of NSPI standards. Public pools may be diving or nondiving. If diving, they shall be further classified into types as an indication of the suitability of a pool for use with diving equipment.

Types VI-XI: Public pools suitable for the installation of diving equipment by type. Diving equipment classified at a higher type may not be used on a pool of lesser type (i.e., Type VIII equipment on a Type VI pool).

Type N: A non-diving public pool (no diving allowed).

APPENDIX B
POOL AND SPA CARE
AND MAINTENANCE

APPENDIX B1: IMPORTANT PHONE NUMBERS

Poison Control Center _____

Ambulance Service _____

Nearest Hospital _____

Family Doctor _____

Pool Dealer _____

Plumber _____

Electrician _____

Fire Department _____

APPENDIX B2: YOUR POOL PROFILE

Pool

Type of Finish _____ Capacity in Gallons _____

Shape _____ Dimensions (length x width x depth _____

Piping Size/Type _____ Date Pool Completed _____

Builder (name, tel. no) _____

Address _____

Heater

Type _____ Serial Number _____

Make/Model _____

Filter

Type _____ Make/Model _____

Backwash Pressure _____ Clean Start-Up Pressure _____

Pump

Make _____ Motor Make _____

Time Clock (hours of operation) _____ Horsepower _____

Chlorination Equipment **Automatic Pool Cleaner**
Make/Model _____ Make Model _____

Diving Board
Length _____ Make/Model _____ Diving Depth _____

What Else Makes Your Pool Different?
(Trees nearby, windy site, heavy use, small children etc.) _____

_____

_____

Courtesy BioLab, Inc, Decatur, Ga.

APPENDIX B3: YOUR POOL CAPACITY

AVERAGE POOL DEPTH

Your pool capacity will determine the initial amount of sanitizer, stabilizer and other chemicals you might need. Use the easy formulas that follow to determine your pool capacity.

Depth of deep end   +   Depth of shallow end
= total feet ÷ 2 = AVERAGE POOL DEPTH

POOL CAPACITY FORMULAS

Oval Pool

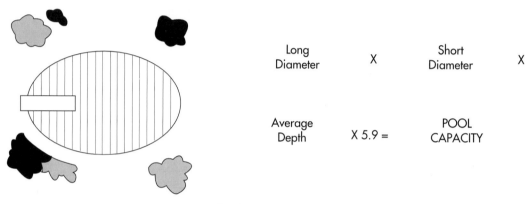

| Long Diameter | X | Short Diameter | X |
| Average Depth | X 5.9 = | POOL CAPACITY | |

Rectangular/Square Pool

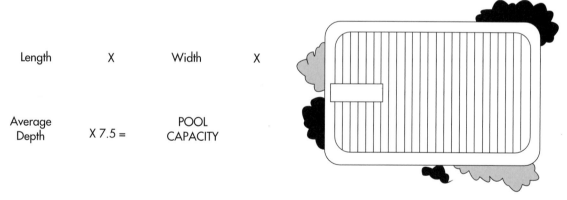

| Length | X | Width | X |
| Average Depth | X 7.5 = | POOL CAPACITY | |

Circular Pool

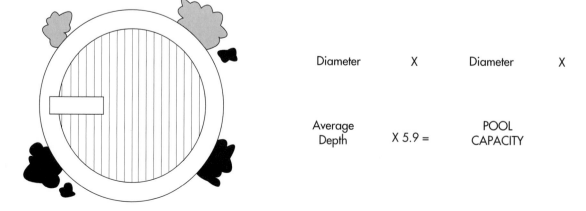

| Diameter | X | Diameter | X |
| Average Depth | X 5.9 = | POOL CAPACITY | |

APPENDIX B4: SERVICE TECHNICIAN'S RECORD FORM

Customer name _____

Pool volume _____

Technician _____

Initial observations:

Date								
Time								
Weather								
Water level								
Inlet check								
Debris in pool								
Algae								

Water chemistry measurements:

Water temperature								
pH								
Total alkalinity								
Calcium								
Cyanuric acid								
Saturation index								

Chemical adjustments made:

Add chlorine								
Automatic feeder setting								
Add sodium bicarbonate								
Add cyanuric acid								
Add algicide								
Other								

Maintenance:

Skim								
Brush								
Vacuum								
Scrub tile								
Empty skimmer baskets								
Empty filter strainer								
Empty pump lint trap								
Filter PSI								
Filter backwash								
Pump primed								
Add/drain water								
Water leaks								

Notes:

APPENDIX B5: PROBLEM/INCENTIVE LOG

DAY: M T W T F S S		DATE:
POOL:		CODE:
	POOL OPENED LATE	LIST TIME:
	GUARD ARRIVED LATE	LIST TIME:
	POOL CLOSED EARLY	LIST TIME:
	HEALTH INSPECTION	PASS OR FAIL
	GUARD NOT IN CHAIR/WATCHING POOL	
	GUARD NOT IN UNIFORM	
	FAIR OR POOR ON FIELD REPORT	
	FAIR OR POOR ON EVALUATION	MIDSEASON END
	FAILURE TO OBTAIN SUB FOR TIME OFF	
	ASSISTED STAFFING	
OTHER/COMMENTS:		
EMP #: NAME:		
EMP #: NAME:		
EMP #: NAME:		
EMP #: NAME:		
COMPLETED BY:		ENTERED BY:

Courtesy American Pool Service, Beltsville, Md.

APPENDIX B6: SWIMMING POOL OPENING— RECORD FORM

☐ Review the pool's winterizing record form and any recommendations made during winterizing service.
☐ Remove pool cover, clean cover, treat with cover conditioner and store.
☐ Note condition of cover: _____
☐ Storage Location: _____

1. Pool structure check:
☐ Surface interior finish—plaster
☐ condition & stains
☐ Liner condition
☐ Title & grouting

☐ Coping
☐ Deck
☐ Drains
☐ Fence/gate
Notes: _____

Notes: _____
_____

☐ Other accessories: _____
_____
_____

2. Drain & flush lines remove plugs from plumbing:
☐ All pipes & hoses
☐ Skimmer line
☐ Main drain line
☐ Return lines

3. Drain & flush equipment; replace equipment drain plugs:
☐ Pump
☐ Filter
☐ Heater

4. Electrical preparations:
☐ Install GFCI's
☐ Replace pool light in housing
☐ Check electrical panel & grounding
☐ Replace electrical fuses
☐ Turn on electricity

5. Opening preparations:
☐ Fill pool with water to skimmer level
☐ Reinstall skimmer basket
☐ Reinstall pump motor (or remove weatherproof cover)
☐ Turn on LP gas
☐ Set pool heater for thermostat

☐ Set pool timer for filtering.

6. Start & check all equipment:
☐ Motor
☐ Pump
☐ Filter
☐ Heater (check for air locks)
☐ Time clock
☐ Automatic cleaning equipment
☐ Piping/valves

7. Install accessories:
☐ Ladder
☐ Hand rails
☐ Diving board
☐ Safety line
☐ Ropes
☐ Safety equipment
☐ List equipment for repair:
_____
_____

8. Clean pool:
☐ Skim/net
☐ Brush
☐ Vacuum
☐ Scrub tile
☐ Backwash filter if needed
☐ Acid wash if plaster is excessively stained
☐ Replace test reagents to ensure accurate results

9. Test water chemistry:
☐ pH
☐ Total chlorine (bromine etc.)
☐ Free chlorine
☐ Cyanuric acid
☐ Total Alkalinity
☐ Calcium hardness
☐ Total Dissolved Solids

10. Add chemicals:
☐ Chlorine (Bromine, etc.)
☐ Cyanuric acid
☐ Sodium bicarbonate
☐ Algicide or shock treatment
Others: _____
_____

NOTES:
_____
_____
_____
_____
_____
_____

From NSPI: *Basic pool and spa technology,* ed 2, 1992, The Institute.

APPENDIX B7: WATER AND ENERGY CONSERVATION CHECKLIST

TO SAVE WATER AROUND YOUR POOL AND YARD

☐ 1. **Repair any leaks.**
Even a small leak in either the equipment or the structural shell can cause substantial water. Just 1-1/2 inches a day in a 15-by-30 foot pool wastes approximately 102,000 gallons per year!

☐ 2. **Buy and use a cover.**
Covers reduce water loss due to normal evaporation.

☐ 3. **Clean your filter.**
If possible, manually clean your filter. You'll do a more thorough job and use much less water. The average backwash uses between 250 and 1,000 gallons of water— without completely cleaning your filter.

☐ 4. **Prohibit diving, splashing, and water fights.**
Boisterous play causes large amount of water loss from "splash-out."

☐ 5. **Control filter cycle and chemical use.**
Use the least possible filtration time and test/treat chemically frequently. Regular care will keep the pool/spa cleaner and will avoid the need to drain and refill to correct conditions caused by neglect.

☐ 6. **Reduce heater temperature.**
If you have a heater, reduce the pool/spa heater temperature because warmer water evaporates more quickly.

☐ 7. **Plug the overflow line when swimming.**
If your pool is equipped with an overflow line, this prevents water loss through the line when the pool is in use.

☐ 8. **Watch when filling.**
Keep an eye on the water level when filling the pool/spa. Forgetting to shut off the water can cause costly waste.

☐ 9. **Turn off tile-spray on automatic pool cleaner.**
This device's splashing causes water loss by evaporation. Overspraying can send water right out of the pool.

☐ 10. **Plant drought-resistant native trees and plants in the yard.**

☐ 11. **Water early and late.**
If allowed, watering of lawns should be done in the early morning or evening, when evaporation is at a minimum.

☐ 12. **Sweep instead of hosing off.**
Sweep decks, patios, driveways, and sidewalks instead of hosing.

TO CONSERVE HEAT:

☐ 1. **Cover your pool.**
The proper cover, kept in place when the pool is not in use, will significantly reduce water lost to evaporation. Also, it cuts heat loss by 50-70 percent. Check with your local NSPI member for the most effective cover for your needs.

☐ 2. **Swim at 78° F.**
The ideal swimming temperature for recreational purposes is 78°. If you have requirements that call for a warmer temperature, such as children or elderly people using the pool, adjust the temperature to those specific needs, but no higher. Lowering the water temperature from 82° to 78°—a mere 4°—will reduce energy consumption by 40 percent, with a corresponding cost savings.

From NSPI: *Basic pool and spa technology*, ed 2, 1992, The Institute.

☐ 3. **Only heat when you use.**

If you use your pool only on weekends or special occasions, don't heat between uses. Turn your heater off or set your thermostat at 68° or lower depending on the period between uses. Turn your heater on the night before or the morning of the day of use depending on the heat use. If you go away on a trip, turn your heater off.

☐ 4. **Shelter your pool.**

Protect the surface of your pool from wind—but not from sunlight— by careful positioning of trees, plantings, fences, and cabanas. The difference between a fully sheltered pool and one exposed to a "mild breeze" of 7 miles per hour can be 400 percent higher energy usage.

☐ 5. **Maintain your heater.**

Have your pool service company do an annual heater inspection. A properly maintained heater is an energy-efficient appliance. Have your pool site inspected to see if an active solar collector system should be a good investment for you.

☐ 6. **Backwash only when needed.**

Be sure to follow your filter manufacturer's instructions concerning backwashing. Backwashing more frequently than necessary wastes water while failing to backwash when needed wastes energy.

TO CONSERVE ELECTRICITY

☐ 1. **Use a timeclock.**

Use a timeclock to manage the daily operating period of the circulation pump and of the pool cleaner booster pump.

☐ 2. **Control filtration.**

Reduce filtration time to 6 hours per day. Depending on your previous usage, this can save you 50 percent or more of the energy used for filtration. If your water should lose clarity, increase filtration time in one-half-hour increments until the pool water is sparkling.

☐ 3. **Control use of automatic cleaner.**

As with filtration, establish a minimum cleaning time (2-4 hours daily) and expand this time on unusually heavy load situations. Be sure to run the cleaner only when the filter is running. If you have a pool cover, follow the pool cleaner manufacturer's instructions about operating the cleaner in conjunction with a cover.

☐ 4. **Clean strainer frequently.**

Be sure to remove foreign matter from the pump strainer baskets and the skimmer regularly. Water will circulate more efficiently.

☐ 5. **Use pool lighting when needed.**

Lighting should always be used for safety—when people are in and around the pool after dark. Use of pool and patio lighting "just for atmosphere" should be reduced.

TO CONSERVE CHEMICALS

☐ 1. **Disinfect in the evening.**

Add chlorine or other disinfectant in the evening while the filter is operating. With reduced filtration time, it is particularly important to maintain an adequate disinfectant residual at all times.

☐ 2. **Keep chemistry balanced.**

Keep pool water chemistry in balance and check regularly. Maintain pool pH between 7.2 and 7.8. Maintain spa pH between 7.2 and 7.6.

☐ 3. **Stabilize outdoor pool water.**

Keep outdoor pool water stabilized to reduce chemical consumption. Maintain a minimum of 30 ppm of stabilizer.

☐ 4. **Trim foliage.**

Trim back excess foliage around pool and keep deck areas clean to reduce chemical and filtering requirements.

APPENDIX B8: WATER LOSS PROCEDURE CHECK LIST

SIGNS AND SYMPTOMS OF SWIMMING POOL/SPA LEAKS

Normal water loss will occur from evaporation due to wind and heat. If your pool or spa loses 1/4" of water or more from its normal level in 24 hours you may have a leak.

To detect water loss, the pool/spa should be set to its normal operating level, marked with a permanent pen, and then checked in 24 hours. To prove that your water loss is not due to evaporation, do this simple check. Place a bucket of water (from the pool) in the pool, mark the water level in both, and leave for 24 hours. If the water level in the pool drops more than the bucket's, you have a leak.

High water bill (if pool has an automatic refill).

Algae or discoloration in the pool or spa water. This indicates an imbalance in the chemicals. This can occur then the water level doesn't stay constant, due to a leak. Consult a local pool service expert.

Loose or falling tiles or cracking of the cement pool deck indicates a possible leak because the surrounding ground is becoming unsettled.

Pool settling into the ground, cracks or gaps in bond beam.

If the pool has an automatic filler that is constantly releasing water.

You notice standing water, soft mushy spots, or uneven grass growth around the pool area.

Poor suction and/or bad circulation may indicate a leak.

NORMAL ACCEPTED LOSS & EVAPORATION: (1 to 1-3/4" per week, depending on region & pool/spa situation.)

ESTIMATED LOSS: Per day:
              Per week:

WATER BILL REFLECTS: Gallons per Month:
                        Est. Domestic Use:
                        Est. Pool Loss:

POOL BUILDER:
APPROX. YEAR BUILT:
SIZE: Depth: Gallonage:
Concrete: Vinyl: Fiberglass:
ANY PREVIOUS LEAKS?
WHERE:
ANY CRACKS IN POOL SHELL, TILE, SKIMMER, GROUTING:
WHERE:
AT WHAT LEVEL IN THE POOL DOES THE WATER STOP:
IS THERE HYDROSTATIC PRESSURE UNDER THE POOL:

ESTIMATE TO REPAIR LEAKS ARE STRICTLY ON A TIME AND MATERIAL BASIS. OUR LABOR CHARGE IS $_____PER TRIP AND/OR PER HOUR PER WORKER. ANY CHECKING THAT YOU CAN DO INITIALLY WILL DECREASE THE COST. REMEMBER, YOU MAY HAVE MORE THAN ONE LEAK. WE CANNOT GUARANTEE THAT THE REPAIR OF THE OBVIOUS LEAK WILL INCLUDE REPAIR OF EVERY LEAK.

From NSPI: *Basic pool and spa technology,* ed 2, 1992, The Institute.

APPENDIX **B9**: LIFEGUARD APPLICATION

Name:_____Social Security#_____-_____-_____

Address:_____Phone #:_____

Required Certifications	issued at	expiration date
Lifeguarding (ARC/YMCA)	_____	_____
CPR (NSC/ARC/AHA)	_____	_____
First Aid Training (type:_____)	_____	_____
Lifeguard Training (ARC/YMCA)	_____	_____
Supplemental Training		
CPO (NSPF/YMCA)	_____	_____
WSI (ARC/YMCA)	_____	_____
SCUBA (PADI/YMCA/NAUI)	_____	_____
OTHER: _____	_____	_____
_____	_____	_____

PREVIOUS LIFEGUARDING/SUPERVISION EXPERIENCE

position	place	supervisor	date
_____	_____	_____	_____
_____	_____	_____	_____
_____	_____	_____	_____

Reference Listing

Name	Title	Phone
_____	_____	_____
_____	_____	_____
_____	_____	_____
_____	_____	_____

Interviewed by:_____ date:_____

Applicant Status: hired (full time):_____hired (substitute):_____

pending:_____stipulations:_____

Courtesy Berry Associates, Chestertown, Md.

APPENDIX B9: EVALUATION

Personnel: Lifeguard / Lifeguard Supervisor

Lifeguard being evaluated_____ by_____Aquatic Coordinator

Observation Period:_____to_____ Date of Evaluation_____

_____

Key: "OK" = Satisfactory   "X" = Needs Improvement

CATEGORIES   RATING   COMMENTS

I.   PERSONALITY   _____
     A. Exercises prudent judgment   _____
     B. Maintains personal hygiene   _____
     C. Maintains poise and composure _____
     D. Maintains a professional attitude _____

II. PREPARATION   _____
     A. Holds current ALS certificate _____
     B. Holds current CPR certificate _____
     C. Holds current FA certificate   _____
     D. Holds current Lifeguard Training
         certificate   _____
     E. Attends all in-service meetings _____

III. TASK RELATED SKILLS   _____
     A. Communicates with peers   _____
     B. Communicates with superiors   _____
     C. Operates within the framework
         of the CSC Policy Manual   _____
     D. Understands emergency
         procedures and is able to
         execute them   _____
     E. Keeps abreast of current safety
         techniques

IV. SAFETY SKILLS   _____
     A. Demonstrates an advanced level
         of fitness   _____
     B. Demonstrates an ability to
         perform rescue techniques   _____
     C. Demonstrates an advanced level
         of CPR and resuscitation ability _____

APPENDIX B9: DAILY ACTIVITY SHEET

Submitted by_____To:_____

Date:_____

Swim Center Staff   Position   Hours on Duty

_____   _____   _____
_____   _____   _____
_____   _____   _____
_____   _____   _____
_____   _____   _____
_____   _____   _____

Chemical Readings
Ideal

	9am	11am	1pm	3pm	5pm
pH 7.2-7.8					
FAC 1.0-1.5					
TA 80-120ppm					
CH 150-300ppm					
H2o Temp. 26c/80f					

		Programming/Pool Load				
Hour	Activity	Guests	Classes	Events	Members	Total
7am						
8am						
9am						
10am						
11am						
12n						
1pm						
2pm						
3pm						
4pm						
5pm						
6pm						
7pm						
8pm						
9pm						
Program Totals						

Special Events:

Courtesy Berry Associates, Chestertown, Md.

Continued

APPENDIX B9: AQUATIC STAFF IN-SERVICE TRAINING FORM

Date:_____Time:_____Group: (circle one)   lifeguards
instructors
management

In service topic:_____

Staff Present: _____   _____   _____

_____   _____   _____

_____   _____   _____

_____   _____   _____

_____   _____   _____

In-Service Trainers Present:_____

_____

Specific Topic Areas/Skills: _____

_____

_____

_____

_____

Comments:

APPENDIX B9: ACCIDENT REPORT FORM

DIRECTIONS: Fill out both sides this form completely and accurately. Place this copy on the Aquatic Director's desk. Copies will be made and sent to the offices checked below.

Personal Information:

1. Name: _____ Age:_____

    Home Address: _____

    Phone:_____

2. In Guest: Sponsor's Name:_____

3. Date of Accident:_____ Time:_____

4. Pool activity at time of accident: mark with an (X)

    Sport practice_____   Recreation Swim_____
    Activity Class (name)_____   Pool load at time of accident:_____

5. What specifically was the person doing at the time of the accident?
    _____
    _____

6. Was there supervision at the time of the accident?   yes_____   no_____
    By whom?_____

7. Part of the body injured:_____
    _____

8. Type of injury sustained: _____

9. Detailed description of accident: _____

10. What First Aid was administered?_____

11. Was EMS notified?   yes_____   no_____

12. Person taken to hospital: yes_____   no_____Taken by:_____

13. Did person refuse medical assistance?   If yes, Victims signature_____

14. Did person return to activity?   yes_____   no_____   Time_____

Report submitted by:_____ Title:_____

Report received by: _____ Title: Aquatic Coordinator

Courtesy Berry Associates, Chestertown, Md.

continued

APPENDIX B9: TRAINING FORM: OSHA BLOODBORNE PATHOGENS STANDARD

In the fall of 1991, OSHA enacted regulation 29 CFR 1910.1030 Bloodborne Pathogens. The OSHA regulation endeavors to appreciable diminish occupationally acquired infections with Hepatitis B Virus (HBV), Human Immunodeficiency Virus (HIV), and other bloodborne diseases that have public health significance. The effective date of the new regulation was June 15, 1992 with various provisions phased in within 60 to 120 days following that date. The following, summarizes the major requirements.

Scope of the Regulation
Public Swimming Pools are impacted by this regulation; specifically employees whose work duties may reasonably be anticipated to involve skin, eye, mucous membrane, or parenteral contact with blood or other potentially infectious materials.

HBV vaccination, and post-exposure evaluation/follow-up
Public Swimming Pools must make HBV vaccination available free of charge to all employees considered immediate care first aid responders under the scope of the regulation. This fee is to be absorbed by the employing facility or firm for lifeguards. These entities must provide such vaccination within 10 working days of initial job assignment, unless the employee has already received HBV vaccine. Because of an array of privacy and religious concerns, OSHA does not mandate that the employee receive the vaccination; however, employees declining the vaccination must sign the official HBV Vaccine Declination. The employee may relinquish the declination at any time, and then the employing facility or firm must provide HBV vaccine at no cost to the employee.

Employees reporting an exposure incident (specific eye, mouth, other mucus membrane, non-intact skin, or parenteral contact with blood or other potentially infectious material that resulted from the performance of job duties) are to be provided free of charge a confidential post-exposure medical evaluation and subsequent medical follow-up including port-exposure prophylaxis and counselling. Public Swimming Pools must provide for collection of blood to establish HBV and HIV serological status from the exposed employee and, if applicable, the source individual.

Exposure Control Plan
Public Swimming Pools must establish and begin implementation of a written Exposure Control Plan by June 15, 1992.

Information and Training Requirements
All lifeguards, swim coaches or other employees falling under the scope of the regulation must participate in a training program ASAP and at least annually thereafter. After that date new employees must receive training at the time of initial assignment.

By signing this information form, the following employees acknowledge that they have read the OSHA Bloodborne Pathogen Standard and further, understand their rights and limitations as employees who may be impacted by this regulation.

Date of Training Session:_____Session Leader:_____

Employee:_____Date:_____
Employee:_____Date:_____
Employee:_____Date:_____
Employee:_____Date:_____

Courtesy Berry Associates, Chestertown, Md.

APPENDIX B9: Swimming Pool Emergency Phone List

_____ Aquatic Coordinator_____

_____ Facility Manager   _____

_____ Owner/Operator   _____

Emergency Medical System   Dial 911

Local Police   _____

Special Situation Procedures

Situation: Intoxicated person
Procedure: Ask the person to leave the pool area. Call local police

Situation: Thievery
Procedure: Call local police immediately.

Situation: Indecent exposure
Procedure: Diplomatically suggest covering up or leaving the pool area.
             In the event of willful exposure, call local police immediately.

Situation: Abuse, disorders
Procedure: In the event that a patron loses control and uses physical or verbal
             abuse, call local police and have the individual removed from the
             pool.

Situation: Fire
Procedure: Pull the fire alarm, evacuate the pool area and locker rooms and dial
             911 to report the fire.

Situation: Power failure (evenings)
Procedure: Clear the pool area and check the pool bottom. If normal power is
             not restored in 10 minutes call the Coordinator to help secure the
             facility.

Situation: Electrical Storms (summer)
Procedure: Prohibit access to pool until storm passes

Courtesy Berry Associates, Chestertown, Md.

continued

APPENDIX B9: EMPLOYEE MSDS TRAINING

Date:_____   Trainer/Instructor:_____

_____

Topics:

- Special handling procedures for swimming pool chemicals

- Storage practices for swimming pool chemicals

- Potential health related hazards

- Swimming pool chemical interactions

> Common swimming pool chemicals
> Sodium Hypochlorite
> Calcium Hypochlorite
> Bromine
> Muriatic Acid
> Sodium Bisulfate
> Sodium Bicarbonate
> Sodium Bicarbonate
> Test Kit reagents

- General Protection Practices

- Emergency Care

Employees present for training session:

_____   _____

_____   _____

_____   _____

_____   _____

Training Verified by:_____Date: _____

Forward one copy to your insurance carrier

Courtesy Berry Associates, Chestertown, Md.

APPENDIX B10: YOUR SPA PROFILE

Spa/Hot Tub

Type of Finish_____ Capacity in Gallons_____

Shape_____ Dimensions (length x width x depth_____

Piping Size/Type_____ Date Spa Installed_____

Supplier/Installer (name, tel. no)_____ Brand/Model_____

Address_____

Heater

Type_____ Serial Number_____

Make/Model_____

Filter

Type_____ Make/Model_____

Backwash Pressure_____Clean Start-Up Pressure_____

Pump

Make_____Motor Make_____

Time Clock (hours of operation)_____ Horsepower_____

Sanitation Equipment

Make/Model_____

What Else Makes Your Spa Different?

(Indoor/Outdoor, trees nearby, windy site, heavy use, small children, air blower, etc.)

_____

_____

_____

Courtesy BioLab, Inc, Decatur, Ga.

APPENDIX B11: SPA INSTALLATION— SITE CHECK LIST

☐ Check local building and safety codes and obtain permits before starting installation.

☐ Make sure chosen installation site is not too close to trees or foliage where falling leaves or pine needles may fall into the spa, or roots may cause excavation problems.

☐ Check for adequate run-off drainage. Don't block designed run-off areas. Don't install a spa in such an area.

☐ Make sure spa and equipment sites are accessible and properly ventilated.

☐ Determine direction of the prevailing wind. If not protected from wind, operating expenses for heating will go up.

☐ Determine if difference in elevation between spa and equipment is too great.

☐ Check for overhead wires.

☐ Check for underground cables and septic tanks.

☐ Check for easy access from house to spa.

☐ Check any gates that provide entry. They must be self-latching and elf-closing.

☐ Check for proper fencing, if required.

☐ Check depth of fill dirt that may lie over a base. Check the types of base (rock or bolder).

☐ Check possible obstacles to piping, including plumbing and utility lines, concrete, sprinkler lines, walks, etc.

☐ Check for privacy from surrounding areas.

☐ Check that required permits are in order, or make appropriate additions.

☐ Make sure there is access to electrical service and that there is available power.

☐ Check that there is access to the gas lines and meter, if required.

From NSPI: *Basic pool and spa technology*, ed 2, The Institute.

APPENDIX B12: SPA SERVICE RECORD FORM

Customer name_____

Customer address_____

Spa volume_____

Initial observations:

Date	
Time	
Technician	

Water chemistry tests:

Water temperature	
pH	
Sanitizer level	
Ozone	
Total dissolved solids	
Iron	
Copper	
Other	

Chemical adjustments:

Add sanitizer	
Automatic feeder setting	
Add sodium bicarbonate	
Add cyanuric acid	
Add calcium	
Add mineral remover	
Add calcium remover	
Add algicide	
Shock treatment	
Other	

Maintenance:

Vacuum spa	
Clean tile	
Backwash filter	
Change filter cartridge	
Clean filter	
Drain/refill spa	
Clean/polish spa	

Equipment check:

Spa Pac	
Pump/motor	
Filter	
Heater	
blower	
Jets	
Chemical feeder	
Ozonator	
Control Panel	
Timer	
GFCI	
Light	
Cover	

Notes:_____

From NSPI: *Basic pool and spa technology*, ed 2, 1992, The Institute.

APPENDIX C
POOL CHEMISTRY

APPENDIX C1: TESTS

IMPORTANT NOTES

1. **Rinse sample tubes thoroughly before and after each test.**
2. **Obtain sample approximately 18" below surface of water.**
3. **Hold bottle vertically when dispensing.**
4. **Protect kit from direct sunlight and temperature extremes.**
5. **Read precautions on all labels carefully. KEEP OUT OF REACH OF CHILDREN.**

Free Chlorine (FC) Test

1. Fill test cell to mark with water to be tested.
2. Add 5 drops R-0001 DPD Reagent #1 and 5 drops R-0002 DPD Reagent #2. Cap and mix.
3. Wipe dry and place in comparator WITH FROSTED SIDE FACING OPERATOR.
4. Match color in test cell with a color standard. Record as parts per million (ppm) free chlorine (FC).
5. Save sample for total chlorine (TC) test.

Total Chlorine (TC) Test

1. Use treated sample from FC test.
2. Add 5 drops R-0003 DPD Reagent #3. Cap and mix.
3. Wipe dry and place in comparator WITH FROSTED SIDE FACING OPERATOR.
4. Match color. Record as ppm total chlorine (TC).

Combined Chlorine (CC) Test

1. Subtract FC from TC. Record as ppm combined chlorine (CC). Formula: TC-FC = CC. Refer to Chlorine Tables for adjustment.

NOTE: Use test cell #4025 for high chlorine (to 10 ppm).

Bromine Test

1. Fill test cell to mark with water to be tested.
2. Add 5 drops R-0001 DPD Reagent #1 and 5 drops R-0002 DPD Reagent #2. Cap and mix.
3. Wipe dry and place in comparator WITH FROSTED SIDE FACING OPERATOR.
4. Match color in test cell with a color standard. Record as parts per million (ppm) bromine. Refer to manufacturer's instructions for proper adjustments.

NOTE: Use test cell #4025 for high bromine (to 10 ppm).

Courtesy Taylor Technologies, Sparks, Md.

pH Test

1. Fill test cell (#4024) to 11.5 mL mark with water to be tested.
2. Using a 1.0 mL pipet (#4030), add 0.5 mL R-1003J Phenol Red Indicator. Cap and mix.
3. Wipe dry and place in comparator WITH FROSTED SIDE FACING OPERATOR.
4. Match color in test cell with a color standard. Record as pH units. If sample color is between two values, pH is average of the two.
5. Save sample for either acid demand test (if pH needs to be LOWERED), or base demand test (if pH needs to be RAISED).

Acid Demand Test

1. Use treated sample from pH test.
2. Add R-0853 Acid Demand Reagent dropwise, mixing and comparing after each drop, until desired pH is reached on comparator. Keep count of drops added. Refer to Acid Demand Tables for correct amount of acid to add to LOWER pH.

Base Demand Test

1. Use treated sample from pH test.
2. Add R-0862 Base Demand Reagent dropwise, mixing and comparing after each drop, until desired pH is reached on comparator. Keep count of drops added. Refer to Base Demand Tables for correct amount of soda ash to add to RAISE pH.

NOTE: pH Indicator, Acid Demand and Base Demand Reagents used for Midget and Slide Comparator Systems are not interchangeable with 2000 Series Comparator Blocks. That is: reagent R-0004, R-0005, and R-0006 cannot be substituted for reagents R-1003J, R-0853, and R-0862.

Total Alkalinity Test

1. Fill sample tube (#9198) to 25 mL mark with water to be tested.
2. Add 2 drops R-0007 Thiosulfate N/10. Swirl to mix.
3. Add 5 drops R-0008 Total Alkalinity Indicator. Swirl to mix. Sample should turn green.
4. Add R-0009 Sulfuric Acid .12N dropwise, swirling and counting after each drop, until color changes from green to red.

5. Multiply drops in Step 4 to 10. Record as parts per million (ppm) total alkalinity as calcium carbonate. Refer to Total Alkalinity Tables for adjustment.

Calcium Hardness Test
1. Fill sample tube (#9198) to 25 mL mark with water to be tested.
2. Add 20 drops R-0010 Calcium Buffer. Swirl to mix.
3. Add 5 drops R-0011L Calcium Indicator Liquid (or 1 level dipper R0011P Calcium Indicator Powder). Swirl to mix. Sample will turn red if calcium hardness is present.
4. Add R-0012 Hardness Reagent dropwise, swirling and counting after each drop, until color changes from red to blue.
5. Multiply drops in Step 4 by 10. Record as parts per million (ppm) calcium hardness as calcium carbonate. Refer to Calcium Hardness Tables for adjustment.

Total Hardness Test
1. Fill sample tube (#9198) to 25 mL mark with water to be tested.
2. Add 10 drops R-0854 Total Hardness Reagent. Swirl to mix. Sample should turn red.
3. Add R-0012 Hardness Reagent dropwise, swirling and counting after each drop, until color changes from red to blue.
4. Multiply drops in Step 3 by 10. Record as parts per million (ppm) total hardness as calcium carbonate.

Magnesium Hardness Test
1. Subtract CH from TH. Record as ppm magnesium hardness (MH). Formula: TH-CH=MH.

Cyanuric Acid Test
1. Fill CYA dispensing bottle (#9194) to 15 mL mark with water to be tested.
2. Add R-0013 Cyanuric Acid Reagent to neck. Cap and mix for 30 seconds. Sample will turn cloudy if cyanuric acid is present.
3. Slowly transfer cloudy solution to CYA view tube (#9193), while looking down through solution, until black dot on bottom of CYA view tube just disappears.
4. Read CYA view tube at liquid level. Record as parts per million (ppm) cyanuric acid.

Copper Test
1. Fill 11.5 mL test cell (#4024) to 11.5 mL mark with water to be tested.
2. Using a 1.0 mL pipet (#4030), add 0.5 mL R-0860 Copper Reagent #1. Using a separate 1.0 mL pipet, add 0.5ml: R-0861 Copper Reagent #2. Cap and mix.
3. Wipe dry and place in comparator WITH FROSTED SIDE FACING OPERATOR. WAIT 5 MINUTES.
4. Match color in test cell with a color standard. Record as parts per million (ppm) copper.

Iron Test
1. Fill 11.5 mL test cell (#4024) to 11.5ml mark with water to be tested.
2. Using a 1.0 mL pipet (#4030), add 0.5 mL R-0851 Iron Reagent #1. Cap and mix. WAIT 2 MINUTES.
3. Using a separate 1.0 mL pipet, add 1.0 mL R-0852 Iron Reagent #2. Cap and Mix.
4. Wipe dry and place in comparator WITH FROSTED SIDE FACING OPERATOR.
5. Match color in test cell with a color standard. Record as parts per million (ppm) iron.

APPENDIX C2: CHEMICAL OPERATIONAL PARAMETERS

These guidelines set forth the suggested operational parameters for the proper chemical treatment and maintenance of swimming pool waters.

Chemical treatment alone will not produce sanitary pool water. A filtration system in proper operational condition is also required to attain sparkling clear, polished sanitary water.

A. Disinfectant Levels	Minimum	Ideal	Maximum	Comments
1. Free chlorine (ppm)	1.0	1.0-3.0	3.0	Hot weather/heavy use may require operation at or near maximum levels. Regular superchlorination is recommended (see E-1).
2. Combined chlorine (ppm)	None	None	0.2	High combined chlorine results in reduced chemical efficacy. Take remedial action to establish break point chlorination. See E-1. Other signs of combined chlorine: • Sharp chlorinous odor • Eye irritation • Algae growth
3. Bromine (ppm)	2.0	2-4	4.0	
4. Iodine (ppm)	Levels not established			NOTE: Local health department officials should be consulted before use.

B. Chemical Values

	Minimum	Ideal	Maximum	Comments
1. pH	7.2	7.4-7.6	7.8	If pH is: Too High: • Low chlorine efficiency • Scale formation • Cloudy water • Eye discomfort Too Low: • Rapid dissipation of disinfectant • Plaster and concrete etching • Eye discomfort • Corrosion of metals • Vinyl liner damage

Courtesy NSPI: *Basic pool and spa technology*, ed 2, 1992, The Institute.

Continued

	Minimum	Ideal	Maximum	Comments
2. Total alkalinity (buffering)(ppm) as $CaCO_3$	60	80-100 for calcium hypochlorite, lithium hypochlorite, and sodium hypochlorite 100-200 For sodium dichlor, trichlor, chlorine gas, and bromine compounds	180	If total alkalinity is: Too Low: • pH bounce • Corrosion tendency Too High • Cloudy water • Increased scaling potential • pH tends to be too high
3. Total dissolved solids (ppm)	300	1000-2000*	3000†	These values offered as guidelines rather than absolute values to indicate concern for accumulation of impurities in the course of operation. Excessive high TDS may lead to hazy water, corrosion of fixtures, etc., and can be reduced by partial draining with addition of fresh water.
4. Calcium hardness (ppm) as $CaCO_3$	150	200-400	500-1000+	Operation of pools at maximum hardness will depend on alkalinity (buffering) requirements of the sanitizer used. Minimum alkalinity and lower pH must be used with maximum hardness. (Over 500 ppm.)
5. Heavy metals	None	None	None	If heavy metals, such as copper, iron, manganese, are present: • Staining may occur • Water may discolor • Chlorine dissipates rapidly • Filter may plug • May indicate pH too low, corrosion, etc.

* High inital TDS may indicate poor water quality due to corrosive mineral salts, humus, or organic mater. Consult local waterauthority.
† Increaing TDS indicated build up of impurities to be controlled by partial drain/refill with fresh water.

Continued

C. Biological Values	Minimum	Ideal	Maximum	Comments
1. Algae	None	None	None	If algae are observed: • Shock treat pool (Refer to Section E-3). • Supplement with brushing and vacuuming. • Maintain adequate disinfectant residual. • Use approved algicide according to label direction (Section E-5).
2. Bacteria	None	None	Refer to local code	If bacteria count exceeds local health department requirements: • Superchlorinate and follow proper maintenance procedures. • Maintain proper disinfectant residual.

D. Stabilizer (if used)

	Minimum	Ideal	Maximum	Comments
1. Cyanuric acid (ppm)	10	30-50	150: Except where limited by health dept., requirements often to 100 PPM	If stabilizer is: Too Low • Chlorine residual rapidly destroyed by sunlight Too High: • May exceed local health department regulations • May reduce chlorine efficacy NOTE: Stabilizer is not needed in indoor or brominated pools.

E. Remedial Practices

	Minimum	Ideal	Maximum	Comments
1. Superchlorination frequency	Monthly	Every other week	Weekly when the temperature is over 85°F	NOTE: Some high use pools may need superchlorination three times a week or more as a preventative measure or when combined chlorine is over 0.2 ppm.
2. Superchlorination to establish break point, dosage in ppm	5	10	—	When combined chlorine is over 0.2 PPM or when eye irritation persists. Repeat as needed.
3. Shock treatment (ppm)	10	—	—	Nonchlorine oxidizers are not considered biocidal but may reduce organic contaminants.
4. Clarifying/Floccing frequency	—	When needed	—	Use all clarifiers following manufacturer's directions.
5. Algicides		Follow manufacturer's directions		Use US EPA-registered products.

Continued

	Minimum	Ideal	Maximum	Comments
F. Temperature				If temperature is:
1. Temperature, °F	—	78°-82°	104°	Too Low / Too High

If temperature is:

Too Low
- Bather discomfort

Too High
- Excessive fuel requirement
- Increased evaporation
- Bather discomfort
- Increased scaling potential
- Increased use of disinfectants
- Increased potential for corrosion

	Minimum	Ideal	Maximum	Comments
G. Water Clarity				
1. Water turbidity	—	—	—	If water is turbid:

If water is turbid:
- Disinfectant level may be low
- Filtration system may be inoperative
- Improper chemical balance (Section B)
- Bottom should be clearly visible at the deepest part of the pool.
- Consult remedial practices (Section E).

	Minimum	Ideal	Maximum	Comments
H. Oxidizers				
1. Ozone, low output generators	—	—	0.1	Serves as oxidizer of water contaminants.
Contact concentration, mg/L when ozone is injected and not removed prior to entry into pool.				
Above pool levels	0	0	0.05	Indoor installations should have adequate ventilation.
I. Oxidation Reduction Potential				
1. ORP	650 MV			

When chlorine or bromine is used as the primary disinfectant, ORP can be used as a supplemental measurement of proper sanitizer activity. The use of ORP testing does not eliminate or supersede the deed for testing the sanitizer level with standard test kits, and ORP reading may be affected by a number of factors including (1) pH, (2) probe film, (3) cyanuric acid, and (4) other. Follow manufacturer's recommendations.

APPENDIX C3: CHEMICAL SAFETY SUMMARY

Oxidizers

The precautions for handling all oxidizers are similar. However, it is up to you to familiarize yourself with the requirements for each.

Name of Oxidizer
calcium hypochlorite
lithium hypochlorite
sodium hypochlorite
trichlor
sodium dichlor
1-bromo-3-chloro-5, 5-dimethylhydantoin
potassium peroxymonosulfate

Protective Equipment
- Eye goggles
- Hands—gloves (rubber, neoprene, or PVC)
- Body—Coveralls and impervious boots (rubber)
- Lungs—Provide ventilation where dust is likely. Wear NIOSH/MSA approved chlorine gas/dust mask if dust is excessive.

Handling Precautions
- Do not take internally
- Avoid contact with eyes, skin or clothing.
- Upon contact with skin or eyes, rinse with water.
- Avoid breathing dust.
- Store all containers in a cool, dry place.
- Do not store containers in direct sunlight.
- Do not store near combustible materials.
- Do not mix oxidizers.
- Use clean, dry utensils when handling oxidizers.
- Keep all oxidizer containers off wet floors.

Conditions & Material to Avoid
- Excessive heat. Oxidizers will decompose, releasing toxic gasses and heat.
- Solvents.
- Acids.
- Other pool chemicals such as acids, algicides, clarifiers, sequestering agents, surface cleaners, etc.
- Organic materials.
- Do not mix oxidizers.

- *Do not mix oxidizers with anything but water. Always add chemicals to plenty of water. Never the reverse.*

Acids

Acids are highly corrosive and must be handled with extreme care.

Names of Acids
muriatic acid (hydrochloric acid, dilute)
sodium bisulfate

Protective Equipment
- Eye goggles or full face shield when splashing may occur.
- Hands—gloves (rubber, neoprene, or PVC)
- Body—Coveralls and impervious boots (rubber)
- Lungs—Wear NIOSH/MSA approved chlorine gas/dust respirator for sodium bisulfate.

Handling Precautions
- Do not take internally
- Avoid contact with eyes, skin, or clothing.
- Upon contact with skin or eyes, rinse with water.
- Avoid breathing vapors (muriatic acid) and dust (sodium bisulfate).
- Store all containers in a cool, dry place.
- *Always add acid to plenty of cool water. Never the reverse.*

Conditions & Materials to Avoid
- Avoid contact with strong alkalies such as caustic soda, sodium carbonate, etc.
- Avoid contact with all oxidizers.
- Do not store in wet or moist conditions.
- Do not store in direct sunlight.

Balance Chemicals

Although acids are balance chemicals, they have been treated separately. The chemicals in this section are all basic (high pH) and increase pH, TA, and calcium hardness.

From NSPI: *Basic pool and spa technology,* ed 2, 1992, The Institute.

continued

Names of Balance Chemicals
sodium bicarbonate
sodium sesquicarbonate
sodium carbonate
sodium hydroxide
calcium chloride-dihydrate

Protective Equipment
• Eye goggles.
• Hand—gloves (rubber, neoprene, or PVC)
• Body—impervious boots (rubber)
• Lungs—Wear NIOSH/MSA approved gas/dust mask or respirator where dust, mist, or spray may occur.

Handling Precautions
• Do not take internally
• Avoid contact with eyes, skin, or clothing.
• Avoid breathing dust, spray, or mist.
• Store all containers in a cool, dry place.
• Always keep containers closed.
• *Caution:* Considerable heat is generated when sodium hydroxide or calcium chloride dihydrate is dissolved in water. Use extreme care. Use lukewarm water. Never add to cold or hot water.

Condition & Materials to Avoid
• Avoid contact with acids.
• Avoid contact with small water volumes.
• Avoid contact with organics and oxidizers.
• Do not store near acids.

APPENDIX C4: QUICK FIX FORMULAS

To Fix	Chemical	Added to	Result
To raise total alkalinity	15 lbs of sodium bicarbonate	Add to 100,000 gallons of pool water	Raises total alkalinity 10 ppm
To raise calcium hardness	11 lbs of calcium chloride	Add to 100,000 gallons of pool water	Raises calcium hardness 10 ppm
To raise chlorine residual or 1 US gallon of sodium	1 lb of chlorine gas or 1 1/2 of calcium hypochlorite or pool water hypochlorite	Add to 120,000 gallons (1,000,000 lbs) of	Raises calcium residual 1.0 ppm
To lower chlorine residual	1 lb of sodium thiosulphate	Add to 100,000 gallons of pool water	Lowers chlorine residual 1.0 ppm

APPENDIX C5: REFERENCE CHART OF CHLORINE PRODUCTS

Chlorine Product	Form	Percent Chlorine	pH	Uses	Dangers
Trichlor (TCCA)	Tablets, sticks, granular	90%	2.8-2.9	Disinfection, scrubbing algae spots	Do not touch
Sodium dichlor (SDCCA)	Granular	56-62%	6.8-7.0	Disinfection, shocking, algae spots	Oxidizer, do not touch
Calcium hypo-chlorite (cal hypo)	Granular tablets, briquettes	65-75%	8.4-11.8	Disinfection shocking, cleaning	Oxidizer, do not inhale or touch
Sodium hypochlorite	Liquid (bleach)	10-15%	13	Disinfection, shocking	Oxidizer, corrosive, do not touch
Lithium hypochlorite	Granular	35%	1.07	Disinfection, shocking, scrubbing algae spots	Oxidizer, avoid touching
Gas chlorine	Gas (liquified)	100%	0-1	Disinfection, shocking	Hazardous, do not breathe

* These chemicals increase TDS with each addition of chemicals.
From NSPI: *Basic pool and spa technology,* ed 2, 1992, The Institute.

APPENDIX C6: USE OF ELEMENTAL CHLORINE

General

Chlorine is one of the chemical elements. The gas has a characteristic odor and greenish yellow color and is about two and one-half (2 $\frac{1}{2}$) times as heavy as air. Chlorine is shipped in Department of Transportation specification steel containers; standard sizes contain either 100 or 150 pounds of chlorine. In the cylinder the chlorine has both a liquid and a gas phase. All cylinders are equipped with the Chlorine Institute standard chlorine cylinder valve.

Chlorine is a "hazardous material" subject to Department of Transportation requirements. When used for pool disinfection, chlorine is considered a pesticide and as such is subject to pertinent regulations of the U.S. Environmental Protection Agency.

Users of chlorine must be trained as to the proper procedures for handling chlorine and as to appropriate emergency procedures. Detailed information is available from chlorine suppliers and the Chlorine Institute, 2001 L Street, N.W., Washington, D.C. 20036.

Equipment and Installation

1. Chlorination equipment should be located so that equipment failure or malfunction will have minimum effect on evacuation of pool patrons in an emergency.
2. Elemental chlorine feeders (chlorinators) should be activated by a booster pump using recirculated water supplied via the recirculation system. The booster pump should be interlocked to the filter pump to prevent feeding of chlorine when the recirculation pump is not running.
3. The chlorinator, cylinders of chlorine and associated equipment should be housed in a reasonable gas-tight and corrosion-resisting housing having a floor area adequate for the purpose. Cylinders should always be stored in an upright position and properly secured.
4. All enclosures should be located at or above ground level. The enclosure should be provided with: ducts from the bottom of the enclosure

to the atmosphere in an unrestricted area, a motor-driven exhaust fan capable of producing at least one air change per minute, and louvers of good design near the top of the enclosure for admitting fresh air. Warning signs should be posted on the doors. It is recommended that the doors to the chlorine room should open away from the pool.

5. Electrical switches for the control of artificial lighting and ventilation should be on the outside of the enclosure adjacent to the door.
6. Contents of a chlorine cylinder can be determined only by weight; therefore, facilities should include a scale suitable for weighing the cylinders. Changing cylinder(s) should be accomplished only after weighing proves contents of cylinder to be exhausted. Care must be taken to prevent water suck-back into the cylinder when empty by closing the cylinder valve.
7. Connections from the cylinders to the system depend on the type of chlorinator to be used and should comply with the chlorinator manufacturer's recommendation.
8. It is recommended that an automatic chlorine leak detector and alarm be installed in the chlorinator room.
9. Respirators approved by the National Institute for Occupational Safety and Health (NIOSH) should be provided for protection against chlorine. It is recommended that at least one approved self-contained breathing apparatus be provided. Respiratory equipment should be mounted outside the chlorine enclosure. Occupational Safety and Health Administration (OSHA) regulations require training and maintenance programs for respirators.
10. Containers may be stored indoors or outdoors. Full and empty cylinders should be segregated and appropriately tagged. Storage conditions should: (a) minimize external corrosion, (b) be clean and free of trash, (c) not be near an elevator or ventilation system, (d) be away from elevated temperatures or heat sources.

For additional information, contact The Chlorine Institute, Inc., 2001 L Street, NW, Washington, D.C. 20036, (202) 775-2790, and request a copy of the "Chlorine Manual" and the wall chart entitled "Handling Chlorine Cylinders & Ton Containers."

Continued

Operational Procedures

1. A specific person should be made responsible for chlorination operations and should be trained in the performance of routine operations including emergency procedures and leak control procedures.

2. Chlorine cylinders must be handled with care. Valve protection caps and valve outlet caps should be in place at all times except when the cylinder is connected for use. Cylinders must not be dropped and should be protected from falling objects. Cylinders should be used on a first-in, first-out basis. New, approved washers should be used each time a cylinder is connected.

3. It is recommended that a safety wall chart be posted in or near the chlorine enclosure and a second chart in the pool office near the telephone. Such charts are available from many suppliers and from the Chlorine Institute, 2001 L Street, N.W., Washington, D.C. 20036. The telephone number of the chlorine supplier should be shown on this chart.

4. Although chlorine suppliers make every effort to furnish chlorine in properly-conditioned cylinders, chlorine gas leaks may still occur. Pool personnel should be informed about leak control procedures and consideration should be given to providing a Chlorine Institute Emergency Kit A.

5. Chlorine suppliers are equipped with a Chlorine Institute Emergency Kit A, which contains devices for capping leaks at cylinder valves and some leaks which occur in the cylinder wall. Further information on these kits and training slides demonstrating their use are available from the Chlorine Institute.

6. As soon as a container is empty, the valve should be closed and the lines disconnected. The outlet cap should be applied promptly and the valve protection hood attached. The open end of the disconnected line should be plugged or capped promptly to keep atmospheric moisture out of the system.

7. To find a chlorine gas leak, use a plastic bottle containing 26° BE Ammonia capable of releasing only vapors when squeezed. A white cloud will result if there is any chlorine leakage. Never use water on a chlorine leak.

APPENDIX C7: 30 PPM SHOCK TABLE FOR ALGAE REMOVAL

Available chlorine (%)*	Volume of water						
	250 gals / 946 L	400 gals / 1,514 L	1,000 gals / 3,785 L	5,000 gals / 18,927 L	20,000 gals / 75.708 L	50,000 gals / 189.271 L	100,000 gals / 378.541 L
5	2.36 cups / 558 mL˙	1.89 pts˙ / 893 mL˙	2.36 qts˙ / 2.23 L˙	2.95 gals / 11.20 L˙	11.8 gals / 44.70 L˙	29.5 gals˙ / 112 L	59.0 gals˙ / 223 L˙
10	1.18 cups˙ / 279 mL˙	.94 pts / 447 mL˙	1.18 qts˙ / 1.12 L˙	1.48 gals˙ / 5.58 L˙	5.90 gals˙ / 22.30 L˙	14.8 gals˙ / 55.80 L˙	29.5 gals / 112 L˙
12	.98 cups˙ / 234 mL*	.78 pts / 372 mL˙	.98 qts / 932 mL˙	1.23 gals˙ / 4.65 L˙	4.92 gals˙ / 18.60 L˙	12.3 gals* / 46.50 L˙	24.6 gals˙ / 93.10 L˙
35	2.86 oz / 81.1 g	4.58 oz / 130 g	11.4 oz / 324 g	3.57 lbs / 1.62 kg	14.3 lbs / 6.50 kg	35.7 lbs / 16.20 kg	71.5 lbs / 32.40 kg
60	1.67 oz / 47.3 g	2.67 oz / 76.0 g	6.67 oz / 190 g	2.08 lbs / 950 g	8.34 lbs / 3.79 kg	20.8 lbs / 94.70 kg	41.7 lbs / 19.00 kg
65	1.54 oz / 43.7 g	2.46 oz / 69.9 g	6.16 oz / 175 g	1.92 lbs / 875 g	7.70 lbs / 3.49 L	19.2 lbs / 8.74 kg	38.5 lbs / 17.50 kg
90	1.11 oz / 31.6 g	1.80 oz / 50.5 g	4.45 oz / 126 g	1.39 lbs / 635 g	5.56 lbs / 2.52 kg	1.3.9 lbs / 6.35 kg	27.8 lbs / 12.60 kg
100	1.00 oz / 28.4 g	1.60 oz / 45.5 g	4.00 oz / 114 g	1.25 lbs / 569 g	5.00 lbs / 2.28 kg	12.5 lbs / 5.70 kg	25.0 lbs / 11.40 kg

˙ For correct chlorine product to add refer to "How to use the Treatment Tables."

APPENDIX C8: SPA DISINFECTANTS

	Chlorine	Bromine	Ozone
Most common form(s) for spa application:	Trichlor tablets dichlor (granular)	Organic bromine (BCDMH tablets) 1- and 2- step bromine salts (granular)	Gas; generated on site
Active disinfectant:	hypochlorous acid, hypochlorite ion	hypobromous acid, hypobromite ion, bromamines,	Ozone's "free radicals"
Proper ppm level:	1.0-3.0 residential 2.0-4.0 commercial	2.0-4.0 residential 4.0-6.0 commercial	—
Most effective e pH:	7.2-7.6	7.2-8.2	7.2-8.2
Lasting residual:	YES	YES	NO
Easy to measure:	YES	YES	YES
Requires other disinfectant:	NO	NO	YES
Requires shocking:	YES	YES	NO
Creates odors:	SOMETIMES	SOMETIMES	SOMETIMES
Irritates eyes/skin:	SOMETIMES	NOT USUAL	NOT USUAL
Affects balance:	YES	YES	NOT USUAL
Methods of adding:	Tablets, feeder or floater Dichlor, hand-fed	Tablets, briquettes, feeder or floater Bromide/oxidants, hand-fed	Ozone generator on, pump on

From *Basic pool and spa technology*, ed 2, 1992, The Institute.

APPENDIX D
SAFETY GUIDELINES

APPENDIX D1: CHILD SAFETY ALTERNATIVES FOR POOLS

Product	Purpose	Type, Price
1. Self-closing/ self-latching devices for doors and windows.	To keep all doors and windows leading to the pool area securely closed, limiting access by unsupervised children.	Hinge pin replacement ($8-10) Swing arm ($15-30)
2. Door exit alarm	To warn parent or guardian when a child opens the door. Placed on/near door.	Door announcer/chime ($35-50); Home Security System
3. Fencing	To isolate swimming pool by way of 4-ft. enclosure. To temporarily isolate swimming pool, when children are visiting.	Chain-link ($1.80/ft.) Picket ($3-4.60/ft.) Ornamental (variable) Portable ($8/ft.)
4. Fence gate closer and latch	To close and latch fence gates securely, making pool inaccessible to a child.	Self-latching ($25-35) Adjust. height (N/A)
5. Fence gate alarm	To sound alarm when gate is open.	N/A
6. Infrared detectors	To sound alarm when area around pool perimeter is entered. Wireless detection.	Light-beam ($300-400) Body energy ($200)
7. Safety covers	To cover the pool with a complete and impenetrable barrier blocking access to water.	Manual closing ($800-2,300); Automatic closing
8. Pool alarms	To sound an alarm when something accidentally or without authorization enters the water. Placed in the pool.	Surface water (wave motion; $140); Pressure Waves (acoustic; $350)
9. Child alarms	To sound an alarm when the child exceeds a certain distance or becomes submerged in water. Clipped on the child.	Electronic monitoring system ($300); Clip-on transmitter ($250-$300)

From NSPI: *Basic pool and spa technology*, ed 2, 1992, The Institute.

Appendix D2

IMPORTANT:

WALL ASSEMBLY
INSTRUCTIONS

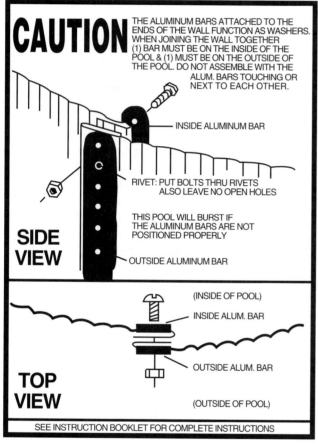

CAUTION

THE ALUMINUM BARS ATTACHED TO THE ENDS OF THE WALL FUNCTION AS WASHERS. WHEN JOINING THE WALL TOGETHER (1) BAR MUST BE ON THE INSIDE OF THE POOL & (1) MUST BE ON THE OUTSIDE OF THE POOL. DO NOT ASSEMBLE WITH THE ALUM. BARS TOUCHING OR NEXT TO EACH OTHER.

INSIDE ALUMINUM BAR

RIVET: PUT BOLTS THRU RIVETS
ALSO LEAVE NO OPEN HOLES

THIS POOL WILL BURST IF
THE ALUMINUM BARS ARE NOT
POSITIONED PROPERLY

SIDE VIEW

OUTSIDE ALUMINUM BAR

(INSIDE OF POOL)

INSIDE ALUM. BAR

OUTSIDE ALUM. BAR

TOP VIEW

(OUTSIDE OF POOL)

SEE INSTRUCTION BOOKLET FOR COMPLETE INSTRUCTIONS

actual size: 4⅝ x 4⅛

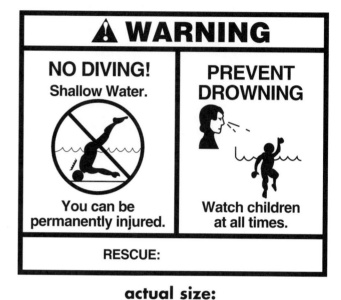

⚠ WARNING

NO DIVING!
Shallow Water.

You can be
permanently injured.

PREVENT DROWNING

Watch children
at all times.

RESCUE:

actual size:
11 x 13⅜
16⅜ x 18½
18⅜ x 24

DEEPER AREA

**Shallow
near the wall.**

actual size: 3⅛ x 6⅜

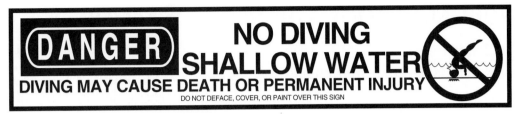

actual size: 2⅞ x 16

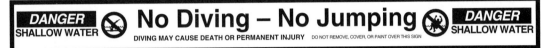

actual size: 1 x 20

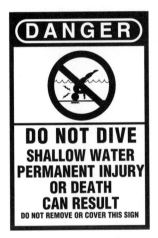

actual size: 3¼ x 2

WARNING

Do not swim
under, through
or behind
this ladder.

Entrapment
may cause
death, paralysis
or
permanent injury.

actual size: 1⁷⁄₁₆ x 1

WARNING

DO NOT
SWIM
UNDER OR
BEHIND
THIS LADDER.
ENTRAPMENT
OR
DROWNING
CAN RESULT!

DO NOT REMOVE OR COVER THIS SIGN

actual size: 3¼ x 2

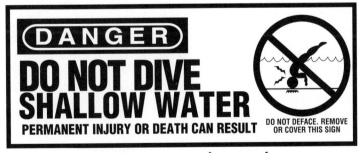

actual size: 5¼ x 15½

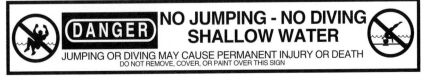

actual size: 3¹⁄₁₆ x 26

APPENDIX D3: POOL CHEMICAL SAFETY

Read the label

Clean-up and disposal—customer checklist

1. Never clean spills with bare hands.
2. Flush a spill with large amounts of water.
3. Do not vacuum a spill.
4. Never use a fire extinguisher on smoking chemicals.
5. Call the fire department immediately for large spills, fire, or disposal assistance.

Transport/storage of pool chemicals—customer checklist

1. Separate your chemicals in cardboard or plastic boxes. Ask your dealer for boxes if you did not bring them.
2. Avoid sudden swerves and stops when driving.
3. Clean spills immediately and properly.
4. Remove chemicals from your car immediately. Don't allow them to sit in the heat of your trunk.
5. Store your chemicals in a locked, dry, cool, well ventilated shed used only for pool supplies.
6. Separate chemicals with cardboard or plastic in storage.

It's Good Business (NSPI Video Outline)

Safety priorities checklist—for pool/spa store owner

1. Safety is YOUR responsibility. Make safe handling and storage or chemicals a priority. Know what to do in an emergency.
2. Either you or someone you're appointed should train all new employees in pool chemical safety.
3. Post the phone number of your fire department and rescue squad by your phone. Make sure your employees know where the numbers are posted.
4. Work with your local fire officials. Let them know your layout and what products you have in your store and warehouse.

Chemical delivery and storage—store checklist

1. Don't order more than you can safely store or sell in a season.
2. Refuse damage goods. Report damage to the supplier for instructions on disposal.
3. Store in a cool, dry, well-ventilated area.
4. Keep the warehouse clean at all times.
5. No smoking in the storage area.
6. Separate incompatible chemicals.
7. Stack at recommended heights.
8. Rotate stock.
9. Label hazardous areas with the proper NFPA 704 placards.

Transportation (NSPI Video Outline)

Proper vehicle loading checklist—business deliveries and service

1. Keep your vehicle clean.
2. Separate incompatible chemicals.
3. Don't carry damaged containers.
4. Put heavy equipment on the rear floor.
5. Anchor your load securely.
6. Carry protective equipment for spills.
7. Post a placard for hazardous loads that exceed limits.
8. If your vehicle weighs more than 10,000 pounds or if your load is placardable, whatever your weight, you also must have a daily vehicle inspection report, your medical cards, and a list of all the regulated material in your load.

APPENDIX D4: CHEMICAL SAFETY

☐ Read the label and instructions.

☐ Use compatible chemicals.

☐ Do not inhale fumes.

☐ Do not over-stock

☐ Drive carefully.

☐ Never combine chemicals.

☐ Don't leave in car.

☐ Store in proper shed.

☐ Separate chemicals in storage.

☐ No smoking.

☐ Mix chemicals at poolside.

☐ Wear gloves and goggles.

☐ Use separate scoops.

☐ Handle with care.

☐ Separate chemicals during transport.

☐ Add chemicals to water.

☐ Mix only exact amounts.

☐ Keep away from children.

☐ Keep dry and off the floor.

☐ Flush with water.

☐ Do not vacuum.

☐ Clean spills properly.

Emergency Numbers

Fire_____

Police_____

Ambulance_____

Physician_____

Poison Center_____

Pool Service Company_____

GLOSSARY

acid A chemical compound that provides hydrogen ions to lower the pH of water. Acids give readings of 6.9 or less on the pH scale. Muriatic acid is a common liquid swimming pool acid. Sodium bisulfate is a common dry swimming pool acid.

acid demand A measurement of acid needed to reduce pH or alkalinity. Usually used with the pH test.

activated carbon Used in the swimming pool industry to remove excess oxidizers, colors, and odors from the water. Usually comes in granular form.

ADA The American Disabilities Act (public law 101-336, passed 1990) gives civil rights protection to approximately 43 million citizens with disabilities similar to those rights provided to individuals on the basis of race, sex, national origin, and religion. It guarantees equal opportunity for individuals with disabilities in employment, public accommodations, transportation, state and local government services, and telecommunications. The law strictly prohibits discrimination in public places against individuals with disabilities.

algae The simplest form of plant life, microscopic and containing chlorophyll, that thrives on sunlight. There are many varieties that enter pools most often by wind or rain. Unsightly and slippery. Easier to prevent than kill. Green, black, and mustard algae are most common in aquatic facilities. There are more than 21,000 known species of algae.

algicide A specialty chemical that aids in killing, controlling and preventing algae. Many varieties of algicides are available; some cause foaming. Quaternary ammonia compounds (Quats) are popular algicides.

algicidal Being capable of **killing** algae

algistat A chemical that inhibits algae growth but is not very effective in killing algae that already exist.

alkaline The property of a compound that allows it to neutralize an acid; in pool water a reading of 7.1 or higher on the pH scale indicates alkaline water. Chemicals added to pool water to raise the pH and offset acidity are known as **alkalies**.

alkalinity The alkaline condition or the pH buffering capacity of water. Determined by the amount of bicarbonate, carbonate, and hydroxide present.

alum A filter aid that when added to a pool's filtration system crates a gelatinous floc on top of the filter bed which helps to precipitate solids out of solutions. The pH must be carefully controlled when alum is used. **Aluminum sulfate** is a common flocculant. Alum is most often used with older, conventional sand and gravel filter systems.

ammonia A hydrogen/nitrogen compound that combines with swimming pool chlorine (FAC) to produce chloramines (CAC) that have obnoxious odors and cause eye burn.

ammonia hydroxide Used for detecting gas chlorine leaks, this ammonia and water alkaline mixture produces a white cloud in the presence of chlorine.

ammonia nitrogen Found on human bodies in the form of sweat, urine, or other waste. Combines with chlorine and bromine to produce chloramines and bromamines, which in turn produce odors and eye burn. Soap showers prior to entering the swimming pool can significantly reduce chloramine production.

ANSI American National Standard Institute develops a variety of standards. **ANSI** in cooperation with **NSPI** publish swimming pool and spa standards.

anthracite (anthrafilt) A filter aid composed of hard coal that can be added to the top of sand filters to help remove chemicals, odors, and tastes.

* Glossaries from both the National Swimming Pool Institute (NSPI) and the National Swimming Pool Foundation (NSPF) were consulted for the Glossary found in this text.

ARC The American Red Cross. National Headquarters are in Washington DC. The ARC offers a variety of comprehensive courses in water safety, CPR, and First Aid.

automatic feeders Electronically controlled pool equipment that monitor and adjust pool chemicals, particularly pH and chlorine levels.

available chlorine Active, unused chlorine that is available to oxidize organic materials and kill bacteria in pool water. This term is used to rating chlorine-containing products as to their total oxidizing power.

backwash A term used to describe one way of cleaning filter media. **Backwashing** calls for the reversing of the flow of water in a filtration system so that dirt trapped in the filter bed is pushed out to waste. Although all filters can be cleaned, not all filters can be backwashed.

backwash cycle The time required to backwash the filter media and elements completely.

backwash rate The flow rate required for effective cleaning of the filter media. Backwash rates are measured in gallons per minute (gpm) per square foot of filter area. The manufacturer's recommendations must be followed for proper backwashing rates.

bacteria One-celled organisms that can either be pathogenic (disease-producing) or nonpathogenic. A **bactericide** is a chemical that kills bacteria.

Baquacil A nonchlorine polymer used as a swimming pool sanitizer and algistat.

barrier A fence, safety cover, wall, or a combination thereof that completely surrounds or covers the swimming pool and obstructs access to the swimming pool.

bather load The number of swimmers in a pool at a given time. Many state codes determine maximum **bather loads** that should not be exceeded. **Swimmer load** is perhaps the more appropriate term; the term **bather** is a remnant from the days when pools were referred to as **baths**.

balanced water Water that is neutral, that is neither corrosive (aggressive) nor basic (scale forming). Balanced water possesses the correct combination of minerals and pH levels.

base or basic A chemical that neutralizes acids, often through hydroxyl ions.

beginners area Those swimming pool areas with a water depth of 3 feet or less.

body coat Diatomaceous earth that builds up on filter elements during the filter cycle. If DE is added to the body coat on a regular basis it is often referred to as a body feed or slurry feed.

breakpoint The process of adding sufficient free available chlorine (FAC) or other nonchlorine oxidants to convert chloramines and ammonia-nitrogen compounds to inert nitrogen gas. All chlorine added after break point is free and uncombined. **Breakpoint chlorination** is necessary to rid a pool of odors and eye burn caused by chloramines.

bridging When the body coat of Diatomaceous Earth filters becomes so thick that the DE coat on adjacent elements touch each other. At this point, filtering is impaired and DE must be removed from the elements.

broadcast A method of introducing granular or powdered chemicals to a pool by spreading them widely over the surface.

brominator A device designed to deliver bromine disinfectant to a swimming pool or spa at a controlled rate.

bromine A swimming pool disinfectant used to kill bacteria and algae. Bromine is often used in hot water spas and hot tubs.

bromamines Produced when free available bromine combines with ammonia and nitrogen wastes brought into the pool by swimmers. Unlike chloramines, bromamines continue to be effective disinfectants.

buffer A combination of weak acids and weak bases and their salts that help to resist changes in pH. Sodium bicarbonate is an example of a popular buffer used in pool water.

calcification Precipitation of calcium carbonate in hard water. Blocks and clogs circulation parts and plumbing.

calcium chloride (CaCl$_2$) A soluble white salt used to raise the calcium hardness of pool or spa water.

calcium hardness The calcium content of the water usually expressed in ppm's Calcium Hardness accounts for approximately 70% of the total hardness. "Soft" water has low calcium hardness and may corrode pool equipment, whereas "hard" water has high levels of calcium hardness and may clog pipes and filters.

calcium hypochlorite A dry, inorganic chlorine that is available in granular form or tablets. It contains 65% active available chlorine. Calcium hypochlorite is flammable and must be handled with care.

cartridge filter A relatively new type of swimming pool filter that utilizes synthetic, porous cartridges to filter water. Cartridge filters are very effective but are often difficult to clean. These filters are used on smaller rather than larger pools. **Depth-type cartridges** rely on the penetration of particles into the medium for removal and provide adequate holding capacity of such particles. **Surface-type cartridges** rely on the retention of particles on the surface of the cartridge for removal.

chelating agents Chemical compounds used to keep metals and minerals in solution so they do not precipitate out in the pool water.

chemical feeder A mechanical device used to dispense pool chemicals into the water. There are many different types of chemical feeders including **diaphragm, piston, erosion, peristaltic, dry, and vacuum.**

chloramines   Produced by free available chlorine combining with ammonia and nitrogenous wastes introduced into pools by swimmers. Renders chlorine less effective and creates odors and eye burn. Must be "shocked" from the pool with large doses of additional free available chlorine. Also known as **combined available chlorine (CAC)**.

chlorinator   A chemical feeder used specifically for dispensing chlorine into pools. **Gas chlorine feeders** are most often referred to as "**chlorinators**."

chlorine   A halogen that is the most popular swimming pool sanitizer and serves as both a disinfectant and oxidizer for swimming pool water. Chlorine is available in many forms, some of which are safe to handle than others. Chlorine kills both bacteria and algae and oxidizes organic debris.

chlorine demand   The amount of chlorine required to disinfect and oxidize all undesirable matter in the pool including ammonia and nitrogenous wastes plus chloramines, bacteria, and algae.

chlorine generator   Equipment that generates chlorine, hypochlorous acid, or hypochlorite on-site for disinfection and oxidation of water contaminants.

chlorine residual   The amount of free available chlorine remaining after the chlorine demand has been satisfied.

clarity   Refers to how clear or transparent water is. Water clarity is determined by how easily objects can be detected underwater at depth. **Water clarity** should not be confused with **water quality**, which refers to bacteria and other contaminants.

clarifier   May also be referred to as a **coagulant** or **flocculant**. A chemical that coagulates and neutralizes suspended particles in water. There are two basic types: inorganic salts of aluminum or iron, and watersoluble organic polyelectrolyte polymers.

colorimetric   A chemical testing procedure by which various shades and hues of colors are compared to determine chemical levels present in pool water. Most chlorine and pH test are colorimetric tests.

coliform   A type of bacteria found in the intestines of warm-blooded animals. When coliform is found in pool water, disease-producing bacteria may also be present. *E* and *B Coli* coliform tests are performed by health officers or certified labs and are generally accepted as a standard of water contamination.

combined available chlorine (CAC)   Also known as chloramines. CAC is produced when inadequate levels of **free available chlorine (FAC)** combine with ammonia and nitrogenous waste introduced into the pool by swimmers. **CAC** is undesirable in pool, causing both odors and eye burn, and is the leading pool problem in busy swimming pools.

comparator   The device used to compare colors during a colorimetric chemical test. Water sample colors are held next to and compared with the comparator colors to determine the chemical level of the sample.

coping   The cap on the pool or spa wall that provides a finishing edge around the pool or spa. It may also be used to secure a vinyl liner to the top of the pool wall. **Coping** can be made of many different materials.

copper   A metal found in some water supplies and also used in many plumbing fixtures. Blue/green water may indicate that high levels of copper exist in the water supply or corrosive water is corroding pool pipes or heater elements.

copper sulfate   Once considered a popular algicide, copper sulfate is rarely used in swimming pools today.

corrosion   The "melting" or "eating-away" of metal parts in swimming pools. Caused by aggressive, acidic, or soft water. This deterioration can be easily prevented by keeping the pH above 7.2 and by maintaining balanced water according to the Saturation Index.

covers   Something that covers, protects, or shelters a swimming pool, spa, or hot tub. There are many different types of pool covers providing a variety of functions. They include **hard top covers** for spas and hot tubs, **winter covers** that keep debris out, **solar covers** that increase water temperature through solar activity, **thermal covers** that insulate and prevent evaporation, and **safety covers** that reduce the risk of drowning of children under 5 years of age.

CNCA   The Council for National Cooperation of Aquatics. A national organization of numerous agencies sharing an interest in improving aquatic safety and education. This organization promotes all phases of aquatics. Headquarters are located in Indianapolis, Indiana.

cyanuric acid (CYA)   A chlorine "conditioner" or "stabilizer" that extends the life of chlorine in outdoor pools. Cyanuric Acid protects chlorine from the dissipating effects of sunlight. Cyanuric acid can be added directly to the pool or it can be purchased already combined with chlorine in tablets or sticks. **Dichlor** and **Trichlor** are commonly used **stabilized chlorines**. CYA levels must be a minimum of 25 ppm in order to extend the life of chlorine but **should not exceed 100 PPM** in pools. According to the Environmental Protection Agency (EPA), high levels of CYA may lead to liver or kidney damage. CYA should not be used indoors.

diaphragm pump A common chemical feeder for pools. This positive displacement pump feeds chemicals to the circulation system at a rate that is easily adjusted. Should be cleaned regularly. This pump is characterized by a diaphragm and check valves.

diatomaceous earth (DE) A fine white powder used as a filter media. **DE** is capable of outstanding filtration, screening out particles as small as one micron in size. DE is composed of fossilized marine life skeletons called diatoms. Because these diatoms are porous, excellent water clarity results when DE filters are used. **Diatomite** is another name for **diatomaceous earth (DE).**

disinfection The process of destroying **bacteria** and **viruses** in order to **prevent disease transmission. Disinfectants** are chemicals used to destroy these contaminants.

diving Entering the water headfirst from a springboard or diving platform. Requires training and supervision. Not to be confused with entering headfirst into shallow water from decks, docks, starting platforms, or others.

diving board A recreational mechanism for entering a swimming pool, consisting of a semirigid board that derives its elasticity through the use of a fulcrum mounted below the board. A jump board is a recreational mechanism that has a coil spring, leaf spring, or comparable device located beneath the board, which is activated by the force exerted in jumping on the board.

diving platform, stationary These are diving devices that are constructed on-site. May include natural or artificial rocks, pedestals, or towers. May be used for recreation or competition, depending upon construction, design, and dimensions.

diving equipment, competitive Includes competitive diving boards, platforms, and related equipment. Fulcrum adjusting diving stands are needed to provide adjustments for competitive diving. Use of this equipment requires training and supervision. All competitive diving equipment must meet **NCAA, US DIVING, OR FINA** standards. **Not intended for aboveground/inground swimming pools.**

DPD (N,N-diethyl-p-phenylene-diamine) The preferred swimming pool colorimetric indicator used in test kits to determine levels of chlorine, bromine, ozone, and some other oxidizers. The darker the shade of red produced by DPD, the more oxidizer present.

dry acid (sodium bisulfate) This granular chemical is safer and easier to use than muriatic acid for **lowering** both **pH** and **total alkalinity.**

effluent Exiting or outflowing water from a pool, pump, or filter.

electrode A sensor used in automatic pool controllers that aids in reading and controlling chemical levels. Electrodes are usually placed inside the pool circulation lines. Silver and copper electrodes may also be used to ionize the water for disinfection and algae control.

electrolysis Electrical current running through water produced by electrically charged ions. Electrolysis can cause corrosion of metal parts in pools.

erosion feeder A simple, canister type chemical feeder that allows a steady, regulated flow of water through the container. Chemical tablets are placed in the erosion feeder where the water current erodes and dissolves the chemical. The erosion rate can be controlled by adjusting the flow rate through the feeder.

equalizer A line that is sometimes added between the bottom of the skimmers and the pool wall to prevent air from being sucked into the filter when the water level is below the skimmer box inlet. When the water level does drop, the equalizer automatically draws water from the pool into the skimmer and back to the filter.

feet of head A measurement of pressure or resistance in a hydraulic system. Feet of head is equivalent to the height of a column of water that would create the some amount of resistance. (100 feet of head equals 43 pounds per square inch.)

filter aid Any chemical or other substance that is added to the water to increase the filters efficiency.

filter cartridge See cartridge filter

filter cycle The length of filtering time between backwashing or other filter cleaning procedures. Longer filter cycles or runs usually mean less work for the pool operators.

filter sand A type of filter media composed of silica, quartz, or similar particles. Filter sand comes in different grades. Manufacturers recommendations must be followed regarding types, grades, and life of filter sand.

filter septum The individual filter membranes found in a DE and some other filtration systems. Can be made of fabric, wire, or similar material. DE clings to the septa in order to trap particles suspended.

filtration The process of removing particulate matter and oils from water as it passes through a porous medium. Many types of filtration are available for swimming pools. A filter usually refers to the mechanical device that traps and strains the suspended particles from the water. Numerous external and internal parts are required for the filter to function properly.

Fireman's switch A mechanism adapted to the time clock that will turn the heater off long enough for it to cool down before the time clock turns the pump off.

flocculant A chemical compound added to some sand filters that aids filtration by creating a foaming, gelatinous mass (called the **floc**) on top of the filter bed, which traps finer particles that might normally pass through the sand. Also referred to as **aggregation**. **Alum** is a common **flocculate**.

flowmeter A device located on a recirculation line that measures flow rate in gallons per minute or liters per minute.

flowrate The rate of flow through a swimming pool recirculation system, most often expressed in gallons per minute. The flowrate is used to determine pool turnovers.

free available chlorine Uncombined, usable chlorine that is free to kill bacteria and algae and oxidize organic material. This is the most active and desirable form of chlorine. Free available chlorine is composed of hypochlorous acid (HOCL) and hypochlorite ion (OCL).

freeboard The clear vertical distance between the top of the filter medium and the lowest outlet of the upper distribution system in a permanent medium filter.

galvanic corrosion The corrosion of metals that takes place when two or more different metals are submerged in an electrolyte.

grab rail Tubular rails used to enter or exit a pool or spa, usually made of stainless steel or chrome plated brass.

gunite A dry mixture of cement and sand, sprayed onto contoured and supported surfaces to build a pool or spa. Water is added to the dry mixture at the nozzle.

gutter The return outlet that surrounds the perimeter of the pool. The gutter is the overflow trough located at the water's edge of most larger pools. Gutters are typically more effective than skimmers.

halogen Fluorine, chlorine, bromine, iodine, and astatine, all of which are found is Group VIIA of the Periodic Table. Most of the halogens are excellent disinfectants.

hair and lint strainer Protects the pool pump by screening out hair, lint, bobbie pins, etc. The removable mesh basket must b e cleaned regularly.

hardness (hard water) Water that contains high levels of calcium and magnesium compounds and other minerals. Hard water produces scale, which in turn clogs pipes, filters, and heaters.

headfirst entry An entry used by an untrained, recreational "diver." Not to be confused with the sport of springboard diving.

hot tub A spa constructed of wood with sides and bottoms formed separately. The whole tub is shaped to join together by pressure from surrounding hoops, bands, or rods; as distinct from spa units formed of plastic, concrete, metal, or other materials.

hydrogen peroxide (H_2O_2) An oxidizing agent that is often used with alternative sanitizers like UV light. Cannot be used by itself and must be handled with extreme care.

hydrochloric acid (muriatic acid) An extremely strong acid used to lower pH as well as a cleaning agent for diving boards, decks, etc. Also produced when chlorine gas is added to water.

hydrotherapy jets A fitting that blends air and water creating a high velocity, turbulent stream of air-enriched water. Used in spas and hydrotherapy pools.

hydrotherapy spa A unit that may have a therapeutic use but which is not drained, cleaned, or refilled for each individual.

hypochlorite A pool chemical containing chlorine used for disinfection and oxidation. Often refers to calcium, sodium, or lithium hypochlorite.

hydrogen The lightest chemical element that is a component of water and a product of many chemical reactions. Can be used to measure acidity and pH.

hydrogen ion The positively charged nucleus of a hydrogen atom. Can be used to measure the acidity of a solution.

hydroxyl ion A negatively charged particle composed of one hydrogen and one oxygen atom.

hypochlorinator Delivers liquid chlorine to a pool at an adjustable rate.

hypochlorous acid (HOCL) Produced when any chlorine type reacts water. **HOCL** is the active disinfectant or **free chlorine** used in the treatment of pools and spas. **HOCL** is an excellent sanitizer, oxidizer, and algicide.

impeller The part (vanes) of a centrifugal pump that spin and move pool water through the circulation system.

indicator A chemical reagent used to produce a color change in a water sample. Phenol red and DPD are two common pool test indicators.

influent Water flowing into a pump, filter, pool, or other vessel.

iodide A chemical compound containing iodine that will be released when placed in pool water. Potassium and sodium iodide are both used for pool disinfection.

iodine A halogen that can be used for swimming pool disinfection but is not common. Although it is an excellent bactericide, iodine is not an effective algicide.

iron When found in high concentrations in water supplies, may precipitate out in red, brown, or murky colors. Staining often begins when the iron content is higher than .3 ppm. Water with high iron levels must either be filtered out before it reaches the pool plant and/or sequestered with a specialty chemical if in the pool itself.

ionization   An electrochemical process using electrodes to convert neutral or noncharged atoms, molecules, or compounds to electrically charged ions. Ionization is used as an alternative sanitizer in some pools to reduce their dependence on chemicals. Staining may accompany ionization.

lifeline   A line running across the surface of the pool dividing shallow and deep ends. Prevents nonswimmers from sliding down the slope into deep water. Floats are normally attached. This safety device may present a hindrance to lap swimming.

lithium hypochlorite (LiOCL)   A dry, granular chlorine that is extremely soluble. This chlorine type is often used as a **shocking** agent but is quite expensive.

logarithm   A mathematical term used in the pool industry to determine the pH scale; the power to which 10 (in the case of pH) must be raised to the reciprocal of the hydrogen ion concentration of pool water.

lower distribution system (underdrain)   Those devices used in the bottom of a permanent medium filter to collect the water during filtering and distribute the water during backwashing.

magnesium hardness   The amount of magnesium found in a water supply or sample; magnesium hardness and calcium hardness equal total hardness.

make-up water (source water)   Outside (fresh) water used to fill or add water to swimming pools.

manometer   An instrument using a column of liquid, usually mercury, to indicate flow rate in gallons per minute.

micron   A unit of measure equalling 1/1000 of a millimeter or 1/1,000,000 of a meter.

microorganism   A microscopic, invisible plant or animal often found in water.

muriatic acid   Also known as hydro-chloric acid or hydrogen chloride, this strong acid is used primarily to reduce total alkalinity and for cleaning chores around the pool. Muriatic acid is extremely corrosive and must be stored and handled with care. A toxic gas is produced when sodium hypochlorite and muriatic acid come in contact with each other. **Sodium bisulfate (dry acid)** is a safer alternative to muriatic acid.

neutral   7.0 on the pH; neither acid nor basic.

nitrogen   An odorless, colorless, tasteless gas found combined in all living tissues. Nitrogen enters the pool combined with body oil, perspiration, and cosmetics and combines with free chlorine to produce chloramines. Chloramines result in odors and eye irritation. Nitrogen compounds also promote algae growth.

NSF   National Sanitation Foundation

NSPI   National Spa and Pool Institute. The major trade organization in the swimming pool industry.

NSPF   National Swimming Pool Foundation. An educational foundation promoting swimming pool research, education, and safety. Also trains Certified Pool Operators.

organic wastes   Introduced to pools by swimming entering the water and the surrounding environment. Include perspiration, urine, saliva, body oil, cosmetics, suntan lotion, etc. Extremely difficult to filter from pool water. Chemical oxidation is usually required to rid a pool of organic waste.

organisms   Animal or plant life like algae or bacteria that can grow in pool water.

ORP   The oxidation reduction potential produced by strong oxidizing agents in a water solution. **ORP**, or **REDOX**, is a measure of the oxidation level measured in millivolts by an **ORP METER**.

OTO   Orthotolidine (OTO) is a colorimetric indicator used to detect total available chlorine. Darker shades of yellow indicate higher levels of chlorine. Effectively measures total chlorine, but OTO testing does not differentiate between free chlorine from combined chlorine, which is why DPD testing is preferred.

overflow system   Refers to removal or pool/spa surface water through the use of overflows, surface skimmers, and surface water collection systems of various design and construction.

oxidation   The process of changing a compound or molecule from a lower to a higher positive oxidation state. For example, the carbon atom of organic swimmer waste is oxidized to carbon dioxide, which has a higher oxidation state. An **oxidizing agent** (like hypochlorous acid) encourages and promotes oxidation.

ozone (O_3)   An artificially on-site produced gas in the swimming pool industry used to disinfect and oxidize pool water. Ozone is a bluish, pungent gas that is a triatomic form of oxygen (O_3). Because of its poor residual properties, ozone is most often used as a supplemental oxidizer.

pathogen   A microorganism-causing disease.

pH   A measure of the acidity, basicity, or neutrality of water. The pH scale runs from 0.0 to 14.0. A pH below 7.0 is considered acid; a pH is considered basic. **Phenol red** (phenolsulfonthalein) is the most common reagent used for the pH test (6.8 to 8.4). Mathematically, pH is defined as the negative logarithm of the hydrogen-ion concentration in water.

polymer An agent used to clump, collect, or flocculate suspended particles in water. Used as a filter aid.

pools A vessel constructed for the purpose of swimming. May be designed specifically for relaxation, recreation, therapy, or competition. NSPI further classifies pools as **aboveground, onground, inground, residential,** and **commercial/public, splasher,** and **wading pools.** Public/commercial pools are further classified into numerous categories.

potable Safe drinking water that is free of bacteria.

potassium peroxymonosulfate One type of nonchlorine shocking agent used to oxidize chloramines and organic waste.

ppm Parts per million. A measurement used in swimming pool testing that indicates the amount of chemical by weight in relation to 1,000,000 parts of water. For example, there are a million pounds of water in a 120,000 gallon pool. Therefore a pound of gas chlorine in a 120,000 gallon pool equals one part per million.

precipitate An insoluble compound produced by a chemical reaction between compounds that are usually soluble. The process in which soluble, invisible compounds in water become insoluble; visible is called **precipitation**. Calcium carbonate and iron are two common pool precipitates.

precoat A thin layer or coating of DE placed on the filter septum to start a filter cycle.

pressure differential The difference, usually measured in PSI, between two gauges.

PSI Pounds per square inch. Used to describe pressure in filter tanks or indicate head pressure.

pump A mechanical device, usually powered by an electric motor that causes hydraulic flow and pressure for the purpose of filtration, heating, and circulation of pool and spa water. Typically, a **centrifugal pump** design is used for pools and spas.

pump curve Characteristics of a pump graphically displayed that is invaluable in selecting and testing pump performance. Considers pump power, resistance, and flow variables.

quaternary ammonium compound ("Quat") An organic compound of ammonia used as an algistat and germicide in pool and spa water. May cause foaming. Concentrations of 3 to 5 ppm are usually recommended for quats.

racing start The method of entry used by a competitive swimmer from the pool deck or from a starting platform to begin a race. Not to be confused with the sport of springboard diving.

rate of flow (flow rate) The amount of water passing through a circulation system measured at a given point on the system. Usually measured in gallons per minute (gpm) on a flow meter. Rate of flow is important in producing good water quality and clarity.

reagent Used for chemical testing; may come in tablets, liquid, or powder.

recirculation system The "closed loop" system used in swimming pools to filter, heat, and chemically treat the water. Composed of numerous parts including pipes, pumps, and filters.

residual The amount of disinfectant or other chemical remaining in the swimming pool water. Although chlorine and bromine have good residual properties, some other disinfectants do not.

return inlet The aperture or fitting through which through treated water under positive pressure returns to a pool or spa.

RID factor Three factors adversely affecting the performance of lifeguards. Failure to **RECOGNIZE** victims, **INTRUSION** of unnecessary, non-lifeguarding tasks, and **DISTRACTION** from the task of protecting swimmers. Developed by Frank Pia.

ring buoy A common lifesaving device that is circular and buoyant. Normally has a long line attached and is meant to be thrown to a distressed swimmer.

sand filter A swimming pool filter using specially graded sand or sand and gravel as the filter media to trap dirt and filter the water.

saturation index An extremely important tool used to check water balance. If used regularly, can help to prevent corrosion and scale. The saturation index is a simple mathematical formula that measures the interrelation of temperature, calcium hardness, total alkalinity, and pH to determine if water is acidic, basic, or neutral.

scale A precipitate composed mostly of calcium carbonate found on pool surfaces and other parts like the heater and filter. Often caused by high pH, high mineral content, or extremely basic water.

sequestering agent A specialty chemical added to swimming pools to keep metals and minerals in solution in order to prevent staining, scaling, and cloudy water.

shelf life The length of time a material (like a pool chemical) can be stored yet still remain suitable for its intended use. Many pool chemicals deteriorate when stored improperly (left uncovered or stored in sunlight, humidity, or in elevated temperatures).

skimmer A swimming pool outlet that functions like a gutter but is much smaller in size. Allows water to continually return from the surface of the pool to the filter system for cleaning and treating. A **skimmer weir** is a one-way door or flap in the skimmer box that continually adjusts to varying water levels so that the skimming action is continuous.

shocking Producing high levels of chlorine or nonchlorine oxidizer to rid a pool of all chloramines and other organic wastes. Often refers to **superchlorination** or **breakpoint**.

slip resistant A surface that has been treated or constructed is such a way as to significantly reduce the chance of the user slipping. The slip-resistant material must not cause an abrasion hazard.

slurry feed A liquid (water and DE mixed) body feed for DE filters fed to the filtration system by means of a slurry feeder. A slurry feed adds media to the filter elements or septa, thereby extending the filter cycle or "run."

soda ash (Na$_2$CO$_3$) A white powder (sodium carbonate) used to raise pH and total alkalinity in most swimming pools.

sodium bicarbonate (NaHCO$_3$) A strong, basic solution (pH 13) used to raise pH in some pools.

sodium hypochlorite (NaOCL, liquid chlorine) A popular swimming pool disinfectant that is 10% to 12% available chlorine with a pH of 13 and is lost in sunlight.

sodium thiosulfate A chlorine neutralizer that has many applications. It may be added directly to the pool to lower high chlorine levels resulting from superchlorination. Often sodium thiosulfate is added to cells for chemical tests like pH and total alkalinity to prevent faulty reading.

soft water Water that has low (less than 100 PPM) or insignificant levels of dissolved calcium and magnesium content.

spa A hydrotherapy unit of irregular or geometrical shell design. Typically contains water heated between 99° and 104° F. A public spa is operated by a owner, licensee, or concessionaire regardless of whether a fee is charged for use. Residential spas are basically used in the home. NSPI further classifies spas.

stabilizer Cyanuric acid (CYA) added to pool water or chlorine to protect outdoor pools and spas from the dissipating effects of the UV rays from the sun. The process of adding cyanuric acid to "save" or "stretch" chlorine is called **stabilization.** CYA levels should be at least 25 ppm to save chlorine but must not exceed 100 ppm.

sterilization The complete killing of all microorganisms by either heat or chemical disinfection.

superchlorination (shock treatment) Introducing extremely high levels of chlorine or some other "nonchlorine" shocking agent to destroy chloramines. This is also referred to as breakpoint and normally requires 10 times the chloramine count in free available chlorine. Superchlorination may also be used to kill algae. At busy pools superchlorination or "shocking" should be performed regularly.

surface skimming action Includes perimeter type overflows, surface skimmers, and surface water collection systems of various designs and construction.

swimmer load The total number of swimmers in the pool at a given time or period of time.

tamperproof Tamperproof equipment means that tools are required to alter or remove parts.

test kit A device used to monitor specific chemical residual or demands in pool or spa water.

titration A chemical testing procedure by which an indicator is added to a given test sample followed by the addition of a titrating solution that brings about a color change (endpoint). The number of titrating drops added to the sample to produce a color change is used to calculate the amount of chemical in solution. Calcium hardness and total alkalinity tests are often titration tests.

total alkalinity (TA) The total amount of carbonates, bicarbonates, and hydroxides in pool water. Total alkalinity buffers and controls pH. Low TA results in pH bounce, making it difficult to stabilize pH levels. High TA makes it difficult to change pH levels. Total alkalinity levels may be maintained between 80 ppm and 150 ppm, but the TA level must be compatible with the chemical disinfectant used and the pool shell.

total available chlorine (TAC) Total available chlorine is the sum of free-available (good) chlorine (FAC) and combined available (bad) chlorine (CAC).

total dissolved solids (TDS) A measure of the total amount of dissolved matter in water, including calcium, magnesium, carbonates, bicarbonates, metallic compounds, and others.

turbidity Cloudiness or lack of clearness (visibility) in water. Usually results from suspended particles in the water. Can be caused by a variety of reasons including low disinfectant levels, inadequate filtration, high chloramine levels, DE in the pool, unbalanced water, etc. When pool water becomes so turbid that the bottom is not easily recognized, the pool should be closed immediately.

turnover rate The number of times a quantity of water equal to the pool volume passes through the filtration system in 24 hours. Larger pools often have a 6-hour (four turns) turnover or 8-hour (three turns) turnover, whereas smaller pools like spas may have a 30-minute turnover.

trichlor (trichlor-s-triazinetrione) A stabilized or organic chlorine that contains three available chlorine atoms. Trichlor has an available chlorine content of 89% and has a pH of 2.9, which is very acidic.

underdrain The plumbing at the bottom of most sand filters tanks that collects the filtered swimming pool water and returns it to the pool. The underdrains also distribute backwash water up through the filter bed for cleaning during the backwash cycle.

underwater light A lighting fixture located in the wall of some swimming pools below the surface of the water. A "wet niche" light is found immersed totally in pool water, whereas a "dry niche" light is housed in the pool wall behind a water proof window. The advantage of the dry niche light is that it can be repaired or replaced out of the water.

upper distribution system Those devices designed to distribute the water entering a permanent medium filter in a manner so as to prevent movement or migration of the filter medium. This system shall also properly collect water during filter backwashing unless other means are provided.

vacuum filter Any pool filter where the pump follows the filer (effluent side) and "pulls" the water through the filter. Conversely, a pressure filter is preceded by pump (influent side) that "pushes" water through the filter. Pressure systems usually have hair and lint strainers, whereas most vacuum systems do not.

velocity The rate of water movement in feet per second.

vinyl liner That plastic membrane constructed of vinyl or vinyl compounds that acts as a container for pool water.

voids Spaces of gaps within a filter media.

weir The device included with a through-the-wall skimmer that controls the amount of surface water (flow) drawn into the skimmer and filtration system.

winterizing The procedure of preparing pools and spas for freezing weather. Includes chemical treatment of the standing water, plus physical and chemical treatment of the standing water, plus physical and chemical protection of the pool or spa and its equipment against freezing.

INDEX